Urologic Surgery: An Issue of Urologic Clinics

Urologic Surgery: An Issue of Urologic Clinics

Editor: Chris Patterson

AMERICAN
MEDICAL PUBLISHERS
www.americanmedicalpublishers.com

AMERICAN
MEDICAL PUBLISHERS
www.americanmedicalpublishers.com

Cataloging-in-Publication Data

Urologic surgery : an issue of urologic clinics / edited by Chris Patterson.
p. cm.
Includes bibliographical references and index.
ISBN 979-8-88740-546-9
1. Genitourinary organs--Surgery. 2. Urinary organs--Surgery. 3. Urology.
4. Surgery, Operative. 5. Genitourinary organs--Diseases--Treatment.
6. Urinary organs--Diseases--Treatment. I. Patterson, Chris.
RD571 .U76 2023
61746--dc23

American Medical Publishers,
41 Flatbush Avenue,
1st Floor, New York,
NY 11217, USA

ISBN 979-8-88740-546-9 (Hardback)

Contents

Preface

Urologic surgery is a surgical specialty that deals with the medical conditions or diseases of the male and female urinary tracts. It is involved in treating diseases of several organs, such as kidneys, ureter, urethra, bladder, penis, testes, prostate, scrotum, etc. There are a number of different urologic surgeries that include vasectomy, cystoscopy, prostate procedures, ureteroscopy, lithotripsy, etc. Vasectomy is a common urologic surgery which is used for birth control in men on a permanent basis. Ureterostomy is a procedure for changing the path that urine takes when exiting the body. Prostate biopsy helps in diagnosing prostate cancer. This book is compiled in such a manner that it will provide an in-depth knowledge about the theory and practice of urologic surgery. It includes contributions of experts and researchers which will provide innovative insights into this field. The book will prove immensely beneficial to medical professionals and students involved in the area of urologic surgery at various levels.

After months of intensive research and writing, this book is the end result of all who devoted their time and efforts in the initiation and progress of this book. It will surely be a source of reference in enhancing the required knowledge of the new developments in the area. During the course of developing this book, certain measures such as accuracy, authenticity and research focused analytical studies were given preference in order to produce a comprehensive book in the area of study.

This book would not have been possible without the efforts of the authors and the publisher. I extend my sincere thanks to them. Secondly, I express my gratitude to my family and well-wishers. And most importantly, I thank my students for constantly expressing their willingness and curiosity in enhancing their knowledge in the field, which encourages me to take up further research projects for the advancement of the area.

Editor

1

Multivariate analysis of early surgical management factors affecting posttraumatic penoscrotal avulsion injury: A level I trauma center study

Min Ji Kim, Dong Hwan Lee, Dong Ha Park and Il Jae Lee*

Abstract

Background: To conduct an accurate evaluation of patients presenting with posttraumatic penoscrotal injuries, and to formulate a treatment algorithm based on this assessment.

Methods: We conducted a retrospective chart review study. Patients with penoscrotal defects admitted to our level I trauma center from 2017 to 2019 were evaluated. The Braden scale score was used for wound evaluation and the Korean patient classification system (KPCS) was used for assessment of severity. Univariate and multivariate analyses were performed for potential risk factors associated with early surgical management.

Results: In total, there were 58 male patients, and the average Braden scale score was 12.08 ± 2.54, with the scrotum (36.20%), and the penile shaft (32.76%) being popular sites for injuries. The wounds requiring surgical treatment were 20.68% ($n = 12$), with local flaps (33.33%) being most commonly used. The significant predictors of advanced wounds which required surgical treatment were old age ($p = 0.026$, odds ratio [OR] 8.238), orthopedic combined injuries ($p = 0.044$, OR 1.088), intubation ($p = 0.018$, OR 9.625), restraint ($p = 0.036$, OR 0.157) and blood transfusion ($p < 0.001$, OR 2.462).

Conclusion: In multiple trauma patients, penoscrotal defects caused by high-speed trauma are an important matter of concern. Specifically, patients with combined skeletal injuries or requiring respiratory care were prone to advanced wounds. We proposed a five-category algorithm to manage such patients, which included severity of the patient's condition, respiration, hemodynamic status, comorbidity, and immobilization. Additionally, inter-departmental cooperation and active intervention by plastic surgeons is needed for the comprehensive treatment of such injuries.

Keywords: Penoscrotal avulsion, Trauma, Wound management, Quality improvement, Wound and injury

Background

In multiple severe trauma patients, high-speed mechanism injuries in accidents can cause penoscrotal defects. The importance of this region for the body's urologic and sexual functions is well known, and the preservation of

*Correspondence: i00325@live.co.kr
Department of Plastic and Reconstructive Surgery, Ajou University School of Medicine, 164, World cup-ro, Yeongtong-gu, Suwon 16499, Republic of Korea

the structure and function of the penoscrotal region is integral to the patient's quality of life [1]. In some disease involving penoscrotal defects such as Fournier's gangrene, the physician has to focus on wound management, often necessitating early referral to a reconstructive specialist [2]. However, severely trauma patients admitted to a level I trauma center differ from patients suffering from a single disease. Recently, cancer-related mortality has decreased by 20% (1991–2009); however, trauma-related mortality has increased by 24% (1990–2010) [3, 4]. These patients are managed according to a structured resuscitation protocol. Furthermore, these multiple trauma patients may present with an edematous perineum, hiding a penoscrotal avulsion injury. In such critical conditions, such wounds that are not immediately obvious, can easily be overlooked even by plastic surgeons.

For the management of penoscrotal avulsion injuries, a comprehensive evaluation of the patient's status is needed. Surgical reconstruction of a penoscrotal lesion is not simple. The goal is to provide wound healing, adequate function, and an acceptable appearance [5]. To date, recent studies have underestimated such injuries; thus, information regarding these injuries is scarce. The purpose of this study was to provide an accurate evaluation of trauma patients with penoscrotal injuries and to propose a treatment algorithm based on this assessment.

Methods

We retrospectively recruited patients who were admitted to our level I trauma center, with trauma-related penoscrotal defects between 2017 and 2019. The following demographic information was collected; age, sex, cause of injury, combined injuries, management protocols including respiratory care, intubation, nutrition, restraint, range of motion, and whether or not they were alive at presentation. The wound characteristics were evaluated according to severity, anatomical lesion, defect size, management technique, operative details, and complications. The Braden scale score was used for wound evaluation, and the KPCS (Korean patient classification system) was used for the assessment for patient severity [6–9]. The Braden Scale assesses risk using six different risk factors: sensory perception, the ability to respond meaningfully to pressure-related discomfort; moisture, defined as the degree to which skin is exposed to moisture; activity, degree of physical activity; mobility, defined as the ability to change and control body position; nutrition, usual food intake pattern; and friction and shear [6, 10, 11]. The Braden scale is widely used to evaluate the risk of sores. It has several components to enable various aspects of wound evaluation. However, it can be used to evaluate other wounds apart from sores. KPCS consisted of 12 areas, 50 nursing activities, and 73 items (factors for general nursing care) [12]. It was developed based on the Workload management system for nurses (WMSN) of the USA. There are many reports of its validity and reliability; therefore, this classification has been included in the basic tools used in tertiary hospitals in Korea [13–15]. Wound dimension was assessed using ImageJ (National Institutes of Health, USA) [16]. For each photographic image, measurements were calibrated using pixels at the margin of the wound comparing with the entire genital area. The wound size was calculated using the percentage of the total genital area according to pixel count. Statistical analysis was performed using Statistical Package for the Social Sciences (SPSS) for Windows version 18.0 (SPSS Inc., Chicago, IL, USA). Data are presented as means ±2 standard deviations. Statistical significance was accepted at $p < 0.05$. Factors that predicted surgically demanding and advanced wounds were identified through a univariate analysis. A surgically demanding wound is defined as an open wound that cannot be expected to heal completely with conservative dressing treatment. Such wounds are expected to require surgical intervention to enable healing. Advanced wounds are a sub-category of surgically demanding wounds. These wounds require surgical treatment, but the focus of treatment is tissue reconstruction. Therefore, simple wounds that require only debridement are excluded from this category. Variables with a p-value< 0.05 were included in the multivariate analysis. Backward-stepwise logistic regression analysis was performed to identify risk factors for trauma-related advanced penoscrotal defects. The need for informed consent was waived by the Institutional Review Board because of the retrospective nature of the study. However, photographic authorization and release consent were obtained from all participants, including parental consent for adolescent patients. This study strictly adhered to Declaration of Helsinki principles.

Results

A total of 58 patients were included in this retrospective study. All the patients were male and had an average age of 59.72 years (range, 40–78). Mean follow-up period was 13.74 months (range, 5.5–22).Intensive care unit patient severity, as assessed by KPCS, had mean values of 4.41 ± 1.22. Wound severity assessed by Braden scale had an average of 12.08, and high-risk patients for whom scale was lower than 12 were 65.52%. The most common cause of injury was a fall, followed by traffic accidents, each contributing to 37.93 and 22.41% of the injuries, respectively. Wound extension was classified on the basis of anatomical sites, and scrotum and shaft were the most commonly injured sires, at 36.20 and 32.76% respectively [17]. On comparing with the total genital area, the involved penoscrotal defect portion was 55.80 ± 30.45% (Table 1).

Comorbidities were classified into nine areas: brain, orthopedic, spine, facial, vascular, lung, intraorgan, and soft tissue comorbidities and acute respiratory distress syndrome. The most common combined injury was orthopedic injury (65.62%), followed by intraorgan injury (37.93%), and spine injury (34.48%). Extensive soft tissue injuries were found in 20.69%, but these injuries did not involve genital wounds. Among 58 patients, 75.85% survived, however, 15 patients died in spite of active resuscitation at a professional trauma center. The rate of ventilator assistance was 44.83, and 91.38% of the patients received a blood transfusion during the hospital stay. Some hemodynamic indicators were evaluated; the collected mean hemoglobin level was 11.41 ± 1.80 and the mean creatinine level was 1.22 ± 0.83 (Table 2).

Among the 58 patients, 12 received surgical wound management. The remaining 47 patients were treated with conservative management, which included aseptic dressing, negative pressure vacuum dressing, and growth factor ingredient medication-assisted dressing.

Table 1 Patient demographics

Variable	Values
No. of subjects	58
Age (years)[a]	59.72 ± 19.25
Sex (n)	
M	58
Severity[b]	4.41 ± 1.22
Braden scale[a]	12.08 ± 2.54
Braden scale (n, %)	
≤ 18	38 (65.521)
Cause of injury (n, %)	
Fall	22 (37.93)
Traffic accident	13 (22.41)
Motorcycle accident	9 (15.51)
Rolling injury	4 (6.90)
Crushing injury	5 (8.62)
Others	5 (8.62)
Site of lesion (n, %)	
Glans	2 (3.44)
Corona	1 (1.72)
Foreskin	8 (1.38)
Shaft	19 (32.76)
Root	7 (12.07)
Scrotum	21 (36.20)
Size of defect (% of total genital area)[a]	55.80 ± 30.45
Follow up months[a]	13.74 ± 8.20

[a] Mean ± 2SD

[b] Korean Patient Classification System for Nurses

Table 2 General comorbidities and hemodynamic status in the study population

Variable	Values
Combined injury (n, %)	
Brain injury	15 (25.86)
Orthopedic injury	38 (65.62)
Spine injury	20 (34.48)
Facial bone injury	7 (12.07)
Vascular injury	15 (25.86)
Lung injury	19 (15.51)
Intraorgan injury	22 (37.93)
Extensive soft tissue injury (except genital)	12 (20.69)
Acute respiratory distress syndrome	10 (17.24)
Intubation (n, %)	26 (44.83)
Absolute bed rest (n, %)	8 (13.79)
Restrain (n, %)	24 (41.37)
Total parenteral nutrition (n, %)	25 (43.10)
Transfusion (n, %)	53 (91.38)
Initial hemodynamic status[a]	
Hb	11.41 ± 1.80
Albumin	3.32 ± 0.69
Bun	17.42 ± 8.87
Creatinine	1.22 ± 0.83
Survival (n, %)	44 (75.86)
Expire (n, %)	15 (25.86)

[a] Mean ± 2SD

The operative options ranged from debridements and local flaps to skin grafts and free flaps (Figs. 1, 2). The most common modality used was local flap in 33.33% of patients, followed by debridement in 25%, and free flap in 25%. Severe complications were not noted, and only minor complications, including partial necrosis, were noted (Table 3).

Univariate analysis identified several clinical variables associated with the development of a surgically demanding advanced wound. Age, Braden scale, orthopedic injury, intraorgan injury, extensive soft tissue injury, intubation, absolute bed rest, restraint, transfusion, hemoglobin, blood urea nitrogen, and survival status were found to be associated with advanced wounds. Multivariate logistic regression analysis of these variables showed that old age ($p = 0.026$, OR 8.238), orthopedic combined injury ($p = 0.044$, OR 1.088), intubation ($p = 0.018$, OR 9.625), restraint ($p = 0.036$, OR 0.157), and transfusion ($p < 0.001$, OR 2.462), were significant predictors of advanced wounds which would require surgical treatment (Table 4).

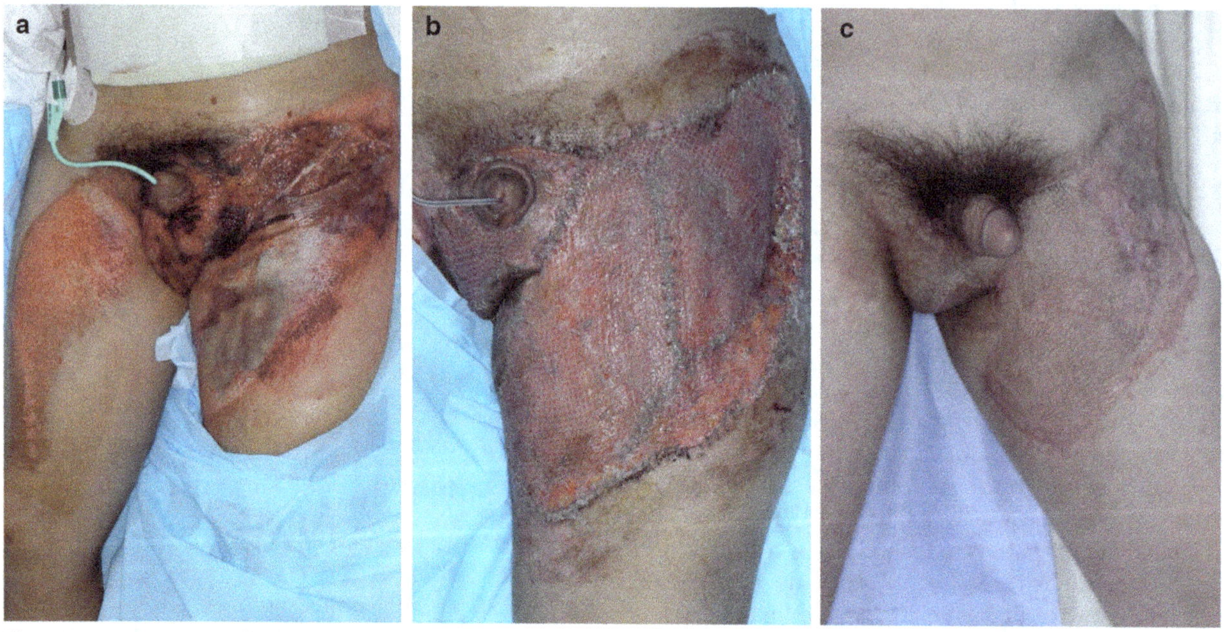

Fig. 1 Representative case of a penoscrotal injury where successful surgical reconstruction was achieved. **a** The 36-year-old male pedestrian with no underlying conditions was hit by a vehicle and admitted for soft tissue injury involving the scrotum and thigh, an ankle fracture, and a pelvic bone fracture. He was transfused for massive blood loss, but not intubated. The urologist confirmed that the wound did not invade the testicles and he had no problems with sexual function and urination. **b** After several debridements, he underwent a split-thickness skin graft. **c** One year later, he had discomfort due to scar contracture in his inguinal area, and the scar contracture was released with a Z-plasty. According to the five-category algorithm, he had orthopedic injury, required restraint, and transfusion—a total of three factors that could signify an advanced wound

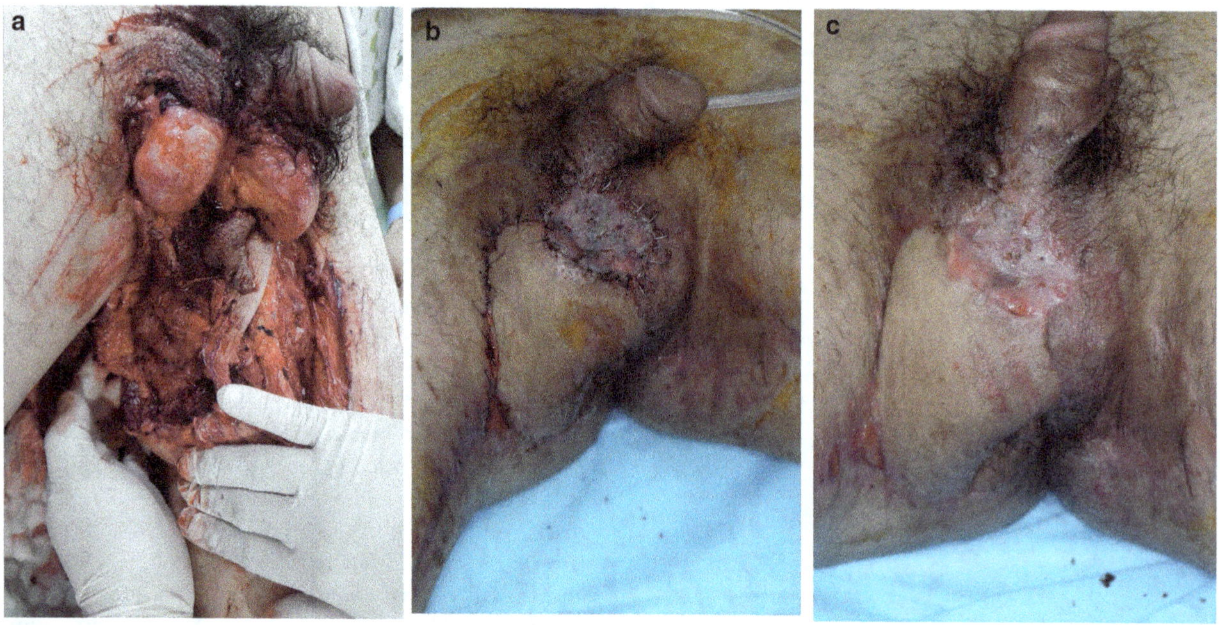

Fig. 2 Representative case of penoscrotal injury where successful surgical reconstruction was achieved. **a** A 34-year-old man with no underlying disease admitted for soft tissue injuries including the scrotum, bilateral thighs, and perineum, because his thigh rolled into a rolling machine. His vital signs were stable. There was no testicular and anal injury. **b** After several debridements, a medial circumflex artery perforator-based local flap rotation, and split-thickness skin grafting were performed. **c** After 1 month, the wound was well healed. According to the five-category algorithm, he had intubation, required restraint, and transfusion—a total of three factors that could signify an advanced wound

Table 3 Outcome of surgical, non-surgical management of penoscrotal defect

Variable	Values
Conservative management (n, %)	47 (81.03)
Surgical management (n, %)	12 (20.68)
Operative option	
Debridement	3 (25.00)
Local flap	4 (33.33)
Skin graft	2 (16.67)
Free flap	3 (25.00)
Surgical complication	
Infection	–
Partial necrosis	3 (25.00)
Total necrosis	–

Discussion

The development of high-speed machines and an advanced building industry has changed the presentation of trauma patients and it leads to associated industrial accidents as well as traffic accidents. Such trauma can involve every part of the body, including the penoscrotal area. Owing to their concealed anatomical locations, such injuries can go easily undetected, further delaying treatment. There are few comments on the mechanism of development of penoscrotal injuries in a trauma patient, besides a direct injury of the perineal area from the trauma. In rotation machines, the capturing force of the machine creates torsion and leads to traction of the area [18, 19]. In falls, direct trauma to the falling side causes friction burns which lead to soft tissue injuries. If the scrotal skin loss is less than 50%, it can often be closed immediately after the trauma [19]. The depth of injury can involve damage to the cavernous bodies, spongy body, or testes [20]. Following blood loss, infection and lymphedema can lead to the development of an irreversible wound.

In this study, our final proposal was an assessment algorithm for trauma-related penoscrotal avulsion injury (Fig. 3). We composed a five-category algorithm, based on our multivariate clinical risk evaluation. The categories were patient severity, respiration, hemodynamic status, comorbidities, and immobilization. In this algorithm, the main factors that contribute to advanced penoscrotal injury are composed of patient stability, immobilization,

Table 4 Variables associated with surgical management of trauma-induced penoscrotal defect

Variables	Univariate analysis		Multivariate analysis		
	Odds ratio	p-value	Odds ratio	95% CI	p-value
Age	1.019	0.006[a]	8.238	0.000, 10.944	0.026[a]
Severity	0.727	0.210	–	–	–
Braden scale	0.548	0.047[a]	2.462	1.497, 4.049	0.877
Cause of injury	1.205	0.057	–	–	–
Brain injury	0.339	0.142	–	–	–
Orthopedic injury	0.460	0.048[a]	1.088	0.008, 1.932	0.044[a]
Spine injury	0.374	0.145	–	–	–
Facial injury	0.693	0.683	–	–	–
Vascular injury	1.019	0.978	–	–	–
Lung injury	0.577	0.394	–	–	–
Intraorgan injury	1.231	0.018[a]	3.087	0.010, 9.724	0.402
Extensive soft tissue injury	1.933	< 0.001[a]	6.772	1.258, 13.578	0.210
ARDS	2.617	0.284	–	–	–
Intubation	2.903	0.021[a]	9.625	1.466, 63.549	0.018[a]
Absolute bed rest	6.429	0.028[a]	1.657	0.147, 3.488	0.344
Restrain	0.253	0.042[a]	1.157	0.028, 0.888	0.036[a]
Total parenteral nutrition	5.040	0.155	–	–	–
Transfusion	2.201	0.001[a]	2.462	1.497, 4.049	< 0.001[a]
Hb	0.229	0.001[a]	1.050	0.733, 1.502	0.791
Albumin	1.821	0.285	–	–	–
BUN	1.254	0.020[a]	0.818	0.691, 0.969	0.351
Creatinine	0.002	0.060	–	–	–
Expire	0.039	0.022[a]	2.007	0.261, 3.988	0.157

[a] Statistically significant; *ARDS* acute respiratory distress syndrome, *BUN* blood urea nitrogen

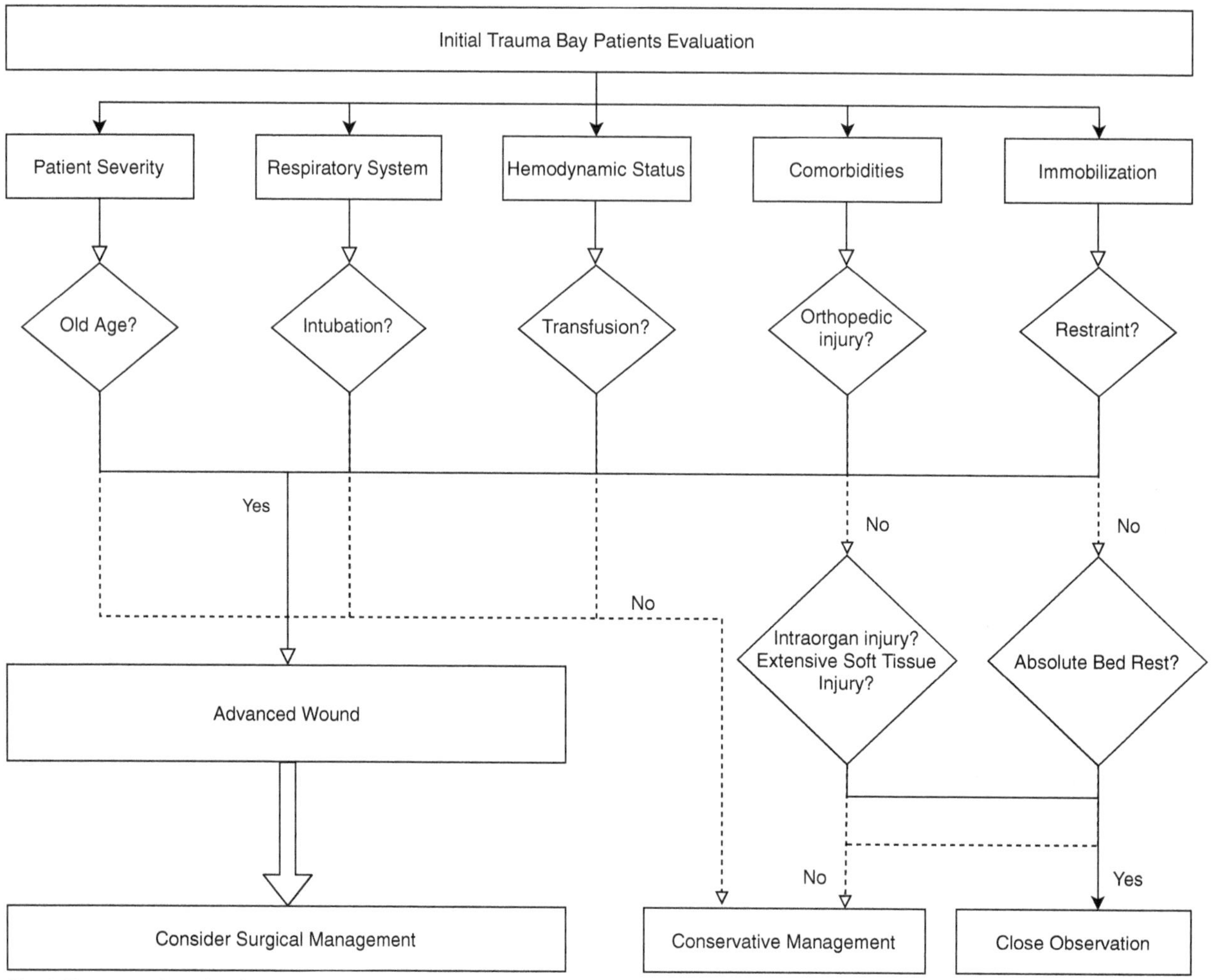

Fig. 3 Treatment algorithm for posttraumatic penoscrotal injury

and oxygen insufficiency. Orthopedic injury and restraint contribute to immobilization, and this can lead to delayed wound healing and wound deepening. Insufficient respiration and blood loss contribute to oxygen insufficiency, which leads to wound necrosis and aggravation of the edema. Through this algorithm, we want to emphasize that such patients should not simply be referred to the plastic surgeon. Initially, the critical care team should get involved with the wound evaluation and discuss management with other teams. The categorized component starts from the initial patient evaluation. Initially in the emergency room, a comprehensive wound approach is required for successful reconstruction. During the patient's hospital stay, there might be further possibilities for the critical care team to get involved. However, our study stated that when the algorithm is first applied, we simply need to check the wound status to determine whether the wound is likely to progress into an advanced wound.

The details of the treatment algorithm are described below. Firstly, in multiple trauma patients, the initial hemodynamic status should be assessed. Various laboratory findings and hemodynamic indicators help us decide whether resuscitation treatments should be started immediately or later. Hemodynamic instability should be considered first; if the patient is persistently unstable, stabilization without active wound management should be considered. Massive blood loss usually requires transfusion; thus, integration of transfusion management should be considered. The next step is the severity of the patient's condition, which should be considered with respect to their age. Respiratory care with intubation, in our experience, increased the risk of penoscrotal injury with a highly advanced wound status; thus, active surgical management should be considered. In multiple trauma patients, their additive injury status leads to further problems. Thus, a categorized evaluation is needed. In particular, combined orthopedic injuries were associated with high rates of advanced penoscrotal wounds which required special attention. Moreover, intraorgan injuries and extensive soft tissue injuries are often associated with advanced penoscrotal wounds; however, no statistical significance was noted in our study. Finally, based on these five categories of evaluation in trauma patients, we aim to detect penoscrotal wounds earlier and start active interventions.

Why is the early diagnosis of surgical prone penoscrotal defects in trauma patients important for reconstruction? Extensive penoscrotal defects ultimately require surgical reconstruction. However, anatomically the lesion penoscrotal area, there is a presence of circumferential muscle and its flexible skin texture has to be dealt with in a very particular attention. Especially erectile function should be reproduced via functional reconstruction. These days, sensate flap reconstruction is possible, hence one should not delay a referral. In our study, the most common surgical option was a local flap. The range of local flaps includes skin advancement using inguinal to upper thigh skin, local fasciocutaneous flaps, and musculocutaneous flaps. The next step for a successful reconstruction is choosing a reconstructive option. This decision is best made after the serial debridement. Once we follow the penoscrotal defect from the initial status without infection, the debrided necrotic tissue can help the surgeon make the decision. Once healthy granulation tissue is observed, we can apply the skin graft, which works best on the scrotum and shaft. As these areas have very thin epithelium this vacuum-assisted treatment is very helpful. However, complex anatomical lesions and wounds extended to the inguinal area are limited with respect to formation of granulation tissue. In this case, we used local flap advancement by using the surrounding abdominal or thigh soft tissue. However, in cases of exposed tendon or vessel, a free flap is required. Functionally and aesthetically pleasing reconstructions are now possible. However, while choosing an appropriate method of surgical reconstruction, we need to take the patient's overall status into consideration.

The limitations of our research are as follows. Owing to the nature of a level I trauma center, the severity of the patients' condition is relatively high, which could have contributed to the higher mortality seen in our study compared to those in other studies. The resuscitation rates such as respiratory resuscitation and transfusion rates were also very high. However, the mortality itself was not directly associated with the severity of the penoscrotal injury. Therefore, there was a limitation in the association between the nature of the trauma center itself with the severity of the wounds. Through this study, we hope that the discovery algorithm used to detect penoscrotal injuries in traumatic patients, will now include more than just an assessment of wound complexity.

Conclusions

In multiple trauma patients, due to the requirement of comprehensive management, penoscrotal defects caused by trauma are prone to going undetected. However, the functional and psychological importance of this area demands definitive attention and care from the physician, especially for patients with combined skeletal injuries or those on respiratory care who are likely to have advanced wounds warranting surgical treatment. We proposed a five-category algorithm to manage penoscrotal injuries in trauma patients. Inter-departmental cooperation and active intervention by plastic surgeons is needed for comprehensive treatment. We hope the proposed algorithm will help in the early detection of trauma-related penoscrotal injuries and promote early referral for their active surgical or non-surgical management.

Abbreviations

KPCS: Korean patient classification system.

Acknowledgements

The authors would like to thank everyone who participated in the management and for taking care of the trauma patients in Ajou trauma center.

Authors' contributions

MJK wrote the original draft. DHL and DHP performed data curation. IJL was involved in visualization. MJK and IJL was responsible for project administration. All authors read and approved the final manuscript.

References

1. Tran NV. Scrotal and perineal reconstruction. In: Seminars in plastic surgery. Thieme Medical Publishers, 2011. p. 213.
2. Chen S-Y, et al. Fournier gangrene: a review of 41 patients and strategies for reconstruction. Ann Plast Surg. 2010;64(6):765–9.
3. Benjamin EJ, et al. Heart disease and stroke statistics—2018 update: a report from the American Heart Association. Circulation. 2018.
4. Jung KW, et al. Cancer statistics in Korea: incidence, mortality, survival, and prevalence in 2016. Cancer Res Treat. 2019;51(2):417.
5. Lee SH, Rah DK, Lee WJ. Penoscrotal reconstruction with gracilis muscle flap and internal pudendal artery perforator flap transposition. Urology. 2012;79(6):1390–6.
6. Iranmanesh S, Rafiei H, Sabzevari S. Relationship between Braden scale score and pressure ulcer development in patients admitted in trauma intensive care unit. Int Wound J. 2012;9(3):248–52.
7. Brindle CT, et al. Outliers to the Braden scale: identifying high-risk ICU patients and the results of prophylactic dressing use. World Counc Enteros Ther J. 2010;30(1):11.
8. Song YJ. The south Korean health care system. Japan Med Assoc J. 2009;52(3):206–9.
9. Lee JH, et al. Application of different prognostic scoring systems and comparison of the FAB and WHO classifications in Korean patients with myelodysplastic syndrome. Leukemia. 2003;17(2):305–13.
10. Baldwin KM, Ziegler SM. Pressure ulcer risk following critical traumatic injury. Adv Wound Care. 1998;11(4):168–75.
11. Griswold LH, Griffin RL, Swain T, Kerby JD. Validity of the Braden scale in grading pressure ulcers in trauma and burn patients. J Surg Res. 2017;219:151–7.

12. Bong M, Kim K, Kim L, Jeong Y, An Y. Availability of patient classification using clinical data. In: NI 2012: 11th international congress on nursing informatics, June 23–27, 2012. Montreal: American Medical Informatics Association; 2012.
13. Seago JA. A comparison of two patient classification instruments in an acute care hospital. J Nurs Adm. 2002;32(5):243–9.
14. Molter NC, Molter NC. Workload management system for nurses: application to the burn unit. J Burn Care Rehabil. 1990;11(3):267–74.
15. Yoo C-S, Kwon E-O, Kim S-H, Cho Y. Reliability, validity, and conversion index of the workload management system for critical care nurses (WMSCN). J Korean. Crit Care Nurs. 2009;2:48–57.
16. Chang AC, Dearman B, Greenwood JE. A comparison of wound area measurement techniques: visitrak versus photography. Eplasty. 2011;11.
17. Keays MA, Dave S. Current hypospadias management: diagnosis, surgical management, and long-term patient-centred outcomes. Can Urol Assoc J. 2017;11(1–2 Suppl1):S48.
18. Tripathi FM, et al. Traumatic avulsion of penile and scrotal skin. Br J Plast Surg. 1982;35(3):302–3.
19. Masters FW, Robinson DW. The treatment of avulsions of the male genitalia. J Trauma Acute Care Surg. 1968;8:430–8.
20. Finical SJ, Arnold PG. Care of the degloved penis and scrotum: a 25-year experience. Plast Reconstr Surg. 1999;104(7):2074–8.

2

External validation of the R.I.R.S. scoring system to predict stone-free rate after retrograde intrarenal surgery

Cong Wang[1], ShouTong Wang[1], Xuemei Wang[2] and Jun Lu[1*]

Abstract

Background: The R.I.R.S. scoring system is defined as a novel and straightforward scoring system that uses the main parameters (kidney stone density, inferior pole stones, stone burden, and renal infundibular length) to identify most appropriate patients for retrograde intrarenal surgery (RIRS). We strived to evaluate the accuracy of the R.I.R.S. scoring system in predicting the stone-free rate (SFR) after RIRS.

Methods: In our medical center, we retrospectively analyzed charts of patients who had, between September 2018 and December 2019, been treated by RIRS for kidney stones. A total of 147 patients were enrolled in the study. Parameters were measured for each of the four specified variables.

Results: Stone-free status was achieved in 105 patients (71.43%), and 42 patients had one or more residual fragments (28.57%). Differences in stone characteristics, including renal infundibulopelvic angle, renal infundibular length, lower pole stone, kidney stone density, and stone burden were statistically significant in patients whether RIRS achieved stone-free status or not ($P<0.001$, P: 0.005, $P<0.001$, $P<0.001$, P: 0.003, respectively). R.I.R.S. scores were significantly lower in patients treated successfully with RIRS than patients in which RIRS failed ($P<0.001$). Binary logistic regression analyses revealed that R.I.R.S. scores were independent factors affecting RIRS success ($P=0.033$). The area under the curve of the R.I.R.S. scoring system was 0.737.

Conclusions: Our study retrospectively validates that the R.I.R.S. scoring system is associated with SFR after RIRS in the treatment of renal stones, and can predict accurately.

Keywords: Urolithiasis, Retrograde intrarenal surgery, Prognosis, Scoring system

Background

With the continuous improvement of flexible ureteroscope equipment, such as endoscope miniaturization, improved deflection angles, enhanced optical quality, and ancillary tools, more and more urologists have become inclined to use retrograde intrarenal surgery (RIRS) to treat kidney stones [1, 2]. Although the current urolithiasis guidelines recommend RIRS for renal stones smaller than 20 mm, with the accumulation of experience of the surgeon and the preoperative judgment of the difficulty of the operation, more surgeons have engaged RIRS to resolve renal stones larger than 20 mm and achieved excellent results [3, 4].

The ensuing question is how to choose the surgical method before surgery, RIRS or percutaneous nephrolithotomy (PCNL), and the postoperative stone-free rate (SFR) is a significant factor. To solve this problem, in 2017, Xiao et al. published the R.I.R.S. scoring system with four different parameters: kidney stone density,

*Correspondence: 842320@163.com
[1] Department of Urology, Shanghai General Hospital, Nanjing Medical University, No.100, Haining Road, Hongkou District, Shanghai 200080, China
Full list of author information is available at the end of the article

inferior pole stones, stone burden, and renal infundibular length (RIL). In this system, each parameter is assigned a different point according to different situations. The total score can range from 4 to 10 points. The higher the score, the more complicated the stone. Although the R.I.R.S. scoring system showed reliable predictive power in the preliminary research results, and there is still a lack of retrospective validation. The purpose of this article is to validate this scoring system and evaluate its validity [5].

Methods

This retrospective study was supported by our Institutional Review Board (IRB No. 2018KY192-3). At the urology department of Shanghai General Hospital, case data from patients undergoing RIRS treatment for kidney stones between September 2018 and December 2019 were retrospectively analyzed. A total of 158 patients who had not been evaluated by computed tomography urography (CTU) before the RIRS and 48 patients who had not completed treatment were excluded. Other exclusion criteria were pelviureteric mass and musculoskeletal or renal malformation. At the end of the evaluation, a total of 147 patients were enrolled in the study (Fig. 1).

In our study, all patients were evaluated by CTU before the RIRS. Patients were evaluated with a kidney ureter bladder (KUB) X-ray or non-contrast computed tomography (NCCT) 1 month after RIRS. Stone-free status was defined as no detectable stone on KUB or NCCT, or fragments of less than 2 mm were also deemed negligible stones [6]. The patients' preoperative characteristics were recorded. These were including age, gender, hypertension, diabetes mellitus status, body mass index (BMI), urine culture, history of surgery, stone location, and laterality of each stone. CTU also assessed number of stones, renal stone density, inferior pole stone, RIL, RIW, RIPA and stone burden. We divided the patients into three groups by their R.I.R.S. scores: 4–5 was mild, 6–8 was moderate, and 9–10 was severe. Using the data we collected, we also calculated the Resorlu-Unsal Stone Score (RUSS) score.

Patients and procedures

All patients completed relevant examinations before surgery to exclude contraindications to operation. All patients were treated with single-dose antibiotics before RIRS. Sensitive antibiotics were used in patients with positive urine culture until negative. An experienced urologist performed all surgeries in the lithotomy position under general anesthesia. All patients were treated with a ureteral access sheath during the operation, promoting the removal of stones and reducing the renal pressure [7]. A flexible ureteroscope was then used for holmium laser lithotripsy via ureteral access sheath (UAS), and the fragments were removed using a stone extractor [8]. When the operation took longer than 90 min, it was stopped to prevent complications. A double j-stent was placed after the operation and was removed about postoperative 1 month.

Data and statistical analysis

Data analysis was accomplished using the SPSS statistical software package (v25.0; IBM, US). Continuous variables were expressed as mean and standard deviation (SD) or median (Q3–Q1; interquartile range); categorical variables were expressed as percentages. Continuous variables were examined using a Student's t test or Mann–Whitney U test. Chi-square test and Fisher's exact test were used to compare the pairs of categorical variables. The two-tailed P value < 0.05 was considered statistically significant. Binary logistic regression analysis was used to identify independent predictors of stone-free status after RIRS treatment. We evaluated the predictive ability of the R.I.R.S. scoring system based on the area under the curve (AUC) from the receiver operating characteristic (ROC).

Results

147 patients participated in this study. 105 (71.43%) achieved stone-free status, and 42 patients (28.57%) had one or more residual fragments. The age, gender, mean BMI, and laterality of stones were similar between the groups (P: 0.494, P: 0.949, P: 0.139, P: 0.085, respectively). The stone characteristics such as renal infundibulopelvic angle (RIPA), inferior pole stone, RIL, kidney stone density, and stone burden have statistically significant differences whether RIRS achieved stone-free status or not ($P < 0.001$, $P < 0.001$, P: 0.005, $P < 0.001$, P: 0.003). Compared with patients who failed RIRS, patients who successfully applied RIRS had a significantly lower scoring system ($P < 0.001$). Preoperative patient characteristics and stone parameters are shown in Table 1. The SFR was significantly decreased over getting score in R.I.R.S. score system ($P < 0.001$), group of this score ($P < 0.001$) and RUSS ($P < 0.001$, Table 2). The binary logistic regression analysis revealed that the R.I.R.S. scoring system and RIPA, lower pole stones, RIL, kidney stone density, and stone burden were considered as independent factors affecting the success of RIRS (P: 0.033, P: 0.001, P: < 0.001, P: 0.007, P: 0.001, P: 0.006). The binary logistic regression analysis results are shown in Table 3.

Discussion

As we know, PCNL has always been the gold standard for the treatment of kidney stones larger than 20 mm [9], but in recent years, patients have rising need for non-invasive surgery. This is why more and more large medical centers are performing ultra-guided surgery.

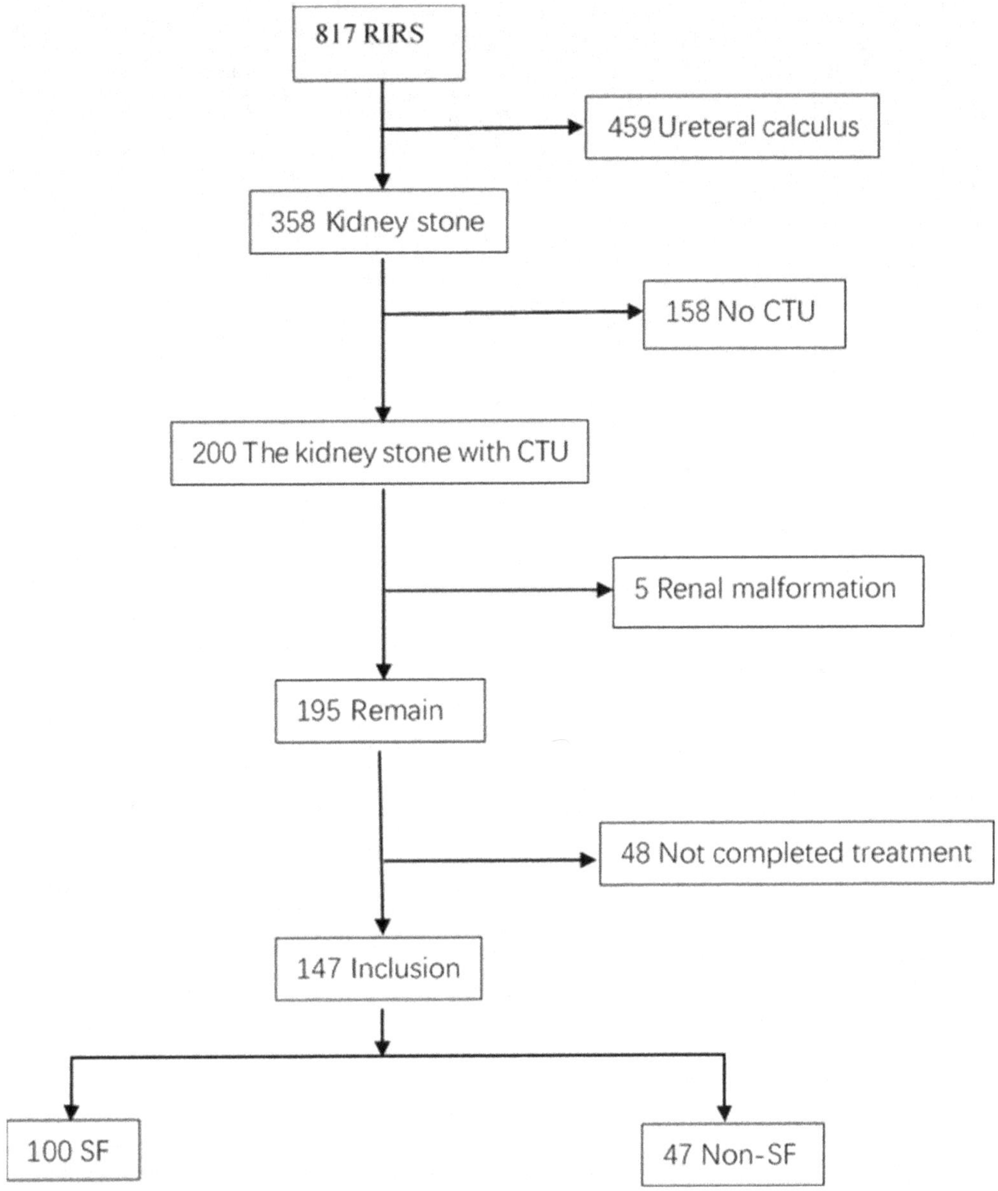

Fig. 1 Flowchart of the enrolled patients

RIRS is less invasive than PCNL and has a lower incidence of complications. RIRS has a higher stone removal rate and fewer additional operations than shockwave lithotripsy (SWL) [10]. The disadvantages of RIRS are its expense and the fragility of the ureteroscope, which adds to the cost of peripherals, including extraction baskets, laser fiber, and access sheaths. The best treatment should balance the benefits, potential complications, and total costs [11]. For this reason, accurate preoperative evaluation and preoperative planning of patient information are crucial.

The RUSS was summarized by Resorlu et al. in 2012 through a single-center retrospective analysis of 207 patients with kidney stones undergoing flexible surgery. Its parameters include stone size, number of stones, lower pole stones with RIPA $<45°$, and abnormal renal anatomy (horseshoe kidney or pelvic kidney). Stone-free status is defined as an absence of stones or residual fragments ≤ 1 mm under computed tomography (CT) examination 1 month after surgery. The final total SFR $=86\%$ [12]. This scoring system has been externally verified by many scholars, proving its effectiveness in predicting

Table 1 The demographic and clinical data of the 147 patients and the stone characteristics used to calculate the R.I.R.S. score

	No. of the patient (%)	SF	Non-SF	*P* value
No. of the patient (%)	147	105 (71.43%)	42 (28.57%)	
Gender				0.949[a]
Male	116 (78.91%)	83 (71.55%)	33 (28.45%)	
Female	31 (21.09%)	22 (70.97%)	9 (29.03%)	
Age	52.00 (61.00–40.00; 21)	53.00 (59.50–38.50; 21.00)	50.00 (63.25–42.25; 21.00)	0.494[d]
Hypertension				0.544[a]
Yes	27 (18.37%)	18 (66.67%)	9 (33.33%)	
No	120 (81.63%)	87 (72.50%)	33 (27.50)	
Diabetes mellitus				0.120[a]
Yes	10 (6.80%)	5 (50.00%)	5 (50.00%)	
No	137 (93.20%)	100 (72.99%)	37 (27.01%)	
BMI (kg/m^2)	24.39 (26.82–22.20; 4.62)	24.49 (27.12–22.67; 4.44)	23.66 (24.93–21.67; 3.26)	0.139[d]
History of surgery				0.088[a]
Yes	29 (19.73%)	17 (58.62%)	12 (41.38%)	
No	118 (80.27%)	88 (74.58%)	30 (25.42%)	
Laterality				0.085[a]
Left	78 (53.06%)	51 (65.38%)	27 (34.62%)	
Right	69 (46.94%)	54 (78.26%)	15 (21.74%)	
RIPA (°)	38.40 ± 23.03	43.70 ± 22.52	25.15 ± 18.75	< 0.001[c]*
Inferior pole stone				< 0.001[b]*
Yes	91 (61.90%)	53 (58.24%)	38 (41.76%)	
No	56 (38.10%)	52 (92.86%)	4 (7.14%)	
RIL (mm)	24.72 (27.31–20.95; 6.36)	24.00 (26.07–20.09; 5.98)	26.47 (28.05–23.39; 4.66)	0.005[d]*
RIW (mm)	8.15 (10.86–6.47; 4.39)	8.56 (10.70–6.52; 4.18)	7.48 (11.47–6.16; 5.31)	0.839[d]*
Stone burden (mm)	13.21(20.00–10.00;10.00)	12.21 (17.36–9.84; 7.52)	15.93 (25.00 –10.75;14.25)	0.003[d]*
Number of stone				0.352[a]
Single	106 (72.11%)	78 (73.58%)	28 (26.42%)	
Multiple	41 (27.89%)	27 (65.85%)	14 (34.15%)	
Renal stone density (Hu)	1403.19 ± 281.40	1330.59 ± 255.41	1584.69 ± 263.16	< 0.001[c]*
Urine culture				0.762[a]
Positive	36 (24.49%)	25 (69.44%)	11 (30.56%)	
Negative	111 (75.51%)	80 (72.07%)	31 (27.93%)	
R.I.R.S. score	7.39 ± 1.31	7.07 ± 1.18	8.19 ± 1.29	< 0.001[d]*

BMI Body mass index, *RIPA* renal infundibulopelvic angle, *RIL* renal infundibulopelvic length, *RIW* renal infundibular width

*Statistical significance was set at $P < 0.05$

[a] Chi-square test

[b] Fisher's exact test

[c] Student's t test

[d] Mann-Whitney U test

postoperative SFR [11]. This scoring system is the most widely used scoring system at present, but it was found that the stone composition is closely related to SFR during the research process. Because the stone's composition cannot be known before the operation, this parameter is not included in the scoring system. However, some scholars discovered that the composition of stones is closely related to their density [13]. Therefore, to render this scoring system more accurate and reasonable, the density of stones should be used in scoring systems.

The R.I.R.S. score is a simple and comprehensive scoring system summarized by Xiao et al. in 2017 in a retrospective analysis of 382 kidney stone patients undergoing RIRS surgery. It contains four parameters, namely stone density, stone burden, RIL, and whether the stone is located in the lower calyx (if it is located in the lower

Table 2 The SFR after RIRS according to the R.I.R.S. scoring system and RUSS

R.I.R.S. score	SFR (%)	R.I.R.S. score group	SFR (%)	RUSS	SFR (%)
4	100% (1/1)	Mild (4–5)	90% (9/10)	0	85.00% (51/60)
5	88.89% (8/9)			1	70.91% (39/55)
6	86.67% (26/30)	Moderate (6–8)	80.19% (85/106)	2	72.22% (13/18)
7	81.08% (30/37)			3	14.29% (2/14)
8	74.36% (29/39)	Severe (9–10)	35.48% (11/31)		
9	41.67% (10/24)				
10	14.29% (1/7)				
Total	71.43% (105/147)				
Linear-by-linear association	$P<0.001$		$P<0.001$		$P<0.001$

Table 3 Binary logistic regression analysis of potential independent predictors for postoperative stone-free outcomes

	P value	Exp (B)	95% CI
Inferior pole stone	< 0.001*	0.56	0.011–0.273
RIPA	0.001*	0.942	0.910–0.976
RIL	0.007*	1.165	1.042–1.303
Renal stone density	0.001*	1.004	1.002–1.006
Stone burden	0.006*	1.121	1.034–1.216
R.I.R.S. score	0.033*	0.438	0.205–0.935

RIPA renal infundibulopelvic angle, *RIL* renal infundibulopelvic length, *RIW* renal infundibular width, *CI* confidence interval

*Statistical significance was considered at $P<0.05$

calyx, RIPA should be considered). Stone-free status is here defined as no stones detectable under KUB, or only stones smaller than 2 mm 1 month after surgery. SFR = 73.6% [5]. The patients enrolled in this scoring system had undergone CTU examinations before surgery and performed three reconstructions, which can accurately measure all the stones' data, including RIPA, RIW, RIL, and other renal anatomical structures. The total score can range from 4 to 10 points. The higher the score, the more complicated the stone and the lower the rate of stone clearance after surgery. It is a simple and comprehensive scoring system. However, many medical centers do not use CTU as a routine preoperative inspection. This may be one drawback of this scoring system; it cannot be widely promoted.

Establishing an accurate diagnosis and determining the best treatment and surgery plan, preoperative imaging is a crucial step [14]. In our center, patients undergo routine preoperative CTU examinations to better understand the patient's urinary tract conditions and the characteristics of stones. NIKESH et al. suggested that CTU should be the standard imaging examination before PCNL because CTU can provide high-resolution spatial imaging and multiplanar reconstruction to accurately indicate the complexity, size, number and distribution of stones, renal pelvis structure and the anatomical relationship with other structures, and so reduce surgical complications and improve SFR and prevent unnecessary increases in the radiation burden [15]. Saskia et al. [16] suggest that CTU is vital before performing an endourologic procedure because CTU can show the anatomy of the renal pyelocaliceal system. Therefore, we recommend that the CTU examination is necessary before RIRS.

We found that the R.I.R.S. scoring system is easy to repeat because the CTU can evaluate all parameters. The RIPA is the most demanding parameter in the evaluation. In our experience, angles can be quickly and effectively assessed after a few learning curves. In this study, we propose evaluating the findings of Xiao et al. [5] and retrospectively validate the R.I.R.S. scoring system in 147 patients treated with RIRS at a single tertiary center by an experienced endourologist. We have found that the R.I.R.S. scoring system is an independent predictor of postoperative stone-free status. It provides high prediction accuracy (AUC = 0.737, Fig. 2).

R.I.R.S. scoring system seems to be a reliable preoperative tool for estimating the probability of stone-free status after RIRS. The practical value of this tool is mainly reflected in two points: patient consultation and research. By quantitatively estimating the complexity of stones, doctors can inform patients of the probability of successful treatment, and quantitative estimates can increase accurate data exchange between researchers.

To obtain a certain number of samples in a short time, this study chose to conduct a retrospective study, so it is inevitable that there are some limitations. First, the patient did not use a unified imaging method to detect the postoperative situation. To reduce the patient's radiation and economic burden, we generally use KUB to evaluate the patient's stone removal, and if there is suspected stone, further CT examinations are performed. This will

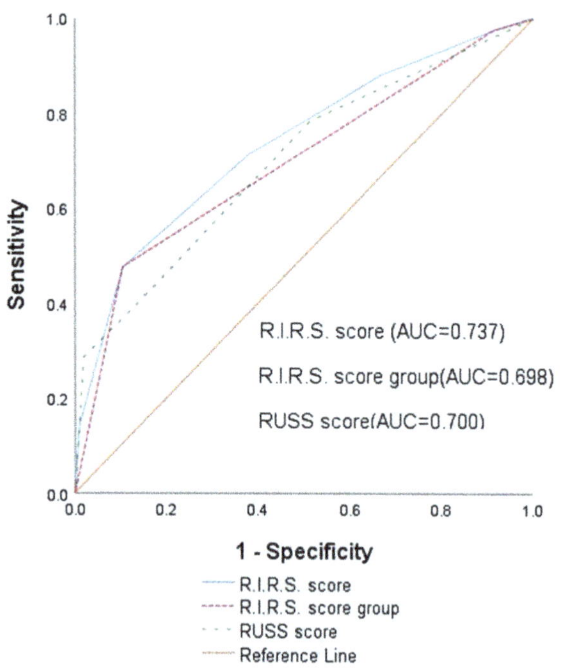

Fig. 2 Receiver operating characteristic curves of the original and three-tiered R.I.R.S. score groups and RUSS

lead to a certain error in the stone-free rate and lead to a certain degree of bias in the research results. Secondly, this study excluded patients who did not undergo CTU examination and patients who did not complete the entire operation, which may lead to selection bias. Finally, we are a single-center small sample size study. Our work's accuracy could not be compared with prospective, multi-center, and large-sample because of these limitations.

Conclusion

This study retrospectively validates that R.I.R.S. scoring system is a simple system that may predict postoperative stone-free rate after RIRS, and can provide high prediction accuracy.

Abbreviations

RIRS: Retrograde intrarenal surgery; SFR: Stone-free rate; RIPA: Renal infundibulopelvic angle; RIL: Renal infundibulopelvic length; CSD: Cumulative stone diameter; CTU: Computed tomography urography; NCCT: Non-contrast computed tomography; BMI: Body mass index; UAS: Ureteral access sheath; RIW: Renal infundibular width; CI: Confidence interval; KUB: Kidney ureter bladder; PCNL: Percutaneous nephrolithotomy; CT: Computed tomography; SWL: Shock wave lithotripsy.

Acknowledgements

The authors appreciate all our participants for their contribution in this study.

Authors' contributions

CW: data management, and manuscript writing and editing. STW: data management, data analysis, and data collection. XMW: data collection. JL: protocol and project development, data management, and manuscript editing. All authors read and approved the final manuscript.

Author details

[1] Department of Urology, Shanghai General Hospital, Nanjing Medical University, No.100, Haining Road, Hongkou District, Shanghai 200080, China.
[2] Department of Urology, Shanghai General Hospital, Shanghai Jiao Tong University School of Medicine, No.100, Haining Road, Hongkou District, Shanghai 200080, China.

References

1. Van Cleynenbreugel B, Kilic O, Akand M. Retrograde intrarenal surgery for renal stones—part 1. Türk Üroloji Dergisi/Turk J Urol. 2017;43(2):112–21.
2. Kilic O, Akand M, Van Cleynenbreugel B. Retrograde intrarenal surgery for renal stones—part 2. Türk Üroloji Dergisi/Turk J Urol. 2017;43(3):252–60.
3. Akman T, Binbay M, Ozgor F, Ugurlu M, Tekinarslan E, Kezer C, Aslan R, Muslumanoglu AY. Comparison of percutaneous nephrolithotomy and retrograde flexible nephrolithotripsy for the management of 2–4 cm stones: a matched-pair analysis. BJU INT. 2012;109(9):1384–9.
4. Breda A, Angerri O. Retrograde intrarenal surgery for kidney stones larger than 22.5 cm. Curr Opin Urol. 2014;24(2):179–83.
5. Xiao Y, Li D, Chen L, Xu Y, Zhang D, Shao Y, Lu J. The R.I.R.S. scoring system: an innovative scoring system for predicting stone-free rate following retrograde intrarenal surgery. BMC Urol. 2017;17(1):1–8.
6. Ghani KR, Wolf JJ. What is the stone-free rate following flexible ureteroscopy for kidney stones? Nat Rev Urol. 2015;12(5):281–8.
7. Traxer O, Thomas A. Prospective evaluation and classification of ureteral wall injuries resulting from insertion of a ureteral access sheath during retrograde intrarenal surgery. J Urol. 2013;189(2):580–4.
8. Schatloff O, Lindner U, Ramon J, Winkler HZ. Randomized trial of stone fragment active retrieval versus spontaneous passage during holmium laser lithotripsy for ureteral stones. J Urol. 2010;183(3):1031–6.
9. Türk C, Petřík A, Sarica K, Seitz C, Skolarikos A, Straub M, Knoll T. EAU guidelines on interventional treatment for urolithiasis. Eur Urol. 2016;69(3):475–82.
10. Preminger GM. Management of lower pole renal calculi: shock wave lithotripsy versus percutaneous nephrolithotomy versus flexible ureteroscopy. Urol Res. 2006;34(2):108–11.
11. Sfoungaristos S, Gofrit ON, Mykoniatis I, Landau EH, Katafigiotis I, Pode D, Constantinides CA, Duvdevani M. External validation of Resorlu-Unsal stone score as predictor of outcomes after retrograde intrarenal surgery. Int Urol Nephrol. 2016;48(8):1247–52.
12. Resorlu B, Unsal A, Gulec H, Oztuna D. A new scoring system for predicting stone-free rate after retrograde intrarenal surgery: The "Resorlu-Unsal Stone Score." Urology. 2012;80(3):512–8.
13. Celik S, Sefik E, Basmacı I, Bozkurt IH, Aydın ME, Yonguc T, Degirmenci T. A novel method for prediction of stone composition: the average and difference of Hounsfield units and their cut-off values. Int Urol Nephrol. 2018;50(8):1397–405.
14. Magrill D, Patel U, Anson K. Impact of imaging in urolithiasis treatment planning. Curr Opin Urol. 2013;23(2):158–63.
15. Thiruchelvam N, Mostafid H, Ubhayakar G. Planning percutaneous nephrolithotomy using multidetector computed tomography urography, multiplanar reconstruction and three-dimensional reformatting. BJU Int. 2005;95(9):1280–4.
16. Weltings S, Hulsbos S, Kieft GJ, Pelger RCM, Roshani H. The anatomy of the renal pyelocaliceal system studied by CTU. Abdom Radiol. 2019;44(2):612–8.

3

Efficacy of transcutaneous perineal electrostimulation versus intracavitary anal electrostimulation in the treatment of urinary incontinence after a radical prostatectomy

R. Pané-Alemany[1], I. Ramírez-García[1,2,3,5*], A. Carralero-Martínez[1], L. Blanco-Ratto[1,4], S. Kauffmann[1,4,6] and E. Sánchez[3]

Abstract

Background: Radical prostatectomy is the gold standard treatment for men with localized prostate cancer. This technique is associated with post-operative urinary incontinence. Pelvic floor physiotherapy is a conservative, painless and economical treatment for this specific situation. Kegel exercises and perineal electrostimulation are common techniques to train pelvic floor muscles. The perineal electrostimulation can be applied to the patient with surface electrodes or by an intra-cavitary anal probe. This study proposes that transcutaneous perineal electrostimulation is as effective as intra-cavitary electrostimulation in reducing urinary incontinence secondary to radical prostatectomy. The main objective is to compare the efficacy of the treatment with transcutaneous perineal electrostimulation versus the same intra-cavitary treatment to reduce the magnitude of urinary incontinence after radical prostatectomy, and the impact on the quality of life.

Methods: This single-blind equivalence randomized controlled trial will include 70 man who suffer urinary incontinence post radical prostatectomy. Participants will be randomized into surface electrodes group and intra-anal probe group. The groups will receive treatment for 10 consecutive weeks. Outcomes include changes in the 24-h Pad Test, and ICIQ-SF, SF-12 and I-QoL questionnaires. Clinical data will be collected at baseline, 6 and 10 weeks after the first session, and 6 months after the end of treatment.

Discussion: The results will allow us to prescribe the most beneficial perineal electrostimulation technique in the treatment of urinary incontinence derived from radical prostatectomy.

Keywords: Male urinary incontinence, Postprostatectomy incontinence, Surface electrodes electrostimulation, Intra-anal probe electrostimulation, Randomized controlled trial

Background

Radical prostatectomy (RP) is the gold standard treatment for men with localized prostate cancer and prostatic hyperplasia. Improvements in anatomical knowledge and surgical techniques have significantly

*Correspondence: inesrg@blanquerna.url.edu
[1] Rehabilitación Abdomino-Pelviana (RAPbarcelona SL), Barcelona, Spain
Full list of author information is available at the end of the article

reduced post-intervention morbidity [1]. However, RP is associated with post-operative urinary incontinence (UI), that can persist for two years or longer and is associated to significant reductions in overall health-related quality of life (QoL) [2–5].

Urinary continence in men depends on the contributions from smooth muscle of the urethra and urethral constriction generated by contraction of three striated muscles: the striated urethral sphincter (SUS); puborectalis/pubovisceralis and bulbocavernosus [6]. RP inherently removes the prostatic segment of the urethra, and its smooth muscle (called the internal sphincter), and may remove or damage the SUS muscle or its innervation [7]. Continence recovery after prostatectomy is likely to require enhanced function of SUS (and other striated muscles) to compensate for the reduced smooth muscle [6, 7].

Pelvic floor muscle training (PFMT) is the most common non-invasive intervention for UI derived from a radical prostatectomy. Available published evidence demonstrates that PFMT with muscular electrostimulation (ES) has a significant positive impact on the early recovery of urinary continence after this intervention [8–10].

The perineal ES can be applied to the patient with surface electrodes or by an intra-cavitary anal probe [11]. Up to now, the most described method of application in the literature has been intra-anal [10, 12]. Each technique stimulates different anatomical points and remains unknown if both have the same effectiveness or one of them has more effect. Intra-cavitary application can be uncomfortable or annoying for patient; nevertheless, perineal surface ES could be a simple therapeutic modality, easy to apply and equal or more effective than intra-cavitary one.

The study hypothesizes that perineal surface ES is as effective as intra-cavitary ES in the reduction of UI secondary to radical prostatectomy. We aim to compare the efficacy of both techniques in reducing the magnitude of UI secondary to radical prostatectomy, and to evaluate its impact on the patients' quality of life. Specifically we plan to estimate the amount (grams) of urine lost in 24 h to evaluate the severity of UI secondary to radical prostatectomy, and to assess the quality of life of the patients participating in the study.

Methods

Study design

This manuscript describes a research protocol for a single blind, equivalence randomized controlled clinical trial. Equivalence trials aim to determine whether one intervention is therapeutically similar to another; equivalence is defined as the treatment effect being between $-\Delta$ and $+\Delta$, Δ meaning the margin of equivalence. If the confidence interval of the outcomes difference between the two studied groups falls within the predetermined margin of equivalence ($-\Delta$ to $+\Delta$), the two types of techniques can be considered equivalent. Participants will be randomly allocated into surface electrodes group (intervention group, IG) and intra-anal probe group (control group, CG). The investigator performing the statistical analyses will be blinded.

Study locations

This trial will take place at RAPbarcelona pelvic floor specialized physiotherapy centre in Barcelona, and at the pelvic floor rehabilitation unit of the Institut Mèdic Tecnologic of Barcelona.

Study population

Patients who consult in one of the two participating centres for UI derived from a radical prostatectomy surgical intervention will be invited to participate during his first physiotherapy visit.

To be eligible, participants must meet the following criteria. Inclusion criteria: having undergone radical prostatectomy, presenting involuntary urine losses after radical prostatectomy intervention (UI grade I, II or III), do not exceeding the year since the surgical intervention, and accepting to participate in the study granting signed informed consent. Exclusion criteria: following a pharmacological treatment for UI, presenting anatomical malformations of the pelvic floor musculature, carrying a pacemaker, presenting anal fistulas, suffering serious psyche disorders, having a history of lower urinary tract infections, requiring radiotherapy as adjuvant treatment, being diagnosed with urethral stricture after surgery, presenting pelvic floor denervation, and suffering neuromuscular diseases.

Investigations

Patients who agree to participate in the study will be cited by telephone and receive ES therapy once a week. At baseline, participants will undergo an initial assessment where data on age, date of surgery, surgical intervention technique and days of catheterization will be collected. The Oxford test (to measure the pelvic floor muscular strength), the 24-h Pad Test (in order to quantify the involuntary loss of urine), the UI questionnaire ICIQ-SF, and the SF-12 questionnaire and the specific I-QoL test (to assess their quality of life) will be evaluated at first visit.

A total of ten treatment physiotherapy sessions will be held on a weekly basis (Table 1).

According to the allocation group, the ES technique will be applied using the Neurotrac Pelvitone® muscular electrostimulator, together with two round surface

Table 1 Treatment sessions

SESSION 1	Collection and recording of baseline data (age, intervention date and intervention technique), Oxford measurement and tests (24-h Pad Test, ICIQ-SF, SF-12, I-QoL) Delivery of the compliance form ES (10 min at 30 Hz and 5 min at 50 Hz) Explanation of the routine for home pelvic floor exercises (10 contractions maintained and 10 fast contractions to be performed three times a day)
SESSION 2	Session protocol: Registration of possible discomfort or adverse effects perceived by the patient Review of the domiciliary exercises routine and record of compliance ES (10 min at 30 Hz and 5 min at 50 Hz)
SESSION 3–5	Session protocol (as described in session 2)
SESSION 6	Collection of 24-h Pad Test data Oxford measurement Record of patient satisfaction with the treatment Session protocol (as described in session 2)
SESSION 7–9	Session protocol (as described in session 2)
SESSION 10	Session protocol (as described in session 2) Oxford measurement Collection of 24-h Pad Test data and completion of ICIQ-SF, SF-12 and I-QoL tests Record of patient satisfaction with the treatment
SESSION 11 (6 months after the end of treatment)	Collection of the 24-h Pad Test, compliance and satisfaction data

electrodes of 32 mm or an Analys Plus® anal stimulation probe of 140 mm.

In both groups, participants will be placed comfortably in a supine position with a pillow under their heads, without pants or underwear, and with the legs bent over two leg supports.

Participants in the IG will receive the treatment through a 32-mm surface electrode attached just above the base of the penis and below the pubis, and another 32-mm surface electrode placed on the perineum (area between the end of the testicles and the anal sphincter).

Patients in the CG will receive the same treatment by means of an anal stimulation probe, which will be placed inside the rectal cavity.

Description of the treatment session (same for both groups)

15 min of perineal ES (with surface electrodes or intra-anal probe according to the allocation to IG or CG, respectively), composed of 10 min of direct current at 30 Hz frequency and a pulse width of 250 microseconds, to train the tonic fibres, and 5 min of alternating current at 50 Hz frequency and a pulse width of 250 microseconds, to train the phasic fibres.

Additionally, Kegel active exercises are going to be performed under the supervision and correction of the physiotherapist in each of the treatment sessions and also carried out at home. This regimen will consist of ten slow and maintained contractions of the perineal musculature (8–10 s) and ten fast contractions (3 s) to be done three times a day (twice in a supine position and once in a sitting or standing position) during the ten weeks the whole treatment lasts.

In each session, treatment adherence and possible adverse effects of the therapy will be identified and recorded in a database designed for the project.

The same treatment protocol will be followed in all sessions. In the sixth session the results of a second 24-h Pad test will be registered, the Oxford test delivered and the satisfaction with the treatment of each patient recorded. In the tenth session, the same tests as in the first session will be re-evaluated.

The indications for the 24-h Pad test will be given in the session previous to the scheduled for the patient to do it at home and bring the results on the following treatment session, excepting for that of session 1 that will be delivered at the time of acceptance in the study.

Six months after the end of the treatment, patients will be contacted by telephone for a final assessment with the purpose of checking whether the possible benefits of the therapy persist.

Outcome measures

Participants will complete four study assessments: baseline, 6 and 10 weeks after first session, and 6 months after the end of treatment.

Primary outcome

Magnitude of urinary incontinence According to the grams of urine collected in a pad with the 24-h Pad Test. This is a quantitative variable (expressed in grams) evaluated in the first, sixth, tenth and eleventh sessions of the study. The Pad test consists of weighing a clean pad in grams (by the same patient), then placing it and weighing it again after an established time (24 h). In case of needing an extra pad before the 24 h are completed, the procedure would be repeated until 24 h were reached. The increase in weight tells us about the severity of incontinence. The values for mild UI are from 1.3 to 20 g, moderate from 21 to 74 g and severe 75 g or more [13, 14].

Secondary outcomes

Severity of the urinary incontinence Assessed with the score obtained in the questionnaire ICIQ-SF, a tool validated and translated into Spanish, specific to the study of UI, used in the basic evaluation of UI from the patient's perspective [15–22]. This is a quantitative variable evaluated in the first, tenth and eleventh sessions of the study.

Quality of life related to health Measured with the SF-12 Quality of Life Scale and the I-QoL questionnaire. The SF-12 health questionnaire is a generic questionnaire. We will use the Spanish adaptation done by Alonso et al. [16, 17] of the SF-12 Health Survey [18, 19]. The SF-12 is a reduced version of the SF-36 Health Questionnaire designed for cases in which this is too long. The SF-12 is answered in an average of ≤ 2 min and the SF-36 needs between 5 and 10 min. It consists of 12 items from the 8 dimensions of the SF-36 physical function, social function, physical role, emotional role, mental health, vitality, body pain and general health status. Higher score means better quality of life. The I-QoL is a specific questionnaire, with only 22 items, that assesses different domains such as avoidance of behaviours, psychosocial impact and feeling of being ashamed. The questionnaire is assessed according to its different scales or globally, so that the higher the scores obtained, the better the quality of life shown [20, 21].

Adverse effects Recorded in each of the treatment sessions through the patient references about his status and evolution.

Adherence to treatment Assessed in each of the treatment sessions, collected through a compliance form designed for the project.

Satisfaction of the participants with the treatment Registered in the sixth and tenth sessions with a scale from 1 to 10 (being 1, not satisfied and 10, very satisfied).

Schedule

	Recruitment	Session 1	Sessions 2–5	Session 6	Sessions 7–9	Session 10	6 months post treatment
Recruitment							
Selection screening	X						
Informed consent	X						
Collection of baseline data		X					
Interventions							
Intervention CG	X	X	X	X	X	X	X
Intervention IG	X	X	X	X	X	X	X
Evaluations							
24-h Pad Test		X		X		X	X
Oxford		X		X		X	
ICIQ-SF		X				X	
SF-12		X				X	
I-QoL		X				X	
Compliance form		X	X	X	X	X	X
Recording of adverse effects			X	X	X	X	X
Treatment satisfaction						X	X

The different achedule phases are shown in italics

Sample size

To estimate the sample size, we use the randomisation and online databases for clinical trials program of the online computer software Sealed Envelope Ltd. 2001–2015 (https://www.sealedenvelope.com/power/continuous-equivalence/).

For this estimate, alpha values of 5% and beta of 20% (power of 80%) were taken into account. Based on data published in the literature [10, 12], and considering an expected difference in the 24-h Pad Test between the two studied groups of 22 g, 32 patients are needed in each arm of the study. The interpretation is as follows: "if there is truly no difference between the control (ES by intra-anal probe) and intervention (ES by surface electrodes) treatment, then 64 patients are required to be 80% sure that the limits of a two-sided 90% confidence interval will exclude a difference in means of more than 22 g".

Assuming that there could be losses to follow-up, the number of individuals to be recruited will be increased by 10% until reaching 70 patients (35 patients per group).

Selection of the sample

The selection of the sample will be done by sampling of consecutive cases, from RAPbarcelona clinic and Institut Médic Tecnològic in Barcelona. In urologists or physiotherapists appointments, patients who underwent radical prostatectomy and presented with UI will be referred to the principal investigator. The protocol will be clearly explained to each of the interested patients who meet all the selection criteria and he will be asked to sign the informed consent if accept participation. After the signature the patient will be allocated to one of the two study groups.

Random allocation of groups

A consecutive inclusion will be done until the desired sample size is reached. The generation of the random sequence will be carried out by the principal investigator using the statistical software Epidat. The randomization list will be delivered to the clinics reception desk and patients will be allocated by telephone at a 1:1 ratio (assignment by third parties).

Each participant will be assigned an identification number created for the study and linked to his treatment group. This number will allow the patient for beginning the treatment sessions. Two physiotherapists previously trained for the application of the study protocol will be in charge of the sessions.

Collection, management and data analysis

Data will be collected in a specific database for this study by the physiotherapists in charge of the application of the technique and sent to a data analyst unfamiliar with the techniques and study groups. The SPSS 24.0 software will be used.

First, a descriptive analysis of the characteristics of the patients included in both study groups, as well as the outcome variables will be carried out. To do this, absolute and relative frequencies (percentages) will be estimated for qualitative variables, and mean or median and standard deviation or range, respectively, depending on the normality of the distribution, for quantitative variables.

In addition, different associations between diverse variables will be analysed.

To check for the equivalence of the study treatments efficacy, intention to treat (ITT) and by protocol (PP) analysis will be performed.

The comparison of results will be done by estimating the differences in a timely manner and with their corresponding 90% confidence intervals (90% CI). Additionally, the adjusted differences will be calculated, following the indications of the CONSORT document [23].

In all cases, the level of statistical significance established will be the usual (5%); Therefore, statistically significant differences will be considered when p values are less than 0.05.

If adverse effects would occur, the physiotherapist together with the principal investigator will decide the continuity of the participant in the study, having his safety and health as a priority.

Discussion

The result of this study will allow us to prescribe the most beneficial ES technique in the treatment of UI derived from radical prostatectomy. If the surface technique is proven equivalent, it would be more comfortable for the patient to receive the treatment.

Abbreviations

RP: Radical prostatectomy; UI: Urinary incontinence; PFMT: Pelvic floor muscle training; SUS: Striated urethral sphincter; ES: Electro stimulation; QoL: Quality of life; ICIQ-SF: International Consultation on Incontinence Questionnaire Short-Form; SF-12: Health Questionnaire Short Form 12; I-QoL: The Incontinence Quality of Life Questionnaire; IG: Intervention group; CG: Control group.

Acknowledgements

None.

Authors' contributions

RPA and IRG were responsible for the study conception and design. ES collaboratively conceptualised the study objectives and methodology and provided a critical revision of the manuscript. ACM, SK and LBR helped conceptualise and design the study. All authors read and approved the final manuscript.

Author details
[1] Rehabilitación Abdomino-Pelviana (RAPbarcelona SL), Barcelona, Spain. [2] Servicio de Fisioterapia, Instituto Médico Tecnológico SL, Barcelona, Spain. [3] Blanquerna School of Health Science-Universitat Ramon Llull, Barcelona, Spain. [4] Fundació Universitària del Bages (FUB), Barcelona, Spain. [5] Universidad Internacional de Catalunya (UIC), Barcelona, Spain. [6] Servicio de Fisioterapia, Womens Salud Y Bienestar de La Mujer SL, Barcelona, Spain.

References

1. Fernández RA, García-Hermoso A, Solera-Martínez M, Correa MT, Morales AF, Martínez-Vizcaíno V. Improvement of continence rate with pelvic floor muscle training post-prostatectomy: a meta-analysis of randomized controlled trials. Urol Int. 2015;94(2):125–32.
2. Penson DF, McLerran D, Feng Z, Li L, Albertsen PC, Gilliland FD, et al. 5-Year urinary and sexual outcomes after radical prostatectomy: results from the prostate cancer outcomes study. J Urol. 2005;173:1701–5.
3. Weber BA, Roberts BL, Mills TL, Chumbler NR, Algood CB. Physical and emotional predictors of depression after radical prostatectomy. Am J Mens Health. 2008;2:165–71.
4. Sanda MG, Dunn RL, Michalski J, Sandler HM, Northouse L, Hembroff L, et al. Quality of life and satisfaction with outcome among prostate-cancer surviviors. N Engl J Med. 2008;358:1250–61.
5. Steineck G, Helgesen F, Adolfsson J, Dickman PW, Johansson J-E, Norlen BJ, et al. Quality of life after radical prostatectomy or watchful waiting. N Engl J Med. 2002;347:790–6.
6. Stafford RE, Ashton-Miller JA, Constantinou CE, et al. A new method to quantify male pelvic oor displacement from 2D transperineal ultrasound images. Urology. 2013;81:685–9.
7. Presti JC, Schmidt RA, Narayan PA, et al. Pathophysiology of urinary incontinence after radical prostatectomy. J Urol. 1990;143:975–8.
8. Marchiori D, Bertaccini A, Manferrari F, Ferri C, Martorana G. Pelvic floor rehabilitation for continence recovery after radical prostatectomy: role of a personal training re-educational program. Anticancer Res. 2010;30(2):553–6.
9. Yamanishi T, Mizuno T, Watanabe M, Honda M, Yoshida K-I. Randomized, placebo controlled study of electrical stimulation with pelvic floor muscle training for severe urinary incontinence after radical prostatectomy. J Urol. 2010;184(5):2007–12.
10. Mariotti G, Sciarra A, Gentilucci A, Salciccia S, Alfarone A, Di PG, et al. Early recovery of urinary continence after radical prostatectomy using early pelvic floor electrical stimulation and biofeedback associated treatment. J Urol. 2009;181(4):1788–93.
11. Ramírez I, Blanco L, Kauffmann S. Rehabilitación del suelo pélvico femenino. Práctica clínica basada en la evidencia. 1ª ed.. Madrid: Editorial Médica Panamericana; 2013.
12. Van KM, Weerdt W, Van PH, Ridder D, Feys H, Baert L. Effect of pelvic floor reducation on duration and degree of incontinence after radical prostatectomy: a randomised controlled trial. Lancet. 2000;355(1):98–102.
13. O'Sullivan R, Karantanis E, Stevermuer TL, Allen W, Moore KH. Definition of mild, moderate and severe incontinence on the 24-hour pad test. BJOG. 2004;111(8):859–62.
14. Karantanis E, Allen W, Stevermuer TL, et al. The repeatability of the 24-hour pad test. Int Urogynecol J Pelvic Floor Dysfunct. 2005;16:63–8.
15. Avery K, Donovan J, Peters TJ, Shaw C, Gotoh M, Abrams P. ICIQ: a brief and robust measure for evaluating the symptoms and impact of urinary incontinence. Neurourol Urodyn. 2004;23(4):322–30.
16. Vilagut G, Ferrer M, Rajmil M, Rebollo P, Permanyer-Miralda G, Quintana JM, Santed R, Valderas JM, Ribera A, Domingo-Salvany A, Alonso J. El cuestionario de salud SF-36 español: una década de experiencia y nuevos desarrollos. Gac Sanit. 2005;19(2):135–50.
17. Alonso J, Regidor E, Barrio G, Prieto L, Rodríguez G. De La Fuente De Hoz L. Valores poblacionales de referencia de la versiónespañola del Cuestionario de Salud SF-36. Med Clin (Barc). 1998;111:410–6.
18. Ware JE Jr, Kosinski M, Keller SD. A 12-Item Short-Form Health Survey: construction of scales and preliminary tests of reliability and validity. Med Care. 1996;34:220–33.
19. Gandek B, Ware JE, Aaronson NK, Apolone G, Bjorner JB, Brazier JE, et al. Cross-validation of item selection and scoring for the SF-12 Health Survey in nine countries: results from the IQOLA Project. International Quality of Life Assessment. J Clin Epidemiol. 1998;51:1171–8.
20. Patrick DL, Martin ML, Bushnell DM, Marquis P, Andrejasich CM, Buesching DP. Cultural adaptation of a quality-of-life measure for urinary incontinence. Eur Urol. 1999;36(5):427–35.
21. Bushnell DM, Martin ML, Summers KH, Svihra J, Lionis C, Patrick DL. Quality of life of women with urinary incontinence: cross-cultural performance of 15 language versions of the I-QoL. Qual Life Res. 2005;14(8):1901–13.
22. Espuña Pons M, Rebollo Alvarez P, Puig Clota M. Validation of the Spanish version of the International Consultation on Incontinence Questionnaire-Short Form. A questionnaire for assessing the urinary incontinence. Med Clin (Barc). 2004;122(8):288–92.
23. Chan AW, Tetzlaff JM, Altman DG, Laupacis A, Gøtzsche PC, Krleža-Jerić K, et al. SPIRIT 2013 statement: defining standard protocol items for clinical trials. Ann Intern Med. 2013;158:200–7.

4

Cerebral oxygenation in 45-degree trendelenburg position for robot-assisted radical prostatectomy: A single-center, open, controlled pilot study

Clemens Wiesinger[1†], Dominik Stefan Schoeb[2*†], Mathias Stockhammer[3], Emir Mirtezani[1], Lukas Mitterschiffthaler[4], Helga Wagner[5], Johann Knotzer[4] and Walter Pauer[1]

Abstract

Background: Within the last decade, robotically-assisted laparoscopic prostatectomy (RALP) has become the standard for treating localized prostate cancer, causing a revival of the 45° Trendelenburg position. In this pilot study we investigated effects of Trendelenburg position on hemodynamics and cerebral oxygenation in patients undergoing RALP.

Methods: We enrolled 58 patients undergoing RALP and 22 patients undergoing robot-assisted partial nephrectomy (RAPN) (control group) in our study. Demographic patient data and intraoperative parameters including cerebral oxygenation and cerebral hemodynamics were recorded for all patients. Cerebral function was also assessed pre- and postoperatively via the Mini Mental Status (MMS) exam. Changes in parameters during surgery were modelled by a mixed effects model; changes in the MMS result were evaluated using the Wilcoxon signed rank test.

Results: Preoperative assessment of patient characteristics, standard blood values and vital parameters revealed no difference between the two groups.

Conclusions: Applying a 45° Trendelenburg position causes no difference in postoperative brain function, and does not alter cerebral oxygenation during a surgical procedure lasting up to 5 h. Further studies in larger patient cohorts will have to confirm these findings.

Keywords: Robotic surgical procedures/adverse effects, Head-down tilt, Robotic surgical procedures/methods, Prostatectomy/adverse effects*, Laparoscopy/adverse effects, Monitoring, Intraoperative

Background

Since Prof. Friedrich Trendelenburg developed the "Raised Pelvic Position" for abdominal and pelvic operations in the 1880s, and its first description by his student Dr. Willy Meyer in 1885, the term "Trendelenburg Position" has become the standard nomenclature to describe a patient lying in supine position [1]. While originally intended to facilitate surgical procedures when treating

*Correspondence: dominik.stefan.schoeb@uniklinik-freiburg.de
†Clemens Wiesinger and Dominik Stefan Schoeb contributed equally to this work
[2] Department of Urology, Faculty of Medicine, Medical Center – University of Freiburg, Hugstetterstr. 55, 79106 Freiburg, Germany
Full list of author information is available at the end of the article

vesicovaginal fistulae [2] and later for other gynecological operations, the patient was placed on a table tilted 45° downwards with legs and feet over the table's edge [1]. This "extreme" form of the Trendelenburg position, however, was later abandoned mostly, and while the "Raised Pelvic Position" served various purposes such as treating venous air embolism [3] or facilitating intestinal surgery in obese patients [4], the angle applied usually did not exceed 30°. Furthermore, while the Trendelenburg position was traditionally employed for the acute treatment of hypotension, clinical studies had not yielded any evidence of this method's beneficial effect on the patient [5]. The original Trendelenburg Position using a 45° angle has recently experienced a revival in the operation theater, with robot-assisted procedures becoming the new standard in minimally invasive surgery. After its first description in 2000 [6, 7], robotically-assisted laparoscopic radical prostatectomy has become the new standard surgical therapy for localized prostate cancer [8] and since then, robotically-assisted surgery has been extended to various other procedures such as hysterectomy [9], proctocolectomy [10], nephrectomy [11], and more.

To perform robot-assisted laparoscopic prostatectomy, an "extreme" 45° Trendelenburg position is often applied, continuing throughout the procedure. In addition to abdominal CO2-insufflation, significantly reduced pulmonary compliance and upper airway edema have been reported [12].

In this study we explore the influence of a prolonged Trendelenburg Position during robotically-assisted radical prostatectomy on intraoperative hemodynamics and cerebral oxygenation, as well as pre- and postoperative cerebral function.

Methods

Patient cohort and study protocol

We enrolled in our study a total of 58 consecutive male patients (study group) who underwent robot-assisted radical prostatectomy (RALP) for localized prostate cancer therapy and 22 consecutive male patients undergoing robot-assisted partial nephrectomy (RAPN) (control group) for suspected kidney-cell carcinoma at the Wels-Grieskirchen Medical Center. We chose the RAPN procedure for our control group since it is a routine, robotically-assisted procedure at our institution, and a horizontal position is maintained during the entire procedure. Preoperative oncological staging and the indication for the above-mentioned surgical intervention were determined according to the current guidelines of the European Association of Urology (EAU) on prostate cancer and renal cell carcinoma. General anesthesia was induced with 150–200 μg of fentanyl and 150–200 mg of propofol then 0.6 mg/kg of rocuronium was administered followed by orotracheal intubation. General anesthesia was maintained with sevoflurane (MAC 0.9–1.2) and continuous infusion of remifentanil (1–2.5 μg/kg/min). Pneumoperitoneum was induced by insufflating CO2 with gas pressure set to 8 mmHg during the whole operation. After pneumoperitoneum was achieved, study patients were positioned in 45° Trendelenburg by tilting the operating table. Control group patients were brought into flank position prior to inducing pneumoperitoneum with the operation table slightly flexed. Once the procedure started, this patient position was maintained during the entire procedure. All surgeries were performed by experienced urologists (>100 robot-assisted procedures) using the da Vinci® Si Surgical System (Intuitive Surgical, Sunnyvale, CA, USA) with the surgeon performing the procedure at a control table located away from the operating table. Patients provided informed consent prior to inclusion in our study, which was approved by our local ethics committee (ethics committee of Upper Austria (Study Nr. O-18-13)); it was therefore conducted in accordance with the ethical standards laid down in the 1964 Declaration of Helsinki and its later amendments. Our sole exclusion criterion was involvement in any other clinical study, but this did not apply since no patients screened met this criterion. The study was designed and conducted in accordance with the consort criteria.

Intraoperative monitoring and data collection

Patient demographics and ASA classification was recorded 24–6 h prior to surgery. In addition, mini-mental status test (MMS) was carried out, and a standard blood workup (hemoglobin, hematocrit, blood coagulation parameters) was obtained. Furthermore, we documented baseline blood pressure and heart frequency. Intraoperative heart frequency (HF), cerebral oxygenation (rSO2), and blood pressure (RR) were obtained and recorded prior to final positioning and consecutively at 10-min intervals throughout the procedure. Also the FiO2 was (=fraction of inspired oxygen) was monitored. To measure rSO2, bilateral cerebral oximetry sensors were placed on the patient's forehead and rSO2 was continuously monitored using near infrared spectroscopy (NIRS) and the INVOS analytics tool for recording. We also recorded total operating time, time in Trendelenburg position and time of robotic actuation. Within 6–24 h after surgery, standard blood panel was repeated and all patients underwent a MMS Test. Complications were classified according to the Clavien Dindo classification and recorded over a 3 months follow up for all included patients.

Statistical evaluation

This trial was designed to explore whether a 45 Degree Trendelenburg Position causes any differences in intraoperative clinical parameters, or changes in the MMS exam result in comparison with patients not in a head-down position. Patients were included in this exploratory study applying the intention-to-treat principle. All statistical calculations were performed by an experienced and licensed statistician (H.W.). Changes in the MMS exam outcome before and after surgery were subjected to the Wilcoxon rank-sum test. To analyze the evolvement of parameters during surgery, we made an exploratory comparison of the different variables at the same time point, followed by a longitudinal analysis of a variable's evolvement, and investigated the change in a given variable compared to its initial value by linear mixed effects models. To analyze changes, the response variable's pre-operation value centered at a reasonable value and that variable's interaction with time were included in the model. All statistical computations were performed using the R statistics software (Version 3.5.2). All tests were two-sided with $p<0.05$ considered to indicate statistical significance, but as this is not a confirmatory trial, significant results can be interpreted only as indicating a potential association.

Results

Patient characteristics and preoperative results

All patients included in our study underwent a complete evaluation, and we observed no drop outs. Median age in our study group was 66, ranging from 48 to 79 years. Our control group's median age was 56 years (45–84). ASA classification showed a median of 2 for both groups. Routine blood panel revealed a median hemoglobin value of 15.3 g/dl (13–17.1) for the RALP group and 14 g/dl (10.20–16.30) for the RAPN group. Median preoperative RR was 137.5 (94–210)/80 (60–110) for our study group and 146.5 (100–180)/80 (60–103) for the control group. The median HF measured 66 bpm (45–92) (RALP) and 70 bpm (60–100) (RAPN). No significant difference was detected in individual preoperative patient characteristics (Table 1) except for the RALP group's higher hemoglobin value.

The preoperative MMS exam revealed a median point value of 30 (IQR = 1) for RALP and a point value of 30 (IQR = 0.75) for RAPN. There was no statistically significant difference here, either ($p=0.29$).

Perioperative results and correlation with patient characteristics

Total median operation time was 180 min (IQR = 56.75; documentation for 2 procedures missing) for the RALP group and 140.5 min (IQR = 76.50) for the RAPN group, thus the study group's surgery time was longer ($p=0.01$). Also, the RALP group's robotic-actuation time (= console time) was significantly longer than the RAPN group's ($p=0.001$). RR values exhibited no difference in systolic values, but the prostate group's diastolic values were significantly higher, although that effect vanished after about 120 min' operation time. However, since the RAPN group's operation time was shorter, we had access to fewer measurements after 120 min, with only 1 measurement at 210 min. Our analysis of any statistical change in systolic RR compared to the initial value showed no group difference either. We noted a significant difference between the RALP and RAPN group in diastolic RR compared to the initial valued ($p=0.00$), with the prostate group's RR values significantly higher 120 min into the operation. Age also seemed to reveal an effect on the change in diastolic RR, with the patients over 60 showing significantly lower values ($p=0.00$). HF during surgery did not differ significantly between groups in either the longitudinal analysis or analysis of change during the operation. We did, however, observe a tendency for older patients (>60 years) to present a lower heart frequency. Intraoperative FiO2 measurements revealed very little variation, with no group difference in the intraoperative change versus the initial value. Although the former was also not associated with patient BMI, higher-BMI patients revealed a generally higher FiO2 ($p=0.01$). The pCO2 (mean overall change: -0.73 ± 0.18; $p<0.001$) value and pO2 (mean overall change: 0.95 ± 0.09; $p<0.001$) and rSO2 value (mean change: -0.18 ± 0.08; $p<0.03$) showed a significantly smaller change in patients with an initially higher value (see also Fig. 1). Patient characteristics demonstrated no significant influence in these values or any difference between study groups.

Table 1 Patient demographics and baseline parameters recorded preoperatively

	RALP	RAPN	p value
Patients total	58	22	–
BMI (kg/m^2)	27.5 (16.41–41.36)	26.7 (21.56–33.95)	0.75
Weight (kg)		79 (48.5–110)	0.57
Height (cm)		171.5 (150–185)	0.45
Hemoglobin (g/dl)		14.00 (10.20–16.30)	**0.0008**
RRsyst (mmHg)		146.5 (100–180)	0.21
RRdiast (mmHg)		80 (60–103)	0.85
HF(bpm)		70 (60–100)	0.08

All data is given as median with range (where applicable), significant p-values are given in bold

RALP robot assisted radical prostatectomy, *RAPN* robot assisted radical nephrectomy

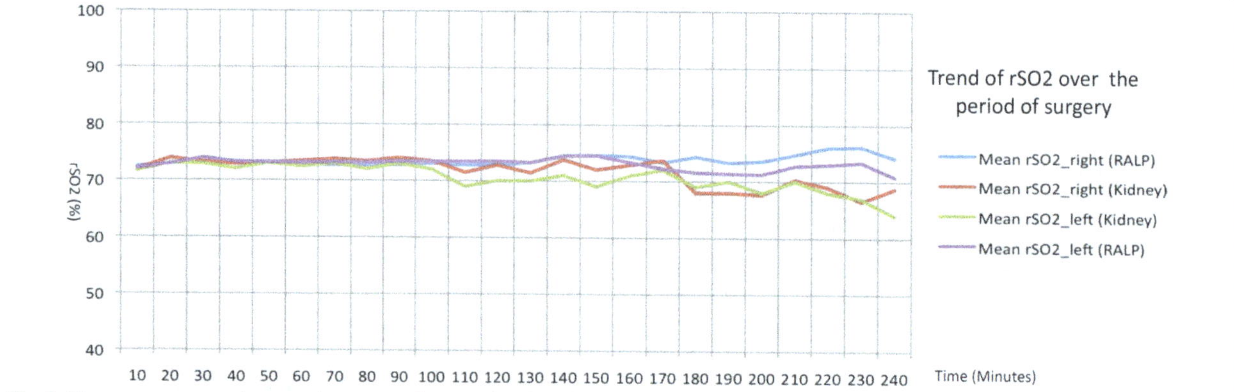

Fig. 1 Mean oxygen saturation over the course of surgery for all performed operations

Postoperative examination and follow up results

Patients were monitored for perioperative and postoperative complications until 3 months after surgery. A total of 22 complications were recorded within the RAPN group and classified according to the Clavien Dindo classification: 10 were classified as category 1, 4 as category 2, 3 as 3a, and 4 as 3b. There were no category 4 or 5 complications. All complications were closely analyzed to determine whether any had been specifically caused by or related to patient positioning, but none were detected.

Postoperative repetition of the MMS exam yielded no significant difference compared to the preoperative value in the RALP group ($p=0.16$) and RAPN group ($p=0.19$), suggesting no negative effect of the operation and intraoperative positioning on cognitive function (Fig. 2).

Discussion

In the current study we compared intraoperatively recorded hemodynamics of patients undergoing Robot-Assisted Radical Prostatectomy and Robot-Assisted Partial Nephrectomy. We documented no relevant preoperative difference in patient characteristics. Analysis of these data, as well as the comparison of both groups showed decreasing blood pressure and slightly elevated pCO2, as well as a slight decrease in pO2 in both groups, as would be expected during a laparoscopic surgical intervention. However, besides slightly higher diastolic blood pressure, hemodynamic monitoring showed no significant difference within the two groups, which suggests that the Trendelenburg position exerted a negligible effect in the RALP group on patients' hemodynamics. In addition, noninvasive cerebral oxygenation monitoring revealed no significant change during the operation, and no difference between our two groups. This finding is supported by other studies applying infrared spectroscopy. In a study by Park et al., intraoperative measurements revealed a statistically significant increase in rSO2 when keeping the pCO2 constant [13]. Other studies report unchanged rSO2, as our data demonstrate [14].Multiple physiological reactions should be considered in this context. On one hand, there is evidence that intracranial

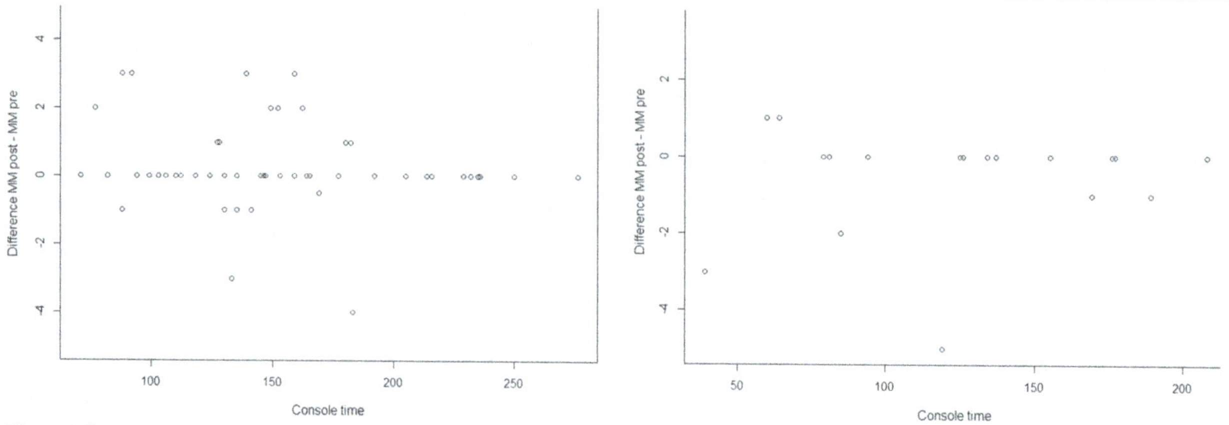

Fig. 2 Difference in point value of pre- and postoperatively Mini Mental Status exam for both groups

pressure rises during Trendelenburg position due to increased venous pressure [15]. This effect is complemented by the increase in intraabdominal pressure due to the pneumoperitoneum, which also increases intracranial pressure by obstructing the venous return [16]. However, pneumoperitoneum also increases cerebral perfusion by raising pCO2 and releasing catecholamine, causing improved cerebral blood flow and in turn potentially higher rSO2 [17]. The net effect of this physiological reactions, as described by Tanaka et al., is a slight increase in cerebral blood volume [18] that was, however, reported to be less than 10%. We found no changes in rSO2 in this study. Our study data indicate that the Trendelenburg position exerts an only slight effect on rSO2, and no signs of impaired cerebral oxygenation.

Follow up of all patients including Mini Mental Status evaluation of the cognitive state also showed no negative effect on the intellectual ability of all operated patients in both groups. In addition, we detected no complications related to the Trendelenburg positioning. We therefore conclude that the Trendelenburg position as applied in Robot-Assisted Radical Prostatectomy is safe for the patient and can be applied during surgical interventions requiring extended operating times. Our study however, has some limitations. First of all, it was exploratory and conducted only on a small cohort; further prospective studies will have to confirm these results. In addition, our control group patients did not undergo the same surgical intervention, since Robot-Assisted Radical Prostatectomy is currently only performed in Trendelenburg position, thus a control group undergoing the same procedure was not possible. Furthermore, our control group included, besides partial nephrectomy, various other Robot-Assisted procedures on the kidney including one radical nephrectomy, one adrenalectomy and a pyeloplasty. As the adrenalectomy was due to a benign hormone-inactive tumor, we cannot rule out that surgical adrenal manipulation might have altered our results.

Conclusions

The 45° Trendelenburg position demonstrated no negative effect on postoperative brain function and did not alter cerebral oxygenation during a surgical procedure lasting up to 5 h in this exploratory study. Further studies in larger patient cohorts will have to confirm these findings.

Abbreviations

ASA: American Society of Anesthesiologists; BMI: Body Mass Index; CA: California; FiO2: Fraction of inspired oxygen; HF: Heart frequency; IQR: Interquartile range; MMS: Mini-mental status; NIRS: Near infrared spectroscopy; RALP: Robotically-assisted laparoscopic prostatectomy; RAPN: Robot-assisted partial nephrectomy; RR: Blood pressure; rSO2: Cerebral oxygenation.

Acknowledgements

Not applicable.

Authors' contributions

CW: Protocol/project development, conduction of experiments, data collection and management, data analysis; DSS, HW: data analysis, manuscript and figure writing/editing; MS, EM, LM: conduct of experiments, data collection and management; JK, WP: Protocol/project development, manuscript and figure writing/editing, supervision. All authors read and approved the final manuscript.

Author details

[1] Department of Urology, Wels-Grieskirchen Medical-Center, Grieskirchner Straße 42, 4600 Wels, Austria. [2] Department of Urology, Faculty of Medicine, Medical Center – University of Freiburg, Hugstetterstr. 55, 79106 Freiburg, Germany. [3] Department of Urology, BHB Salzburg, Kajetanerplatz 1, 5010 Salzburg, Salzburg, Austria. [4] Department of Anesthesiology and Intensive Care II, Wels-Grieskirchen Medical Center, Grieskirchner Straße 42, 4600 Wels, Austria. [5] Medical Statistics and Biometry, Institute for Applied Statistics, Johannes Kepler University Linz, Altenbergerstrasse 69, 4040 Linz, Austria.

References

1. Thiery M. Friedrich Trendelenburg (1844–1924) and the trendelenburg position. Gynecol Surg. 2009;6(3):295–7.
2. Trendelenburg F (1890) Über Blasenscheidenfisteloperationen und über Beckenhochlagerung bei Operationen in der Bauchhöhle. Druck und Verlag von Breitkopf und Härtel
3. Orebaugh SL. Venous air embolism: clinical and experimental considerations. Crit Care Med. 1992;20(8):1169–77.
4. Buchwald H. Three helpful techniques for facilitating abdominal procedures, in particular for surgery in the obese. Am J Surg. 1998;175(1):63–4.
5. Johnson S, Henderson SO. Myth: the Trendelenburg position improves circulation in cases of shock. CJEM. 2004;6(1):48–9.
6. Pasticier G, Rietbergen JB, Guillonneau B, Fromont G, Menon M, Vallancien G. Robotically assisted laparoscopic radical prostatectomy: feasibility study in men. Eur Urol. 2001;40(1):70–4. https://doi.org/10.1159/000049751.
7. Binder J, Kramer W. Robotically-assisted laparoscopic radical prostatectomy. BJU Int. 2001;87(4):408–10.
8. Hakenberg OW. A brief overview of the development of robot-assisted radical prostatectomy. Arab J Urol. 2018;16(3):293–6. https://doi.org/10.1016/j.aju.2018.06.006.
9. Payne TN, Dauterive FR. A comparison of total laparoscopic hysterectomy to robotically assisted hysterectomy: surgical outcomes in a community practice. J Minimal Invas Gynecol. 2008;15(3):286–91.
10. Miller AT, Berian JR, Rubin M, Hurst RD, Fichera A, Umanskiy K. Robotic-assisted proctectomy for inflammatory bowel disease: a case-matched comparison of laparoscopic and robotic technique. J Gastrointest Surg. 2012;16(3):587–94.
11. Gill IS, Sung GT, Hsu TH, Meraney AM. Robotic remote laparoscopic nephrectomy and adrenalectomy: the initial experience. J Urol. 2000;164(6):2082–5.
12. Kilic O, Börgers A, Köhne W, Musch M, Kröpfl D, Groeben H. Effects of steep Trendelenburg position for robotic-assisted prostatectomies on intra-and extrathoracic airways in patients with or without chronic obstructive pulmonary disease. Br J Anaesth. 2014;114(1):70–6.
13. Park E, KOO BN, Min K, Nam S, . The effect of pneumoperitoneum in the steep Trendelenburg position on cerebral oxygenation. Acta Anaesthesiol Scand. 2009;53(7):895–9.
14. Harrison G. The effect of posture on cerebral oxygenation during abdominal surgery. Anaesthesia. 2001;56(12):1181–201.

15. Mavrocordatos P, Bissonnette B, Ravussin P. Effects of neck position and head elevation on intracranial pressure in anaesthetized neurosurgical patients: preliminary results. J Neurosurg Anesthesiol. 2000;12(1):10–4.
16. Halverson A, Buchanan R, Jacobs L, Shayani V, Hunt T, Riedel C, Sackier J. Evaluation of mechanism of increased intracranial pressure with insufflation. Surg Endosc. 1998;12(3):266–9.
17. Abe K, Hashimoto N, Taniguchi A, Yoshiya I. Middle cerebral artery blood flow velocity during laparoscopic surgery in head-down position. Surg Laparosc Endosc Percutaneous Tech. 1998;8(1):1–4.
18. Tanaka N, Yamamoto M, Abe T, Osawa T, Matsumoto R, Shinohara N, Saito H, Uchida Y, Morimoto Y. Changes of cerebral blood volume during robot-assisted laparoscopic radical prostatectomy: observational prospective study using near-infrared time-resolved spectroscopy. J Endourol. 2019;33(12):995–1001.

5

Comparison of functional and oncological outcomes of innovative "three-port" and traditional "four-port" laparoscopic radical prostatectomy in patients with prostate cancer

Ben Xu*†, Si-da Cheng†, Yi-ji Peng and Qian Zhang*

Abstract

Background: To compare the functional and oncological outcomes between innovative "three-port" and traditional "four-port" laparoscopic radical prostatectomy (LRP) in patients with prostate cancer (PCa).

Methods: We retrospectively collected the data of PCa patients treated at our institutions from June 2012 to May 2016. According to the inclusion criteria, a total of 234 patients were included in the study, including 112 in group A (four-port) and 122 in group B (three-port). The perioperatively surgical characteristics, functional and oncological outcomes were compared between groups.

Results: There were no statistical differences in the baseline parameters between these two groups. Compared with group A, the operative time (OT) and estimated blood loss (EBL) were significantly less in group B. On follow-up, the rate of positive surgical margin (PSM), prostate specific antigen (PSA) biochemical recurrence and continence after LRP did not show any statistically significant difference between the groups. An identical conclusion was also received in comparison of overall survival (OS) and biochemical recurrence-free survival (BRFS) between both groups.

Conclusions: Innovative "three-port" LRP can significantly shorten the OT and reduce the EBL compared with the traditional "four-port" LRP. Meanwhile, it does not increase the rate of PSM and PSA biochemical recurrence. "Three-port" LRP could be popularized in the future in view of its superior surgical technique, considerably better functional outcomes and remarkable oncological control.

Keywords: Three-port, Laparoscopic radical prostatectomy, Prostate cancer, Continence, Oncological control

Background

PCa is the second most common cancer in males (15% of newly diagnosed tumors), and the fifth major cause of cancer death worldwide [1]. The incidence of PCa is also increasing in China, which has become the highest incidence tumor in the male genitourinary system [2, 3]. For the localized PCa, RP is still the first-line treatment option, enabling patients to obtain more than 10 years of life expectancy [4].

Since LRP was reported in the 1990s [5], it has been widely applied based on its advantage of less surgical trauma and faster recovery. Moreover, with the emergence of robotic surgical platform, its unique three-dimensional vision, fine intracavitary manipulation and ergonomic design make robot-assisted laparoscopic radical prostatectomy (RARP) widely used throughout the world in the recent 10 years [6–8]. Although RARP can overcome the disadvantages of the traditional LRP and

*Correspondence: xuben_pku@sina.com; zhangqian@bjmu.edu.cn
†Ben Xu amd Si-da Cheng have contributed equally to this paper
Department of Urology, National Urological Cancer Center, Peking University First Hospital and Institute of Urology, Peking University, 8 Xishiku Street, Xicheng District, Beijing 100034, China

shorten the learning curve, it must be admitted that its cost is relatively high [9]. Such huge medical costs thus make it difficult to promote in the developing countries. To make a balance between a low price and more precise manipulation, our center innovatively adopted "three-port" LRP instead of the traditional "four-port" LRP from the year of 2012.

In this investigation, we retrospectively compared the perioperatively surgical parameters between the innovative "three-port" and traditional "four-port" LRP. More importantly, the functional and oncological outcomes including PSM, PSA biochemical recurrence, continence, short-term OS and BRFS were also compared to make this technique more practical and suitable for the future promotion.

Methods

We retrospectively collected the data of PCa patients receiving LRP at our institutions from June 2012 to May 2016. The diagnosis of PCa was confirmed by a transrectal needle biopsy at our institutions 1–8 weeks before the LRP.

From the year of 2012, patients who met the following criteria were included into this trial: (1) All of the patients were confirmed by a transrectal needle biopsy with the assistance of magnetic resonance imaging preoperatively at our institutions; (2) The operation was performed between June 2012 and May 2016; (3) It was operated by a single surgeon (Dr. Qian Z) based on the previous medical records. The exclusion criteria included: (1) The medical record was fragmentary with incomplete perioperative characteristics [age, body mass index (BMI), prostate volume, PSA level, Gleason Score, OT, EBL, drainage indwelling days, hospitalization days, surgical complications, postoperatively pathological stages, and PSM]; (2) Patients who had undergone neoadjuvant androgen deprivation therapy; (3) Patients with preoperatively suspicious lymph node metastatic disease; (4) Patients with previously major abdominal surgery; (5) Patients with history of transurethral resection of the prostate; (6) Patients who received nerve sparing radical prostatectomy; (7) Salvaged LRP after radiation therapy. Patients who met the following criteria were operated by the "three-port" technique: (1) the volume of prostate measured by B-ultrasonography preoperatively was less than 40 ml; (2) B-ultrasonography showed that the middle lobe of prostate did not protrude into the bladder; (3) the BMI was less than 24 kg/m^2. The other patients who were not in conformity with the above requirements were still performed by the "four-port" LRP.

Accordingly, a total of 234 patients were included in the study, including 112 in group A (four-port) and 122 in group B (three-port). Among them, a total of 17 "three-port" patients were intraoperatively converted to "four-port". Five cases had intra-operative bleeding requiring additional suction port while in other 12 the prostate was found to be large and hence needed an additional port for proper exposure and dissection.

The perioperatively surgical characteristics, functional and oncological outcomes were compared between groups. The surgical characteristics included OT, EBL, hospitalization and drainage days. The recovery of urinary control function after operation was evaluated according to the use of daily urine pad, and 0–1 piece of urinary pad per day was defined as a satisfactory urinary continence [10]. The oncological outcomes were evaluated by the parameters of PSM, PSA biochemical recurrence rate, OS and BRFS obtained by the follow-up records. The PSA biochemical recurrence was defined as PSA ≥ 0.2 ng/ml, OS was defined as the time from the end of operation to death or follow-up due to any reason, and BRFS was defined as the time from the end of operation to the occurrence of PSA biochemical recurrence or death or the end of follow-up.

All the data were analyzed by SPSS 20.0 versions. Categorical variables were represented by frequency and percentage. Continuous variables conforming to normal distribution were represented by mean ± standard deviation (SD), and continuous variables not conforming to normal distribution were represented by median and range. Chi-square test or Fisher exact test were used for categorical variables, with t test or Mann–whitney test for continuous variables. Bilateral $P < 0.05$ was defined as a statistically significant difference.

Results

The baseline characteristics of patients in both groups were listed in Table 1. There were none of statistical differences in the baseline parameters between the two groups. The perioperatively surgical data of these two groups were shown in Table 2. The average OT in group A was 105.06 min, and that of the group B was 92.28 min ($P = 0.001$). The average EBL in group A was 121.90 ml, and that of the group B was 103.85 ml ($P = 0.031$). The postoperative hospitalization in group A was 4.54 days, and that of the group B was 4.50 days ($P = 0.812$). The drainage days in group A was 3.47 days, and that of the group B was 3.43 days ($P = 0.743$). Compared with group A, the OT and EBL were significantly less in group B.

The functional and oncological outcomes of the two groups were revealed in Table 3. There was no significant difference in the postoperative T stage and Gleason scores. By analyzing the oncological outcomes of two methods, the mean rate of PSM in the two groups was 32.1% and 32.0% respectively ($P = 1.000$), and the PSA biochemical recurrence rate was 10.7% and 10.7%

Table 1 The patients' baseline characteristics in both groups

	Overall	Group_A	Group_B	*P* value
Cases	234	112	122	
Age [mean (SD)]	66.92 (7.80)	67.07 (8.75)	66.79 (6.85)	0.781
TPSA [mean (SD)]	13.90 (6.43)	14.22 (6.24)	13.60 (6.62)	0.465
Biopsy Gleason scores (%)				0.597
3+3	69 (29.5)	29 (25.9)	40 (32.8)	
3+4	49 (20.9)	28 (25.0)	21 (17.2)	
3+5	14 (6.0)	5 (4.5)	9 (7.4)	
4+3	85 (36.3)	41 (36.6)	44 (36.1)	
4+4	6 (2.6)	3 (2.7)	3 (2.5)	
4+5	11 (4.7)	6 (5.4)	5 (4.1)	
cT stage (%)				0.638
cT2a	11 (4.7)	4 (3.6)	7 (5.7)	
cT2b	32 (13.7)	14 (12.5)	18 (14.8)	
cT2c	160 (68.4)	81 (72.3)	79 (64.8)	
cT3a	28 (12.0)	11 (9.8)	17 (13.9)	
cT3b	3 (1.3)	2 (1.8)	1 (0.8)	

respectively ($P=1.000$). In the evaluation of the degree of urinary control recovery at 3 months, 6 months and 12 months after operation, the satisfied urinary continence in group A was obtained in 92/112 cases (82.1%), 97/112 cases (86.6%) and 102/112 cases (91.1%). The corresponding rate was 94/122 cases (77.0%), 99/122 cases (81.1%) and 104/122 cases (85.2%) in group B. The *P* value for each period between both groups were 0.423, 0.340 and 0.242 respectively. Above all, the similar results were obtained in the rate of PSM, PSA biochemical recurrence and continence after "three-port" or "four-port" LRP without any statistically significant difference ($P>0.05$).

By depicting a curve of OS and BRFS, a more accurate reflection of oncological outcomes was demonstrated in Fig. 1. In the follow-up periods, the OS was 100% with the 71.6% of BRFS in group A, and the OS was 100% with the 73.2% of BRFS in group B. There was no significant difference in OS ($P=0.300$) and BRFS ($P=0.800$) between these two groups.

Discussion

For the early localized PCa, RP is still the most widely used treatment method. With the continuous progress of technology, LRP and RARP both embody the advantages of small trauma, less postoperative pain and rapid postoperative recovery. What's more, RARP has unique advantages such as flexible operation equipment, three-dimensional vision and short learning curve, which has been widely applied by many centers in many developed countries [11]. Several systematic reviews and meta-analysis results had shown that RARP took the advantages of perioperatively surgical data, lower PSM, satisfied urinary continence and sexual function over LRP, but some researchers believed that there existed no dramatic difference in tumor prognosis between LRP and RARP [12–15]. However, it is worth noting that many studies have shown that RARP has a higher cost than LRP due to the increased cost of surgical instruments [9, 14, 16]. Based on the limitation of cost and medical resources, LRP is still an important choice for many underdeveloped and developing countries.

Since it was first reported in 1997 [17], the traditional "four-port" or "five-port" LRP has been widely used in the world. Reviewing the literatures concerning traditional LRP, Rassweiler et al. [18] reported 219 cases with an average OT of 218 min and an average EBL of 800 ml; Hu et al. [19] reported 358 cases with an average OT of 246 min and an average EBL of 200 ml; Ploussard et al. [20] reported 219 cases with an average OT of 175.5 min and an average EBL of 800 ml. Compared with the results above and the traditional "four-port" LRP performed by ourselves, our clinical practice in "three-port" LRP showed that the average OT (92.28 min) and EBL (103.85 ml) were notably improved. It is believed that the improvement of perioperatively surgical data is mainly related to the rationality and advantages of the "three-port" technique. Additionally, it may also be contributed to the fact that the surgeon launched the innovative "three-port" LRP after fully mastering the traditional "four-port" LRP. Retrospectively analyzing our database, nearly 100 cases of traditional "four-port" LRP were completed before the "three-port" LRP was developed in

Table 2 Intraoperatively surgical parameters in both groups

	Overall	Group A	Group B	*P* value
Cases	234	112	122	
OT [mean (SD)]	98.40 (30.27)	105.06 (30.79)	92.28 (28.57)	0.001
EBL [mean (SD)]	112.49 (64.05)	121.90 (67.09)	103.85 (60.11)	0.031
Hospitalization [mean (SD)]	4.52 (1.14)	4.54 (1.34)	4.50 (0.93)	0.812
Drainage days [mean (SD)]	3.45 (0.90)	3.47 (1.01)	3.43 (0.79)	0.743

Table 3 Patient characteristics

	Overall	Group_A	Group_B	*P*
Cases	234	112	122	
pT_stage (%)				0.809
pT2b	16 (6.8)	8 (7.1)	8 (6.6)	
pT2c	125 (53.4)	63 (56.2)	62 (50.8)	
pT3a	56 (23.9)	24 (21.4)	32 (26.2)	
pT3b	37 (15.8)	17 (15.2)	20 (16.4)	
Patho_GS (%)				0.638
3+3	16 (6.8)	7 (6.2)	9 (7.4)	
3+4	70 (29.9)	27 (24.1)	43 (35.2)	
4+3	100 (42.7)	57 (50.9)	43 (35.2)	
4+4	3 (1.3)	1 (0.9)	2 (1.6)	
4+5	30 (12.8)	12 (10.7)	18 (14.8)	
5+3	7 (3.0)	3 (2.7)	4 (3.3)	
5+4	8 (3.4)	5 (4.5)	3 (2.5)	
SurgicalMargin (%)				1
Negative	159 (67.9)	76 (67.9)	83 (68.0)	
Postive	75 (32.1)	36 (32.1)	39 (32.0)	
BioChemicalRecurrence (%)				1
Negative	209 (89.3)	100 (89.3)	109 (89.3)	
Positive	25 (10.7)	12 (10.7)	13 (10.7)	
Continence (%)				
Third month	186 (79.5)	92 (82.1)	94 (77.0)	0.423
Sixth month	196 (83.8)	97 (86.6)	99 (81.1)	0.340
Twelfth month	206 (88.0)	102 (91.1)	104 (85.2)	0.242

2012. However, with the progress of current technology and the visualization of laparoscopic teaching methods, we believe that young doctors can directly perform the "three-port" LRP even though the youths are still in the initial stage of the traditional "four-port" LRP without spending the learning curve. It is not necessary to go through the learning curve process from "four-port" to "three-port" technique. Certainly, it is strongly suggested that the young doctors should perform the "three-port" LRP with the guidance of experienced doctors who have been skilled and proficient in this technique.

PSM is an important index to evaluate the prognosis of PCa after RP, which is closely related to PSA biochemical recurrence and postoperative adjuvant treatment [21]. According to the systematic review, it is uncertain whether RARP has advantages over LRP in controlling the PSM. It has been reported that the rate of PSM in LRP is 12.0–22.2%, while that of RARP is 13.5–22.5% [12, 19, 22, 23]. Our results suggest that the rate of PSM in "three-port" and "four-port" technique were 32.0% and 32.1% without any statistical difference. BCR is another critical index of oncological outcomes closely related to PSM. Our conclusion revealed that the 1-year BCR of "three-port" and "four-port" was both 10.7% similarly compared with the recent literatures [24, 25]. The above results indicated that "three-port" LRP did not significantly increase PSM and BCR, which could be controlled at a better level on the basis of rich surgical experience. Finally analyzed by the description of OS and BRFS, it was further confirmed that "three-port" LRP could guarantee a satisfactory survival rate.

The recovery of urinary control is a considerable aspect to evaluate the functional prognosis after RP. Asimakopoulos et al. [25] reported that the urinary control rates at 3 months, 6 months and 1 year after LRP were 63.3%, 75.0% and 83.3%, respectively. Ploussard et al. [20] reported that the urinary control rates of 1377 patients with LRP at 3 months, 6 months and 1 year were 39.4%, 58.9% and 68.5%, respectively. Porpiglia

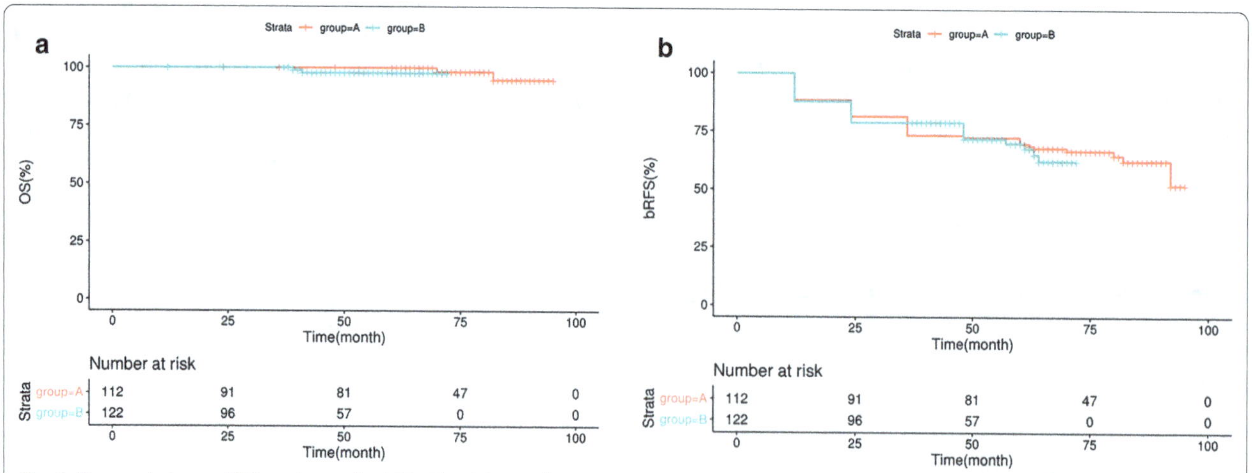

Fig. 1 The survival rate of PCa patients after LRP. **a** The OS rate of PCa patients in group A (red line) and group B (green line). **b** The BRFS rata of PCa patients in group A (red line) and group B (green line)

et al. [26] reported that the urinary control rates of LRP at 3 months, 6 months and 1 year were 61.6%, 73.3% and 83.3%, respectively. Our results stated that the urinary control rates of "three-port" LRP at 3 months, 6 months and 1 year were 77.0%, 81.1% and 85.2% respectively, providing a stable recovery of urinary continence without increasing the incidence of postoperative urinary incontinence.

In conclusion, the "three-port" LRP can significantly shorten the OT and EBL, without increasing the rate of PSM, PSA biochemical recurrence and urinary incontinence. More importantly, it could obtain a considerable outcome in the tumor prognosis. Its main advantages were: (1) more fast recovery by reducing a puncture trocar; (2) avoiding improper traction and auxiliary operation by inexperienced assistants; (3) a triangle layout providing sufficient space, meanwhile reducing the fatigue of the surgeon. Admittedly, it must be addressed that there still existed some defects and disadvantages in the "three-port" LRP: (1) it is mainly suitable for extraperitoneal operation, not for the transperitoneal manipulation. If the extended lymph node dissection plans to be implemented, it needs to be converted to the traditional "four-port" LRP; (2) if the prostate volume is larger, the operator will be limited in a narrow space, and thus the assistant is required to assist in providing an adequate exposure by adding an additional port; (3) if there is much bleeding during the operation, the assistant is still demanded to suck the blood by using an aspirator in the fourth port.

This study was a retrospectively and non-randomized controlled study with inherent selection bias. In this study, the follow-up time of tumor prognosis and functional prognosis is relatively short. In the future, a prospectively randomized controlled study with a large sample and long-term follow-up is needed to further confirm the advantages of "three-port" LRP in functional and oncological outcomes.

Conclusions

In conclusion, innovative "three-port" LRP can significantly shorten the OT and reduce the EBL compared with the traditional "four-port" LRP. Meanwhile, it does not increase the rate of PSM and PSA biochemical recurrence. "Three-port" LRP could be popularized in the future in view of its superior surgical technique, considerably better functional outcomes and remarkable oncological control.

Abbreviations

LRP: Laparoscopic radical prostatectomy; PCa: Prostate cancer; OT: Operative time; EBL: Estimated blood loss; PSM: Positive surgical margin; PSA: Prostate specific antigen; OS: Overall survival; BRFS: Biochemical recurrence-free survival; RARP: Robot-assisted laparoscopic radical prostatectomy; BMI: Body mass index; DVC: Dorsal vein complex; SD: Standard deviation.

Acknowledgements

None.

Authors' contributions

XB and CSD carried out the design of this research, analysis and interpretation of data, and drafted the manuscript. PYJ participated in the collection of data and data analysis. ZQ assisted in the design of this research and project development. All authors read and approved the final manuscript.

References

1. Ferlay J, Soerjomataram I, Dikshit R, et al. Cancer incidence and mortality worldwide: sources, methods and major patterns in GLOBOCAN 2012. Int J Cancer. 2015;136:e359-386.
2. Wong MC, Goggins WB, Wang HH, et al. Global incidence and mortality for prostate cancer: analysis of temporal patterns and trends in 36 countries. Eur Urol. 2016;70:862–74.
3. Chen W, Zheng R, Baade PD, et al. Cancer statistics in China, 2015. CA Cancer J Clin. 2016;66:115–32.
4. Mottet N, Bellmunt J, Bolla M, et al. EAU-ESTRO-SIOG guidelines on prostate cancer. Part 1: screening, diagnosis, and local treatment with curative intent. Eur Urol. 2017;71:618–29.
5. Guillonneau B, Cathelineau X, Barret E, et al. Laparoscopic radical prostatectomy: technical and early oncological assessment of 40 operations. Eur Urol. 1999;36:14–20.
6. Robertson C, Close A, Fraser C, et al. Relative effectiveness of robot-assisted and standard laparoscopic prostatectomy as alternatives to open radical prostatectomy for treatment of localised prostate cancer: a systematic review and mixed treatment comparison meta-analysis. BJU Int. 2013;112:798–812.
7. Zihni AM, Ohu I, Cavallo JA, et al. Ergonomic analysis of robot-assisted and traditional laparoscopic procedures. Surg Endosc. 2014;28:3379–84.
8. Lee GI, Lee MR, Clanton T, et al. Comparative assessment of physical and cognitive ergonomics associated with robotic and traditional laparoscopic surgeries. Surg Endosc. 2014;28:456–65.
9. Forsmark A, Gehrman J, Angenete E, et al. Health economic analysis of open and robot-assisted laparoscopic surgery for prostate cancer within the prospective multicentre LAPPRO trial. Eur Urol. 2018;74:816–24.
10. Lepor H, Kaci L, Xue X. Continence following radical retropubic prostatectomy using self-reporting instruments. J Urol. 2004;171:1212–5.
11. Trinh QD, Sammon J, Sun M, et al. Perioperative outcomes of robot-assisted radical prostatectomy compared with open radical prostatectomy: results from the nationwide inpatient sample. Eur Urol. 2012;61:679–85.
12. Novara G, Ficarra V, Rosen RC, et al. Systematic review and meta-analysis of perioperative outcomes and complications after robot-assisted radical prostatectomy. Eur Urol. 2012;62:431–52.
13. Tewari A, Sooriakumaran P, Bloch DA, et al. Positive surgical margin and perioperative complication rates of primary surgical treatments for prostate cancer: a systematic review and meta-analysis comparing retropubic, laparoscopic, and robotic prostatectomy. Eur Urol. 2012;62:1–15.
14. Huang X, Wang L, Zheng X, et al. Comparison of perioperative, functional, and oncologic outcomes between standard laparoscopic and robotic-assisted radical prostatectomy: a systemic review and meta-analysis. Surg Endosc. 2017;31:1045–60.
15. Cao L, Yang Z, Qi L, et al. Robot-assisted and laparoscopic vs open radical prostatectomy in clinically localized prostate cancer: perioperative, functional, and oncological outcomes: a systematic review and meta-analysis. Medicine (Baltimore). 2019;98:e15770.
16. Bolenz C, Freedland SJ, Hollenbeck BK, et al. Costs of radical prostatectomy for prostate cancer: a systematic review. Eur Urol. 2014;65:316–24.
17. Schuessler WW, Schulam PG, Clayman RV, et al. Laparoscopic radical prostatectomy: initial short-term experience. Urology. 1997;50:854–7.
18. Rassweiler J, Seemann O, Schulze M, et al. Laparoscopic versus open radical prostatectomy: a comparative study at a single institution. J Urol. 2003;169:1689–93.

19. Hu JC, Nelson RA, Wilson TG, et al. Perioperative complications of laparoscopic and robotic assisted laparoscopic radical prostatectomy. J Urol. 2006;175:541–6.
20. Ploussard G, de la Taille A, Moulin M, et al. Comparisons of the perioperative, functional, and oncologic outcomes after robot-assisted versus pure extraperitoneal laparoscopic radical prostatectomy. Eur Urol. 2014;65:610–9.
21. Karakiewicz PI, Eastham JA, Graefen M, et al. Prognostic impact of positive surgical margins in surgically treated prostate cancer: multi-institutional assessment of 5831 patients. Urology. 2005;66:1245–50.
22. Kasraeian A, Barret E, Chan J, et al. Comparison of the rate, location and size of positive surgical margins after laparoscopic and robot-assisted laparoscopic radical prostatectomy. BJU Int. 2011;108:1174–8.
23. Sooriakumaran P, Srivastava A, Shariat SF, et al. A multinational, multi-institutional study comparing positive surgical margin rates among 22393 open, laparoscopic, and robot-assisted radical prostatectomy patients. Eur Urol. 2014;66:450–6.
24. Dahl DM, Barry MJ, McGovern FJ, et al. A prospective study of symptom distress and return to baseline function after open versus laparoscopic radical prostatectomy. J Urol. 2009;182:956–65.
25. Asimakopoulos AD, Pereira Fraga CT, Annino F, et al. Randomized comparison between laparoscopic and robot-assisted nerve-sparing radical prostatectomy. J Sex Med. 2011;8:1503–12.
26. Porpiglia F, Morra I, Lucci Chiarissi M, et al. Randomised controlled trial comparing laparoscopic and robot-assisted radical prostatectomy. Eur Urol. 2013;63:606–14.

6

Analgesic efficacy of intrathecal morphine and bupivacaine during the early postoperative period in patients who underwent robotic-assisted laparoscopic prostatectomy

Jung-Woo Shim[1], Yun Jeong Cho[1], Hyong Woo Moon[2], Jaesik Park[1], Hyung Mook Lee[1], Yong-Suk Kim[1], Young Eun Moon[1], Sang Hyun Hong[1] and Min Suk Chae[1*]

Abstract

Background: The present study was performed to investigate the analgesic efficacy of intrathecal morphine and bupivacaine (ITMB) in terms of treating early postoperative pain in adult patients who underwent robotic-assisted laparoscopic prostatectomy (RALP).

Methods: Fifty patients were prospectively enrolled and randomly classified into the non-ITMB (n = 25) and ITMB (n = 25) groups. The ITMB therapeutic regimen consisted of 0.2 mg morphine and 7.5 mg bupivacaine (total 1.7 mL). All patients were routinely administered the intravenous patient-controlled analgesia and appropriately treated with rescue intravenous (IV) opioid drugs, based on the discretion of the attending physicians who were blinded to the group assignments. Cumulative IV opioid consumption and the numeric rating scale (NRS) score were assessed at 1, 6, and 24 h postoperatively, and opioid-related complications were measured during the day after surgery.

Results: Demographic findings were comparable between patients who did and did not receive ITMB. The intraoperative dose of remifentanil was lower in the ITMB group than in the non-ITMB group. Pain scores (i.e., NRS) at rest and during coughing as well as cumulative IV opioid consumption were significantly lower in patients who received ITMB than in those who did not in the post-anesthesia care unit (PACU; i.e., at 1 h after surgery) and the ward (i.e., at 6 and 24 h after surgery). ITMB was significantly associated with postoperative NRS scores of ≤ 3 at rest and during coughing in the PACU (i.e., at 1 h after surgery) before and after adjusting for cumulative IV opioid consumption. In the ward (i.e., at 6 and 24 h after surgery), ITMB was associated with postoperative NRS scores of ≤ 3 at rest and during coughing before adjusting for cumulative IV opioid consumption but not after. No significant differences in complications were observed, such as post-dural puncture headache, respiratory depression, nausea, vomiting, pruritus, or neurologic sequelae, during or after surgery.

*Correspondence: shscms@gmail.com
[1] Department of Anesthesiology and Pain Medicine, Seoul St. Mary's Hospital, College of Medicine, The Catholic University of Korea, 222, Banpo-daero, Seocho-gu, Seoul 06591, Republic of Korea
Full list of author information is available at the end of the article

Conclusion: A single spinal injection of morphine and bupivacaine provided proper early postoperative analgesia and decreased additional requirements for IV opioids in patients who underwent RALP.

Keywords: Intrathecal, Morphine, Bupivacaine, Robotic-assisted laparoscopic surgery

Background

Robotic-assisted laparoscopic prostatectomy (RALP) is a technically advanced surgical procedure with minimally invasive features that provides a better surgical view and maneuverability than open and/or laparoscopic prostatectomy does [1]. In a large cohort study, RALP seemed to produce a better clinical oncological prognosis, including lower risks of a positive surgical margin, decreased requirement for radiation treatment, and reduced 30-day mortality, compared to open radical prostatectomy [2]. In addition, patients who underwent RALP benefit from favorable functional consequences such as a two-fold higher chance of reaching continence and potency compared to laparoscopic prostatectomy [3]. However, patients who underwent RALP frequently experience considerable pain, particularly during the day after surgery that may result from skin-port incisions, multiple dissections of prostate-involved and surrounding tissues, bladder spasm, and transurethral catheter irritation [4]. Numerous pain control methods, including peripheral and/or central nerve block techniques have been investigated to ameliorate the acute pain that occurs immediately after RALP [5–7].

The analgesic efficacy of intrathecal morphine during open abdominal surgery is better than that of an intravenous (IV) opioid, but the incidence rates of side effects are comparable between the two pain control methods [8]. Another open abdominal surgery study suggested that pain levels assessed using a visual analogue scale at rest and during coughing are more satisfactory after administering intrathecal morphine compared to a ropivacaine wound infusion [9]. Spinal analgesia seems to provide better outcomes in laparoscopy-based minimally invasive surgery than epidural and/or IV analgesia do from the immediate postoperative period until the patient is deemed medically suitable for discharge and during the total hospital stay, in terms of bowel function recovery, pain scores, changes in pulmonary function, and quality of life [10]. A combination of intrathecal morphine and bupivacaine (ITMB) is reported to have additive impacts on early postoperative analgesia in patients undergoing gynecologic surgery [11]. Therefore, ITMB seems to be a potentially acceptable strategy for improving acute pain control after RALP.

The aims of this study were to evaluate pain scores and cumulative IV opioid consumption on day 1 after administering ITMB, and to investigate the association between ITMB and an appropriate analgesic result after adjusting for cumulative IV opioid consumption in patients who underwent RALP. In addition, we compared postoperative complications between patients who did and did not receive ITMB.

Patients and methods

Ethical considerations

This single-center, prospective randomized controlled study was approved by the institutional review board of the ethics committee of Seoul St. Mary's Hospital (approval number: KC19MESI0629 on October 7, 2019) and was performed according to the principles of the Declaration of Helsinki. The study protocol was retrospectively and prospectively registered at a publicly accessible clinical registration site that is recognized by the International Committee of Medical Journal Editors (Clinical Research Information Service, Republic of Korea, approval number: KCT0004350 on October 17, 2019). Written informed consent was obtained from all patients at our hospital who were enrolled between October 2019 and December 2019. Our study adhered to the CONSORT guidelines and includes a completed CONSORT checklist as an Additional file 1.

Study population

Inclusion criteria for this study were: male gender, age 19–75 years, scheduled for elective RALP for prostate cancer, and American Society of Anesthesiologists (ASA) physical status I or II [12]. Exclusion criteria were: emergency cases; age < 19 or > 75 years; ASA physical status of III–V; intraoperative development of hemodynamic instability and/or massive hemorrhage that required rescue management, such as transfusion of blood products or infusion of a strong vasopressor (i.e., epinephrine or norepinephrine); severe nausea and vomiting that required withholding an additional IV opioid infusion within 1 day after surgery; and refusal to participate in the study.

A total of 63 patients were assessed for eligibility in our study; 13 patients with age > 75 years (n = 10) or ASA physical status of III (n = 3) were excluded, and thus, 50 patients were enrolled in this study (Fig. 1). Randomization was performed using sealed, opaque envelopes. An independent colleague randomly grouped the envelopes in blocks of 10 with a 1:1 ratio to produce an equal distribution across the whole study period. The envelopes were stacked and stored. When an enrolled patient arrived in the holding area, the upper envelope was opened by the attending anesthesiologist. The surgical team, physician, and nurses in the post-anesthesia care unit (PACU) and ward as well as researchers were all blinded to the group allocations. The attending anesthesiologist and nurses in the operating room, who were not involved in further patient care or data collection other than filling in medical record forms, were aware of the group allocations.

Surgery and anesthesia

RALP was exclusively performed by expert urologists using a robotic-assisted laparoscopic device (Da Vinci Si System; Intuitive Surgical, Sunnyvale, CA, USA). Patients were positioned in the lithotomy position and the operative field was disinfected and draped. CO_2 gas was insufflated into the abdominal cavity (i.e., pneumoperitoneum) with a pressure of up to 15 mmHg through a 12-mm camera trocar inserted through a periumbilical incision. After inserting the remaining five trocars, including three 8-mm robotic trocars, and 15-mm and 5-mm assisting trocars, intra-abdominal pressure was reduced to 12 mmHg, and the patient was placed in the steep Trendelenburg position at the maximal angle (45°) of the surgical table (Maquet, Rastatt, Baden-Württemberg, Germany); this approach was routinely applied to achieve the optimal surgical view. Intra-abdominal pressure was maintained at 12–15 mmHg during surgery. The surgical position was restored to the supine position and the CO_2 gas was removed at the time of peritoneal closure.

Balanced anesthesia was provided under standard vital sign monitoring, such as the electrocardiogram, systolic and diastolic blood pressure, heart rate, SpO_2, body temperature, and capnography, by attending expert

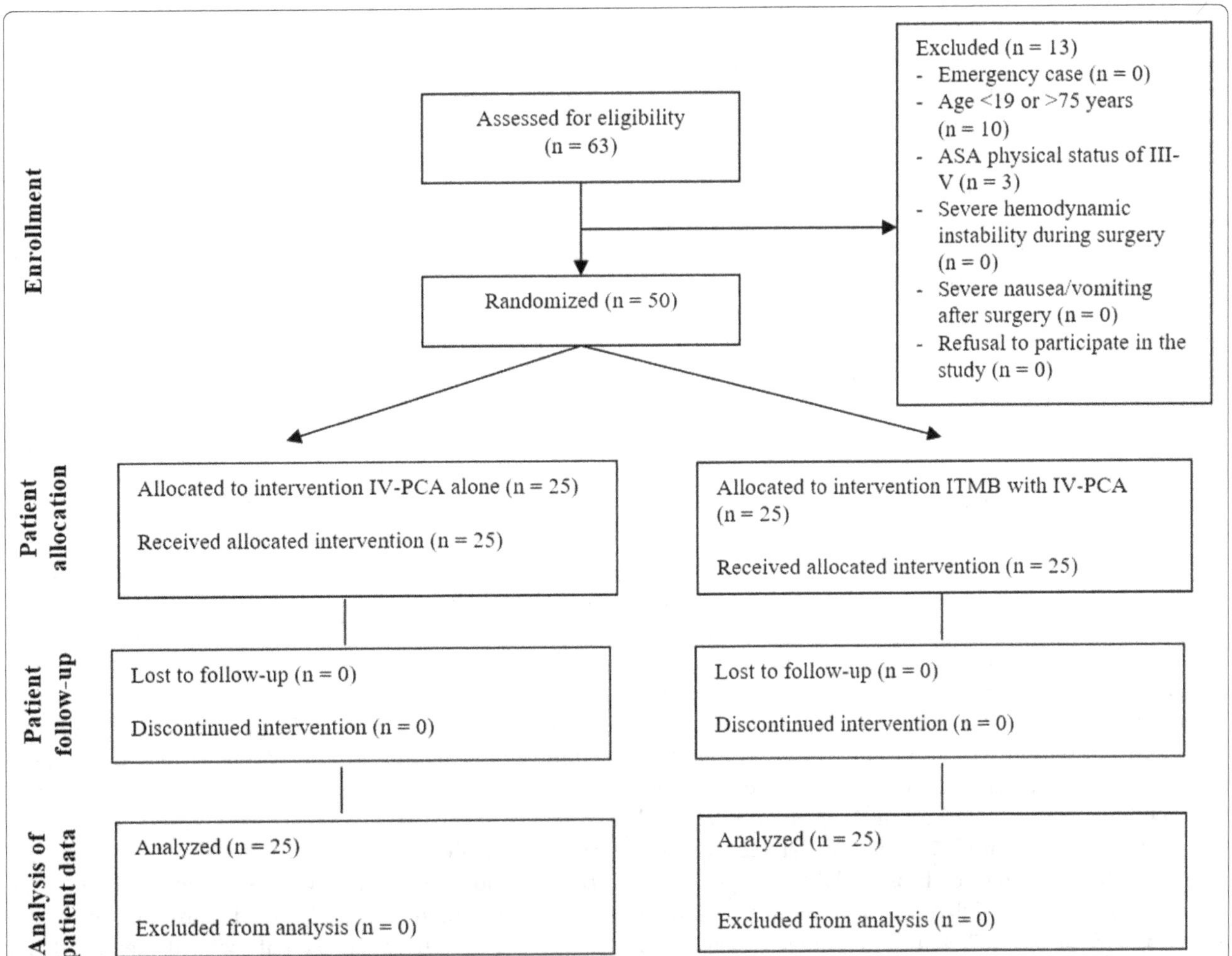

Fig. 1 CONSORT diagram showing how study participants went through the different trial phases. English editing service

anesthesiologists who were aware of the group allocations but were not involved in later patient care or data collection other than the completion of medical records. Propofol (1–2 mg/kg; Fresenius Kabi, Bad Homburg, Germany) and 0.6 mg/kg rocuronium (Merck Sharp and Dohme Corp., Kenilworth, NJ, USA) were infused to induce anesthesia; and 4.0%–6.0% desflurane (Baxter, Deerfield, IL, USA) with medical air/oxygen was provided to maintain anesthesia under a Bispectral Index™ (Medtronic, Minneapolis, MN, USA) of 40–60 to ensure adequate hypnotic depth. Remifentanil (Hanlim Pharm. Co., Ltd., Seoul, Republic of Korea) was continuously infused at a rate of 0.1–0.5 µg/kg/min, as appropriate. Rocuronium was repeatedly administered under train-of-four monitoring (more than one twitch). End-tidal CO_2 was set between 30 and 40 mmHg by adjusting the mechanical ventilator mode. Hypotensive events were defined as systolic blood pressure < 90 mmHg or diastolic blood pressure < 60 mmHg over 5 min, and treated with rescue IV ephedrine (Daewon Pharm. Co., Ltd., Seoul, Republic of Korea) and/or fluid resuscitation therapy based on the discretion of the attending anesthesiologists, as appropriate.

In the PACU, the attending physicians and nurses were not consulted unless surgical issues, such as massive hemorrhage requiring blood product transfusion, or persistent hemodynamic issues, such as hypotension requiring continuous vasopressor (i.e., epinephrine or norepinephrine) infusion or fluid resuscitation therapy during or after surgery, arose. All patients were transferred to the ward at 1 h after surgery.

ITMB intervention

None of the patients received sedative premedication in the operating room to allow immediate identification of any nerve injury during the intrathecal intervention performed prior to the induction of general anesthesia. After establishing standard vital sign monitoring, the patient was positioned in the right or left lateral decubitus position, and the skin over the lumbar region was cleaned with chlorhexidine and draped. The patients received 0.2 mg (0.2 mL) of intrathecal morphine sulfate (BCWORLD Pharm. Co., Ltd., Seoul, Republic of Korea) and 7.5 mg (1.5 mL) of bupivacaine (Mitsubishi Tanabe Pharm. Co., Ltd., Osaka, Japan) using a sterile 25G Quincke type-spinal needle (TAE-CHANG Industrial Co., Ltd., Chungcheongnam-do, Republic of Korea) between lumbar vertebrae 3 and 4. Morphine sulfate and bupivacaine (total 1.7 mL) were administered as a single injection after obtaining cerebrospinal fluid.

The entire study population was randomly assigned and classified into the following two groups: patients who did *vs.* those who did not receive ITMB.

IV opioid administration

All patients undergoing RALP were routinely given IV patient-controlled analgesia (IV-PCA) (AutoMed 3200; Acemedical, Seoul, Republic of Korea), which included 1,000 µg of fentanyl (Dai Han Pharm. Co., Ltd., Seoul, Republic of Korea), 90 mg of ketorolac (Hanmi Pharm. Co., Ltd., Seoul, Republic of Korea), and 0.3 mg of Naseron (Boryung Co., Ltd., Seoul, Republic of Korea). The IV-PCA program consisted of a 2-mL (20 µg of fentanyl) bolus injection and a 0.5-mL (5 µg of fentanyl) basal infusion of the IV-PCA solution with a lockout time of 10 min. The cumulative fentanyl consumption via IV-PCA was assessed at 1, 6, and 24 h after surgery. When patients suffered acute postoperative breakthrough pain (i.e., pain score > 6 on a numeric rating scale [NRS]), pethidine (BCWORLD Pharm. Co., Ltd.) and/or tramadol (YUHAN, Seoul, Republic of Korea) as rescue analgesic IV drugs were administered based on the discretion of the attending physicians in the PACU or the ward, who were blinded to the group assignments. The usage frequencies and doses of the rescue analgesic drugs were recorded. Cumulative IV opioid consumption was calculated from the dose conversion of fentanyl, tramadol, and pethidine into morphine according to the equivalent analgesic dose ratio (i.e., 100 µg of fentanyl = 100 mg of tramadol = 100 mg of pethidine = 10 mg of morphine) [13–15], and assessed at 1, 6, and 24 h after surgery.

Perioperative findings

The preoperative findings included age, height, weight, body mass index (BMI), comorbidities (i.e., diabetes mellitus [DM] and hypertension), history of abdominal surgery, prostate cancer stage [16], laboratory variables (i.e., prostate-specific antigen, hemoglobin, white blood cell [WBC] count, and neutrophil, lymphocyte, and platelet counts). Intraoperative findings included surgical duration, hypotensive events, rescue IV ephedrine dose, total dose of remifentanil, hourly fluid infusion, hourly urine output, and total blood loss volume. The NRS score (1–3, mild pain; 4–6, moderate pain; 7–10, severe pain) at rest and during coughing was assessed at 1, 6, and 24 h after surgery. In our study, an NRS score ≤ 3 was considered an acceptable pain control target. Development of opioid-related complications on day 1 after surgery was assessed, including post-dural puncture headache, respiratory depression, nausea, vomiting, pruritus, and neurologic sequela.

Statistical analysis

The minimum sample size was determined based on the difference in cumulative IV opioid consumption on day 1 after surgery between patients who did and did not receive ITMB. Cumulative consumption was calculated from previous electronic medical records at our hospital (unpublished). The mean cumulative IV opioid consumption (morphine equianalgesic dose) on postoperative day 1 by the patients who received no ITMB (n = 10) and ITMB (n = 10) was 45.01 and 23.23 mg, respectively, and the standard deviation (SD) for 20 patients was 25.49 mg. A minimum sample size of 22 patients in each group was required for $\alpha = 0.05$ and a power of 0.8. Therefore, we recruited 25 patients for each group assuming a dropout rate of 10%.

Values are expressed as the means ± standard deviations, medians with interquartile ranges (IQR) in parentheses, or numbers with percentages in parentheses. The normality of the distribution of continuous data was evaluated using the Shapiro–Wilk test. The perioperative findings were compared between patients who did and did not receive ITMB using the unpaired t-test or the Mann–Whitney U-test and Pearson's χ^2 test or Fisher's exact test, as appropriate. Odds ratios (reported with 95% confidence intervals [CIs] in parentheses) of ITMB with a postoperative NRS score ≤ 3 at rest and during coughing were investigated before and after adjusting for cumulative IV opioid consumption using logistic regression analysis. All tests were two-sided, and a p-value < 0.05 was considered significant. Statistical analyses were performed using SPSS for Windows (*ver.* 24.0; IBM Corporation, Armonk, NY, USA) and MedCalc for Windows software (*ver.* 11.0; MedCalc Software, Ostend, Belgium).

Results

Demographic findings in patients who underwent RALP

In the present study, all patients (n = 50) were rated as ASA physical status I or II and underwent elective RALP. The median age was 64 (62–68) years, and the median BMI was 24.0 (22.6–26.7) kg/m^2. Twelve patients (24.0%) had DM and 19 patients (38.0%) had hypertension. Eleven patients (22.0%) were assessed to be at prostate cancer stage I, 32 patients (64.0%) were at stage II, and 7 patients (14.0%) were at stage III. The median prostate specific antigen level was 7.1 (4.9–10.8) ng/mL; the median WBC count, hemoglobin level, and platelet count were 6.2 (5.0–7.4) × 10^9/L, 14.4 (13.7–15.1) g/dL, and 195.5 (166.3–227.3) × 10^9/L, respectively.

The median surgical duration was 120 (114–135) min. Twenty-one patients (42.0%) experienced transient hypotensive events, and the median dose of rescue ephedrine was 0 (0–5) mg. There were no cases of persistent hypotension requiring continuous vasopressor (i.e., epinephrine or norepinephrine) infusion or fluid resuscitation therapy during or after surgery. The median dose of total remifentanil was 0.4 (0.2–0.5) mg, and the median levels of crystalloid infusion, urine output, and blood loss were 3.8 (2.9–4.9) mL/kg/h, 0.6 (0.4–0.8) mL/kg/h, and 100 (50–100) mL, respectively.

Comparison of pre- and intraoperative findings between patients who did or did not receive ITMB

No significant differences were observed in the preoperative findings between patients who did and did not receive ITMB (Table 1). The total remifentanil infusion dose was lower in patients who received ITMB than in those who did not, and the ITMB group exhibited a higher rate of hypotensive events and required a higher rescue ephedrine dose compared to the no-ITMB group, although the differences were not statistically significant. Other intraoperative findings were similar between the two groups (Table 2).

Analysis of postoperative NRS score and cumulative IV opioid consumption between patients who did and did not receive ITMB

The NRS score and cumulative IV opioid consumption after surgery were compared between the two groups (Table 3). In the PACU (i.e., at 1 h after surgery), incidences of mild pain (i.e., NRS score ≤ 3) at rest and during coughing were higher in the ITMB group (68.0% at rest and 52.0% during coughing) than in the no-ITMB group (12.0% at rest and 4.0% during coughing). In the ward (i.e., at 6 h after surgery), the incidences of mild pain at rest and during coughing were higher in the ITMB group (84.0% at rest and 52.0% during coughing) than in the no-ITMB group (20.0% at rest and 12.0% during coughing). In the ward (i.e., at 24 h after surgery), the incidences of mild pain at rest and during coughing were higher in the ITMB group (92.0% at rest and 52.0% during coughing) than in the no-ITMB group (68.0% at rest and 16.0% during coughing). The median (IQR) cumulative level of IV opioid consumption was significantly lower in the ITMB group than in the no-ITMB group—4.4 (2.9–5.7) versus 12.1 (5.8–14.0) mg, respectively, in the PACU; 8.4 (6.0–10.2) versus 18.5 (12.7–28.4) mg, respectively, in the ward (i.e., at 6 h after surgery); and 18.7 (15.0–24.2) versus 38.4 (26.6–57.1) mg, respectively, in the ward (i.e., at 24 h after surgery).

We also assessed whether there was an association between ITMB and postoperative NRS score ≤ 3 at rest and during coughing in the PACU and ward (Table 4). In the PACU (i.e., at 1 h after surgery), ITMB was significantly associated with postoperative NRS scores ≤ 3 at rest both before ($\beta = 2.746$; odds ratio = 15.583; 95% CI 3.583–67.784; $p < 0.001$) and after adjusting for cumulative IV opioid consumption ($\beta = 2.092$; odds ratio = 8.098; 95% CI 1.258–52.133; $p = 0.028$). ITMB was significantly associated with postoperative NRS scores ≤ 3 during coughing both before ($\beta = 3.258$;

Table 1 Comparison of preoperative findings between the patients who did or did not receive intrathecal morphine and bupivacaine (ITMB)

Group	No ITMB	ITMB	*p*
n	25	25	
Age (years)	65.0 (61.5–68.0)	64.0 (62.0–71.5)	0.853
Height (cm)	170.0 (166.3–172.0)	169.0 (164.1–172.5)	0.69
Weight (kg)	68.0 (61.5–78.0)	67.0 (62.5–75.5)	0.593
Body mass index (kg/m^2)	23.9 (22.7–27.2)	24.1 (22.2–26.5)	0.438
Comorbidity			
Hypertension	7 (28.0%)	12 (48.0%)	0.145
Diabetes mellitus	7 (28.0%)	5 (20.0%)	0.508
History of abdominal surgery	6 (24.0%)	5 (20.0%)	0.733
Prostate cancer stage			0.482
Stage I	4 (16.0%)	7 (28.0%)	
Stage II	18 (72.0%)	14 (56.0%)	
Stage III	3 (12.0%)	4 (16.0%)	
Laboratory variables			
Prostate-specific antigen (ng/mL)	7.0 (4.5–12.4)	7.4 (5.1–10.5)	0.954
Hemoglobin (g/dL)	14.4 (14.0–15.0)	14.5 (13.4–15.3)	0.727
White blood cell count (× 10^9/L)	5.5 (4.7–7.1)	6.9 (5.2–7.8)	0.162
Neutrophils (%)	54.9 (50.7–58.1)	54.8 (51.4–55.0)	0.362
Lymphocytes (%)	33.6 (30.3–36.2)	34.0 (33.5–38.8)	0.299
Platelet count (× 10^9/L)	188.0 (162.5–219.0)	202.0 (170.5–233.5)	0.26

Values are expressed as the mean ± standard deviation, medians with interquartile ranges in parentheses, or numbers with percentages in parentheses

Table 2 Comparison of intraoperative findings between patients who did or did not receive ITMB

Group	No ITMB	ITMB	*p*
n	25	25	
Surgical duration (min)	120 (108–143)	120 (115–130)	1.000
Hypotensive event[a]	8 (32.0%)	13 (52.0%)	0.152
Rescue ephedrine dose (mg)	0.0 (0.0–4.0)	4.0 (0.0–8.0)	0.095
Remifentanil dose (mg)	0.5 (0.4–0.6)	0.2 (0.2–0.3)	< 0.001
Hourly fluid infusion (mL/kg/h)	3.5 (3.0–4.2)	4.3 (2.8–6.0)	0.233
Hourly urine output (mL/kg/h)	0.6 (0.4–0.7)	0.7 (0.4–0.9)	0.322
Blood loss (mL)	100 (50–100)	100 (50–150)	0.449

Values are expressed as the mean ± standard deviation, medians with interquartile ranges in parentheses, or numbers with percentages in parentheses

[a] A hypotensive event was defined as systolic blood pressure < 90 mmHg or diastolic blood pressure < 60 mmHg over 5 min

odds ratio = 26.0; 95% CI 3.032–222.928; $p = 0.003$) and after adjusting for cumulative IV opioid consumption ($\beta = 2.61$; odds ratio = 13.593; 95% CI 1.344–137.478; $p = 0.027$). In the ward (i.e., at 6 h after surgery), ITMB was significantly associated with postoperative NRS score ≤ 3 at rest before ($\beta = 3.045$; odds ratio = 21.0; 95% CI 4.924–89.561; $p < 0.001$), but not after adjusting for cumulative IV opioid consumption. ITMB was significantly associated with postoperative NRS score ≤ 3 during coughing before ($\beta = 2.072$; odds ratio = 7.944; 95% CI 1.884–33.498; $p = 0.005$), but not after adjusting for cumulative IV opioid consumption. In the ward (i.e., at 24 h after surgery), ITMB was significantly associated with postoperative NRS score ≤ 3 at rest before ($\beta = 1.689$; odds ratio = 5.412; 95% CI 1.017–28.791; $p = 0.048$), but not after adjusting for cumulative IV opioid consumption. ITMB was significantly associated with postoperative NRS score ≤ 3 during coughing before ($\beta = 1.738$; odds ratio = 5.687; 95% CI 1.51–21.424; $p = 0.01$), but not after adjusting for cumulative IV opioid consumption.

Comparison of postoperative complications between patients who did or did not receive ITMB

No significant differences in complications, such as post-dural puncture headache, respiratory depression, nausea, vomiting, pruritus, or neurologic sequelae, were detected on day 1 after surgery between the two patient groups (Table 5).

Table 3 Comparison of postoperative numeric rating scale (NRS) score and cumulative intravenous (IV) opioid consumption between patients with/without ITMB

Group	No ITMB	ITMB	*p*
n	25	25	
At 1 h after surgery (in the PACU)			
NRS score at rest			< 0.001
1–3	3 (12.0%)	17 (68.0%)	
4–6	13 (52.0%)	5 (20.0%)	
7–10	9 (36.0%)	3 (12.0%)	
NRS score during coughing			< 0.001
1–3	1 (4.0%)	13 (52.0%)	
4–6	8 (32.0%)	7 (28.0%)	
7–10	16 (64.0%)	5 (20.0%)	
Cumulative IV opioid consumption (mg)[a]	12.1 (5.8–14.0)	4.4 (2.9–5.7)	0.001
At 6 h after surgery (in the ward)			
NRS score at rest			< 0.001
1–3	5 (20.0%)	21 (84.0%)	
4–6	13 (52.0%)	3 (12.0%)	
7–10	7 (28.0%)	1 (4.0%)	
NRS score during coughing			0.009
1–3	3 (12.0%)	13 (52.0%)	
4–6	13 (52.0%)	8 (32.0%)	
7–10	9 (36.0%)	4 (16.0%)	
Cumulative IV opioid consumption (mg)[a]	18.5 (12.7–28.4)	8.4 (6.0–10.2)	< 0.001
At 24 h after surgery (in the ward)			
NRS score at rest			0.034
1–3	17 (68.0%)	23 (92.0%)	
4–6	8 (32.0%)	2 (8.0%)	
7–10	0 (0.0%)	0 (0.0%)	
NRS score during coughing			0.024
1–3	4 (16.0%)	13 (52.0%)	
4–6	18 (72.0%)	11 (44.0%)	
7–10	3 (12.0%)	1 (4.0%)	
Cumulative IV opioid consumption (mg)[a]	38.4 (26.6–57.1)	18.7 (15.0–24.2)	< 0.001

Values are expressed as medians with interquartile ranges in parentheses, or numbers with percentages in parentheses

PACU post-anesthesia care unit

[a] Morphine equianalgesic dose (mg)

Discussion

The main findings of our study are that a low dose of intrathecal morphine (i.e., 0.2 mg) and 0.5% bupivacaine (i.e., 7.5 mg) had a significant analgesic benefit during the first 24 h postoperatively in patients who underwent RALP. Patients who received ITMB reported lower pain levels and required less cumulative IV opioids than those who did not receive ITMB. In the PACU, ITMB seemed to play a predominant role in achieving an optimal analgesic level (i.e., NRS score ≤ 3) at rest and during coughing, independent of cumulative IV opioid consumption. In the ward, ITMB was associated with attenuating pain level. In addition, the incidence rates of nausea/vomiting and pruritus were marginally higher in patients who received ITMB than in those who did not, but no post-dural puncture headache, respiratory depression, or neurologic sequelae occurred in the patients who received ITMB.

RALP is a minimally invasive surgery requiring small incisions; however, patients frequently suffer moderate to severe pain for the first 24 h postoperatively due to visceral irritation and a prolonged pneumoperitoneum with a high CO_2 pressure. Thereafter, patients experience a gradual decrease in pain severity [17, 18]. The intrathecal approach is safe and acceptable for acute postoperative pain control and has several advantages over systemic

Table 4 Association between ITMB and postoperative NRS score ≤ 3 at rest and during coughing in the PACU and ward

	β	Odds ratio	95% CI	p
At 1 h after surgery (in the PACU)				
NRS score ≤ 3 at rest				
IV-PCA alone	Reference			
ITMB and IV-PCA	2.746	15.583	3.583–67.784	< 0.001
ITMB and IV-PCA[a]	2.092	8.098	1.258–52.133	0.028
NRS score ≤ 3 during coughing				
IV-PCA alone	Reference			
ITMB and IV-PCA	3.258	26.0	3.032–222.928	0.003
ITMB and IV-PCA[a]	2.610	13.593	1.344–137.478	0.027
At 6 h after surgery (in the ward)				
NRS score ≤ 3 at rest				
IV-PCA alone	Reference			
ITMB and IV-PCA	3.045	21.0	4.924–89.561	< 0.001
ITMB and IV-PCA[a]	1.713	5.547	0.804–38.249	0.082
NRS score ≤ 3 during coughing				
IV-PCA alone	Reference			
ITMB and IV-PCA	2.072	7.944	1.884–33.498	0.005
ITMB and IV-PCA[a]	− 0.030	0.971	0.133–7.079	0.976
At 24 h after surgery (in the ward)				
NRS score ≤ 3 at rest				
IV-PCA alone	Reference			
ITMB and IV-PCA	1.689	5.412	1.017–28.791	0.048
ITMB and IV-PCA[a]	0.572	1.771	0.219–14.329	0.592
NRS score ≤ 3 during coughing				
IV-PCA alone	Reference			
ITMB and IV-PCA	1.738	5.687	1.51–21.424	0.01
ITMB and IV-PCA[a]	0.776	2.172	0.439–10.745	0.342

IV-PCA intravenous patient-controlled analgesia, *CI* confidence interval

[a] After adjustment for cumulative IV opioid consumption

Table 5 Comparison of complications on day 1 after surgery between patients who did or did not receive ITMB

Group	No ITMB	ITMB	p
n	25	25	
Post-dural puncture headache	0 (0.0%)	0 (0.0%)	1.000
Respiratory depression	0 (0.0%)	0 (0.0%)	1.000
Nausea	2 (8.0%)	6 (24.0%)	0.247
Vomiting	0 (0.0%)	1 (4.0%)	1.000
Pruritus	0 (0.0%)	4 (16.0%)	0.110
Neurologic sequela	0 (0.0%)	0 (0.0%)	1.000

Values are expressed as numbers with percentages in parentheses

and/or epidural pain-relief methods, including less invasiveness, a smaller opioid requirement for providing a similar analgesic effect, and a lower risk of procedural failure [5, 10, 19]. Due to the hydrophilic nature of morphine, the analgesic effect of single-shot intrathecal morphine continuously maintained for 24 h after surgery may be suitable for treating pain due to laparoscopic surgery [20]. As part of multimodal pain management, single-shot intrathecal morphine contributes to optimal pain recovery after minimally invasive surgery [21, 22]. Bae et al. [19] reported that the pain score (i.e., numerical pain score at rest and during coughing) was lower and less morphine was required during the first 24 h after RALP in patients who received 300 μg of intrathecal morphine than in those who did not receive intrathecal morphine. The incidence rates of opioid-related complications (i.e., nausea, vomiting, dizziness, headache, and pruritus) were comparable between patients who did and did not receive intrathecal morphine.

A higher morphine dose (e.g., > 500 μg) ensures a strong analgesic effect, but the probability of complications such as nausea, vomiting, and respiratory depression increases in line with the morphine dose [23, 24]. A relatively low dose of morphine (e.g., 100–400 μg) with a local anesthetic (e.g., bupivacaine) may allow the appropriate analgesic target to be reached without side effects in patients undergoing laparoscopic surgery [5, 25, 26]. Nguyen et al. [26] suggested that a regimen of 0.4 mg of intrathecal morphine and 15 μg of fentanyl with an additional 15 mg of 0.5% bupivacaine significantly decreases IV morphine consumption rate and the pain score compared to using intrathecal opioids alone after laparoscopic liver surgery. An intrathecal mixture of morphine (200 μg in patients ≤ 75 years or 150 μg in patients > 75 years) and 10 mg 0.5% bupivacaine was associated with a lower dose of opioid infusion in patients in the enhanced recovery after surgery program for laparoscopic colonic resection [25]. Sherif et al. [22] reported that the analgesic impact (i.e., visual analogue scale score and total morphine consumption) and recovery outcomes (i.e., time to first ambulation, return of intestinal sounds, and hospital stay) were superior in patients who received 0.3 mL (0.3 mg) of intrathecal morphine and 1.2 mL of 0.5% bupivacaine than in patients who received 0.3 mL of intrathecal saline and 1.2 mL of 0.5% bupivacaine after laparoscopic bariatric surgery. Patients who underwent RALP and received 300 μg of intrathecal morphine and 12.5 mg of bupivacaine exhibited better early postoperative recovery, as represented by the Quality of Recovery-15 questionnaire score on postoperative day 1, than those who received a subcutaneous sham injection or 0.1-mg/kg load of IV morphine loading [5]. The optimal spinal dose of bupivacaine for the recovery of motor function and guaranteed hospital discharge in patients undergoing ambulatory surgery is 7.5 mg; this dose was able to resolve motor block within 5 h and achieve discharge within 6 h in 95%

of patients [27]. Our study suggested that an intrathecal low-dose regimen (i.e., 0.2 mg of morphine and 7.5 mg of 0.5% bupivacaine) may be effective for acute pain control in the PACU (i.e., at 1 h after surgery) and the ward (i.e., at 6 and 24 h after surgery) without fatal complications. In particular, this regimen may be able to provide a significantly better analgesic effect in the PACU patients (i.e., eightfold higher score at rest and 14-fold higher score during coughing after adjusting for IV opioid dose) compared to outcomes from using IV-PCA alone. This regimen did not significantly affect intraoperative hemodynamic factors (i.e., hypotensive events or the requirement for a rescue dose of ephedrine) or the incidence of postoperative complications (i.e., post-dural puncture headache, respiratory depression, and neurological deficit). However, as intrathecal bupivacaine-induced hemodynamic disturbance, such as hypotension, may be aggravated in vulnerable patients, such as those of advanced age, due to hypovolemia or decreased sympathetic tone and baroreceptor activity, it is necessary to meticulously adjust the dose of additive bupivacaine while taking age into consideration [28, 29].

Limitations

This study had some limitations that should be discussed. First, our patients were treated for postoperative pain using numerous IV opioids, including fentanyl in IV-PCA, and pethidine and/or tramadol as IV rescue analgesic drugs. Although cumulative IV opioid consumption was calculated by dose conversion of fentanyl, tramadol, and pethidine into morphine according to the equivalent analgesic dose ratio, these calculated doses may be less precise compared to directly measuring the actual amounts of the IV opioid drugs. Second, we were unable to blind the patients and the attending anesthesiologists to the group assignments. The intrathecal practice was performed before inducing anesthesia to avoid potential neurological complications such as nerve injury. However, there were no patients with surgical or hemodynamic issues required consultation from the attending physicians and nurses in the PACU and ward (who recorded the study data), and therefore, the latter were blinded to the group assignments. Third, the sample size was calculated to allow detection of a difference in cumulative IV opioid consumption on day 1 after surgery between patients who did and did not receive ITMB. However, it might not have been sufficient to compare the groups with regard to differences in postoperative complications, such as the rate of intraoperative hypotensive events. Further studies with larger populations are required to elucidate the association between ITMB and postoperative complications. Fourth, although our regimen, which used a lower dose compared to a previous RALP study [5], led to acceptable analgesic benefits during the first 24 h after surgery, we are unable to determine the optimal doses of ITMB for RALP. As the analgesic mechanisms differ between morphine and bupivacaine [30, 31], further studies are required to investigate the dose–response relationship and synergistic effects between these two analgesic drugs.

Conclusion

A single spinal injection of morphine and bupivacaine provided proper early postoperative analgesia and decreased additional requirements for IV opioids in patients who underwent RALP. The patients who received ITMB were intraoperatively stable and tolerated postoperative spinal practice-related complications. ITMB is considered a critical analgesic modality as part of a multimodal analgesia recovery strategy for RALP.

Abbreviations

RALP: Robotic-assisted laparoscopic prostatectomy; IV: Intravenous; ITMB: Intrathecal morphine and bupivacaine; ASA: American Society of Anesthesiologists; PACU: Post-anesthesia care unit; IV-PCA: Intravenous patient-control analgesia; NRS: Numeric rating scale; DM: Diabetes mellitus; WBC: White blood cell; SD: Standard deviation; IQR: Interquartile.

Acknowledgements

All authors thank Eunju Choi, Hyeji An and Hyunsook Yoo (Anesthesia Nursing Unit, Seoul St. Mary's Hospital, The Catholic University of Korea, Seoul, Republic of Korea) for participation of our study.

Authors' contributions

JWS and MSC designed the study, wrote the manuscript, and analyzed and interpreted the data. JWS, YJC, HWM, JP, HML, YSK, YEM, SHH and MSC collected the data and provided critical comments. All authors revised the manuscript critically for important intellectual content. All authors read and approved the final manuscript.

Author details

[1] Department of Anesthesiology and Pain Medicine, Seoul St. Mary's Hospital, College of Medicine, The Catholic University of Korea, 222, Banpo-daero, Seocho-gu, Seoul 06591, Republic of Korea. [2] Department of Urology, Seoul St. Mary's Hospital, College of Medicine, The Catholic University of Korea, Seoul, Republic of Korea.

References

1. Ficarra V, Novara G, Artibani W, Cestari A, Galfano A, Graefen M, Guazzoni G, Guillonneau B, Menon M, Montorsi F, et al. Retropubic, laparoscopic, and robot-assisted radical prostatectomy: a systematic review and cumulative analysis of comparative studies. Eur Urol. 2009;55(5):1037–63.
2. Pearce SM, Pariser JJ, Karrison T, Patel SG, Eggener SE. Comparison of perioperative and early oncologic outcomes between open and robotic assisted laparoscopic prostatectomy in a contemporary population based cohort. J Urol. 2016;196(1):76–81.
3. Porpiglia F, Fiori C, Bertolo R, Manfredi M, Mele F, Checcucci E, De Luca S, Passera R, Scarpa RM. Five-year outcomes for a prospective randomised controlled trial comparing laparoscopic and robot-assisted radical prostatectomy. Eur Urol Focus. 2018;4(1):80–6.
4. Woldu SL, Weinberg AC, Bergman A, Shapiro EY, Korets R, Motamedinia P, Badani KK. Pain and analgesic use after robot-assisted radical prostatectomy. J Endourol. 2014;28(5):544–8.
5. Koning MV, de Vlieger R, Teunissen AJW, Gan M, Ruijgrok EJ, de Graaff JC, Koopman J, Stolker RJ. The effect of intrathecal bupivacaine/morphine on quality of recovery in robot-assisted radical prostatectomy: a randomised controlled trial. Anaesthesia. 2019.

6. Dal Moro F, Aiello L, Pavarin P, Zattoni F. Ultrasound-guided transversus abdominis plane block (US-TAPb) for robot-assisted radical prostatectomy: a novel "4-point" technique-results of a prospective, randomized study. J Robot Surg. 2019;13(1):147–51.
7. Weinberg AC, Woldu SL, Bergman A, Roychoudhury A, Patel T, Berg W, Wambi C, Badani KK. Dorsal penile nerve block for robot-assisted radical prostatectomy catheter related pain: a randomized, double-blind, placebo-controlled trial. SpringerPlus. 2014;3:181.
8. Ko JS, Choi SJ, Gwak MS, Kim GS, Ahn HJ, Kim JA, Hahm TS, Cho HS, Kim KM, Joh JW. Intrathecal morphine combined with intravenous patient-controlled analgesia is an effective and safe method for immediate postoperative pain control in live liver donors. Liver Transplant. 2009;15(4):381–9.
9. Lee SH, Gwak MS, Choi SJ, Park HG, Kim GS, Kim MH, Ahn HJ, Kim J, Kwon CH, Kim TS. Prospective, randomized study of ropivacaine wound infusion versus intrathecal morphine with intravenous fentanyl for analgesia in living donors for liver transplantation. Liver Transplant. 2013;19(9):1036–45.
10. Levy BF, Scott MJ, Fawcett W, Fry C, Rockall TA. Randomized clinical trial of epidural, spinal or patient-controlled analgesia for patients undergoing laparoscopic colorectal surgery. Br J Surg. 2011;98(8):1068–78.
11. Lui MW, Li TKT, Lui F, Ong CYT. A randomised, controlled trial of rectus sheath bupivacaine and intrathecal bupivacaine, without or with intrathecal morphine, vs. intrathecal bupivacaine and morphine after caesarean section. Anaesthesia. 2017;72(10):1225–9.
12. Mayhew D, Mendonca V, Murthy BVS. A review of ASA physical status - historical perspectives and modern developments. Anaesthesia. 2019;74(3):373–9.
13. Xia J, Paul Olson TJ, Tritt S, Liu Y, Rosen SA. Comparison of preoperative versus postoperative transversus abdominis plane and rectus sheath block in patients undergoing minimally invasive colorectal surgery. Colorectal Dis. 2020;22:569–80.
14. Treillet E, Laurent S, Hadjiat Y. Practical management of opioid rotation and equianalgesia. J Pain Res. 2018;11:2587–601.
15. Pereira J, Lawlor P, Vigano A, Dorgan M, Bruera E. Equianalgesic dose ratios for opioids. A critical review and proposals for long-term dosing. J Pain Symp Manag. 2001;22(2):672–87.
16. Buyyounouski MK, Choyke PL, McKenney JK, Sartor O, Sandler HM, Amin MB, Kattan MW. Prostate cancer—major changes in the American Joint Committee on Cancer eighth edition cancer staging manual. CA Cancer J Clin. 2017;67(3):245–53.
17. Kong SK, Onsiong SM, Chiu WK, Li MK. Use of intrathecal morphine for postoperative pain relief after elective laparoscopic colorectal surgery. Anaesthesia. 2002;57(12):1168–73.
18. Goh YC, Eu KW, Seow-Choen F. Early postoperative results of a prospective series of laparoscopic vs. open anterior resections for rectosigmoid cancers. Dis Colon Rectum. 1997;40(7):776–80.
19. Bae J, Kim HC, Hong DM. Intrathecal morphine for postoperative pain control following robot-assisted prostatectomy: a prospective randomized trial. J Anesth. 2017;31(4):565–71.
20. Rathmell JP, Lair TR, Nauman B. The role of intrathecal drugs in the treatment of acute pain. Anesth Analg. 2005;101(5 Suppl):S30-43.
21. Cheah JW, Sing DC, Hansen EN, Aleshi P, Vail TP. Does Intrathecal morphine in spinal anesthesia have a role in modern multimodal analgesia for primary total joint arthroplasty? J Arthroplasty. 2018;33(6):1693–8.
22. El Sherif FA, Othman AH, Abd El-Rahman AM, Taha O. Effect of adding intrathecal morphine to a multimodal analgesic regimen for postoperative pain management after laparoscopic bariatric surgery: a prospective, double-blind, randomized controlled trial. Br J Pain. 2016;10(4):209–16.
23. Clergue F, Montembault C, Despierres O, Ghesquiere F, Harari A, Viars P. Respiratory effects of intrathecal morphine after upper abdominal surgery. Anesthesiology. 1984;61(6):677–85.
24. Gjessing J, Tomlin PJ. Postoperative pain control with intrathecal morphine. Anaesthesia. 1981;36(3):268–76.
25. Wongyingsinn M, Baldini G, Stein B, Charlebois P, Liberman S, Carli F. Spinal analgesia for laparoscopic colonic resection using an enhanced recovery after surgery programme: better analgesia, but no benefits on postoperative recovery: a randomized controlled trial. Br J Anaesth. 2012;108(5):850–6.
26. Nguyen M, Vandenbroucke F, Roy JD, Beaulieu D, Seal RF, Lapointe R, Dagenais M, Roy A, Massicotte L. Evaluation of the addition of bupivacaine to intrathecal morphine and fentanyl for postoperative pain management in laparascopic liver resection. Reg Anesth Pain Med. 2010;35(3):261–6.
27. Lemoine A, Mazoit JX, Bonnet F. Modelling of the optimal bupivacaine dose for spinal anaesthesia in ambulatory surgery based on data from systematic review. Eur J Anaesthesiol. 2016;33(11):846–52.
28. Salinas FV, Sueda LA, Liu SS. Physiology of spinal anaesthesia and practical suggestions for successful spinal anaesthesia. Best Pract Res Clin Anaesthesiol. 2003;17(3):289–303.
29. Hartmann B, Junger A, Klasen J, Benson M, Jost A, Banzhaf A, Hempelmann G. The incidence and risk factors for hypotension after spinal anesthesia induction: an analysis with automated data collection. Anesth Analg. 2002;94(6):1521–9.
30. Wiffen PJ, Derry S, Moore RA. Impact of morphine, fentanyl, oxycodone or codeine on patient consciousness, appetite and thirst when used to treat cancer pain. Cochrane Database Syst Rev. 2014;5:Cd011056.
31. Lemke KA, Dawson SD. Local and regional anesthesia. Vet Clin North Am Small Anim Pract. 2000;30(4):839–57.

7

One-year urinary and sexual outcome trajectories among prostate cancer patients treated by radical prostatectomy

Lin Yang[1,2,3*], Jung Ae Lee[4], Emily Heer[1], Claire Pernar[5], Graham A. Colditz[3], Ratna Pakpahan[3], Kellie R. Imm[3,10], Eric H. Kim, Robert L. Grubb III[6,7], Kathleen Y. Wolin[8], Adam S. Kibel[9] and Siobhan Sutcliffe[3]

Abstract

Background: To examine one-year trajectories of urinary and sexual outcomes, and correlates of these trajectories, among prostate cancer patients treated by radical prostatectomy (RP).

Methods: Study participants were recruited from 2011 to 2014 at two US institutions. Self-reported urinary and sexual outcomes were measured at baseline before surgery, and 5 weeks, 6 months and 12 months after surgery, using the modified Expanded Prostate Cancer Index Composite-50 (EPIC-50). Changes in EPIC-50 scores from baseline were categorized as improved (beyond baseline), maintained, or impaired (below baseline), using previously-reported minimum clinically important differences.

Results: Of the 426 eligible participants who completed the baseline survey, 395 provided data on at least one EPIC-50 sub-scale at 5 weeks and 12 months, and were analyzed. Although all mean EPIC-50 scores declined markedly 5 weeks after surgery and then recovered to near (incontinence-related outcomes) or below (sexual outcomes) baseline levels by 12 months post-surgery, some men experienced improvement beyond their baseline levels on each sub-scale (3.3–51% depending on the sub-scale). Having benign prostatic hyperplasia (BPH) at baseline (prostate size $\geq$ 40 g; an International Prostate Symptom Index Score $\geq$ 8; or using BPH medications) was associated with post-surgical improvements in voiding dysfunction-related bother at 5 weeks (OR = 3.9, 95% CI: 2.1–7.2) and 12 months (OR = 3.3, 95% CI: 2.0–5.7); and in sexual bother at 5 weeks (OR = 5.7, 95% CI:1.7–19.3) and 12 months (OR = 3.0, 95% CI: 1.2–7.1).

Conclusions: Our findings provide additional support for considering baseline BPH symptoms when selecting the best therapy for early-stage prostate cancer.

Keywords: Localized prostate cancer, Benign prostatic hyperplasia, Radical prostatectomy, Urinary outcome, Sexual outcome

Background

Early-stage, localized prostate cancer can be managed in several ways, including watchful waiting, active surveillance, and curative modalities such as radical prostatectomy (RP), external radiotherapy, and brachytherapy. As each of these modalities has high survival rates [1], the

*Correspondence: Lin.Yang@albertahealthservices.ca
[1] Department of Cancer Epidemiology and Prevention Research, Cancer Research and Analytics, Cancer Care Alberta, Alberta Health Services, 5th Floor, Holy Cross Centre, Box ACB, 2210 - 2 St. SW, Calgary, AB T2S 3C3, Canada
Full list of author information is available at the end of the article

benefits of curative therapies must be carefully weighed against their harms, including their side effects [2–4].

A number of studies have documented the natural history of prostate cancer treatment side effects [5–12]. For RP, in particular, studies indicate that men tend to experience an initial large decline in urinary and sexual function immediately after surgery (i.e., within the first two months), followed by a gradual improvement to near or below baseline levels by the first year post-surgery. One exception to this pattern is voiding dysfunction (or urinary irritation or obstruction). Symptoms of voiding dysfunction have been observed to improve beyond pre-surgical values in a few previous studies, presumably because of relief of urinary obstruction by prostatectomy in men with both prostate cancer and benign prostatic hyperplasia (BPH) [13]. These findings have led AUA, ASTRO, and SUO to recommend surgery over radiation therapy for patients with clinically localized prostate cancer and obstructive, non-cancer-related lower urinary tract dysfunction [14]. However, as this recommendation is Grade C, additional high-quality evidence from randomized controlled trials and prospective observational studies is still needed.

To our knowledge, voiding dysfunction is the only outcome in which improvement beyond pre-surgical values has been explored. Although mean improvement has not been observed in other outcomes, such as sexual function or bother, it is possible that examination of mean trajectories may have obscured improvement or other trajectories experienced by only a subset of participants—for instance, those who use medication and devices to treat their erectile dysfunction (ED) after surgery. Understanding the full range of side effect trajectories would be useful to help set patients' expectations post-surgery and to further aid with treatment decision-making. Therefore, we analyzed data from the prospective Prostatectomy, Incontinence, and Erectile Dysfunction (PIE) Study to describe the full range of urinary and sexual side effect trajectories, the percentage of patients with improvement beyond baseline in each domain, and factors related to improvement in the first year post-surgery (i.e. BPH- and ED-related factors).

Methods

Study population and design

Prostate cancer patients were recruited into the PIE study from 2011 to 2014 at two sites, Washington University School of Medicine and Brigham & Women's Hospital. All men undergoing RP for clinically localized prostate cancer were eligible, except for those who: (1) had previously undergone treatment for prostate cancer, radiation therapy to the pelvis (including bladder, rectum, or prostate), or major pelvic surgery (including penile implant or urinary sphincter); (2) had known urethral stricture or colostomy; (3) were unable to urinate and required indwelling catheterization; and (4) did not speak English. Men who received neo-adjuvant therapy or any additional prostate cancer-related therapies (e.g., radiation or hormonal therapies) during the one-year study follow-up were excluded from the analyses. The PIE study was approved by the institutional review boards at both institutions. All participants provided informed consent.

Urinary and sexual outcomes

Patient-reported urinary and sexual outcomes were assessed at baseline before RP, and 5 weeks, 6 months, and 12 months post-RP by the modified Expanded Prostate Cancer Index Composite-50 (EPIC-50) [15]. This validated scale includes sub-scales for urinary function (i.e., continence), urinary bother, sexual function, and sexual bother. We split the urinary bother scale into two sub-scales to distinguish incontinence-related bother from voiding dysfunction-related bother [16]. For each EPIC-50 sub-scale, a summary score was calculated and then transformed linearly to a 0-to-100 scale, with higher scores indicating better function and less bother.

Demographic and lifestyle factors

Before RP, participants completed a baseline questionnaire including items on age, education, household income, race/ethnicity, insurance status, and marital status, as well as lifestyle factors, such as cigarette smoking history. Self-reported data on frequency of performing pelvic floor (i.e., Kegel) exercises after RP was ascertained on the follow-up questionnaires.

BPH- and ED-related factors

We abstracted data on clinical characteristics from participants' medical charts. These included comorbidities (Charlson Comorbidity Index), prostate cancer characteristics (pre-surgical clinical staging, prostate-specific antigen [PSA] concentration, and post-surgical pathological staging); pre-surgical urological conditions, including BPH (prostate size measured from the RP specimen, International Prostate Symptom Index [IPSS], and self-reported BPH medication use [overall, α-blocker use only, and 5α-reductase inhibitor use with or without α-blockers]); surgical characteristics taken from the operative note (blood loss during surgery, attempted number of neurovascular bundles preserved, type of surgical procedure, and bladder neck reconstruction), and sexual dysfunction therapies (pre- and post-surgical ED medication and device use).

Statistical analysis

To begin to explore and display the distributions of urinary and sexual outcomes over time, we constructed boxplots with lines connecting the mean values from baseline through 12 months. This display is similar to figures presented in previous analyses of post-RP outcomes. Next, we investigated side effect trajectories by calculating the difference in each urinary and sexual outcome between baseline and 12 months for each participant and then by ranking participants according to their magnitude of change for each outcome (i.e., from the minimum to the maximum). To illustrate these trajectories, we selected a sample of participants (i.e., those ranked at the 5th, 25th, 50th, 75th, and 95th percentiles) for each outcome and plotted each participant's change from baseline through 12 months, analogous to a selective "spaghetti plot".

Given that some changes may be too small to be meaningful to patients, we next categorized both short- and long-term changes (from baseline to 5 weeks and 12 months, respectively) into clinically meaningful categories, using sub-scale-specific minimum clinically important difference (MCID) ranges reported by Skolarus and colleagues [17]. The upper bounds of these sub-scale-specific ranges were chosen to obtain conservative estimates: i.e., 9 point change in the urinary domain (7 for voiding dysfunction-related symptoms) and 12-point change in the sexual domain [17]. We used these sub-scale-specific values to create the following categories of change: improved beyond baseline (positive change greater than the MCID), maintained (within the positive to negative values of the MCID), and impaired below baseline (negative change greater than the MCID) [16, 18]. We also used the lower bounds of sub-scale-specific ranges to classify participants in sensitivity analyses.

Multinomial logistic regression was used to explore BPH- and ED-related factors associated with short- and long-term improvement beyond baseline and maintenance in urinary and sexual outcomes (in sub-scales with at least 10 men for stable estimation). Factors considered were individual measures of BPH (pre-surgical prostate size, IPSS score, and reported use of BPH medications, overall and separately by type), as well as a composite BPH outcome (prostate size $\geq$ 40 g [19], IPSS score $\geq$ 8 [20], or medication use), and measures of sexual dysfunction (pre- and post- surgical ED medication and device use). Sensitivity analyses were performed by: (1) adjusting for factors significantly associated with improvement or maintenance in at least one urinary or sexual outcome; (2) using the lower bounds of the EPIC-50 sub-scale-specific MCID ranges to classify participants; (3) excluding men with pre-surgical EPIC-50 scores too high to experience improvement (i.e., higher than the value obtained by subtracting the sub-scale specific MCID from 100); (4) restricting to men with complete data on specific urinary and sexual outcomes at baseline, 5 weeks and 12 months; and (5) repeating the analyses using the 6 month follow-up data.

Results

Participant characteristics

Of the 426 eligible participants who completed the baseline survey, 395 (92.7%) provided data on at least one EPIC-50 sub-scale at baseline, 5 weeks, or 12 months, and were included in the analysis. The majority of included participants (mean age = 60.7 years) were Caucasian (91.9%), had completed at least some college education (83.6%), earned $\geq$ \$75,000 per year (61.4%), were married or living with a partner (82.5%), and had never smoked (62.5%, Table 1). Among participants with data on the Charlson Comorbidity Index (n = 167), 103 (61.7% of 103 and 26.2% of 394) had at least one comorbidity. Considering their prostate cancer-specific characteristics, most participants had clinical stage T1 (78.5%) and pathologic stage T3 (88.9%) disease, with a pre-surgical PSA concentration between 4 and 10 ng/mL. The majority (92.3%) of men underwent a minimally-invasive RP and 65.2% had a bilateral never-sparing procedure.

Changes in urinary and sexual outcomes

With respect to urinary incontinence, most men had high function (mean = 93.1) and bother scores (mean = 95.8, i.e., good function and not much bother) at baseline. Scores for voiding dysfunction-related bother were also high (mean = 74.5), but lower than for incontinence-related bother. With respect to sexual outcomes, baseline levels were lower than for urinary outcomes, and were also lower for sexual function (mean = 56.2) than for bother (mean = 68.9), indicating worse sexual function but not as much bother (Fig. 1a–e). Five weeks after surgery, mean levels of each of these outcomes were markedly decreased. For urinary incontinence-related outcomes, levels recovered to near, but below, baseline 6 months post-surgery and then slowed to a plateau by 12 months. In contrast, for voiding dysfunction-related bother, levels recovered to above baseline 6 months post-surgery and then remained relatively constant through 12 months. Finally, for sexual-related outcomes, mean levels remained well below baseline but continued to improve gradually through 12 months post-surgery.

When individual trajectories of change were examined, a generally similar impression of symptom change was obtained, particularly when viewing the median (50th) percentile trajectories (Fig. 2a–e). However, these displays also highlighted improved (beyond baseline) or maintained outcomes in all domains over time. Improvement was greatest for voiding dysfunction-related bother

Table 1 Socio-demographic, lifestyle, and clinical characteristics of prostate cancer patients in the prostatectomy, incontinence and erectile dysfunction (PIE) study

	N	% or mean (SD)
Socio-demographic and lifestyle factors		
Age (years, mean, SD)	395	60.7 (6.9)
Caucasian (%)	385	91.9
Education (%)	385	
High school degree or less		16.4
Some college		30.9
College degree		23.9
Post graduate		28.8
Household income (%)	365	
< $50,000		18.3
$50,000—< $75,000		20.3
≥ $75,000		61.4
Married or living with a partner (%)	395	82.5
Smoking (%)	385	
Never smoker		62.5
Former smoker		32.7
Current smoker		6.8
Charlson Comorbidity Index (%)	394	
No comorbidities		16.2
Any comorbidities		26.2
Missing		57.6
Prostate cancer- and surgery-related factors		
Clinical T1 stage (%)	381	78.5
Pathological stage (%)	389	
T2		11.1
T3		88.9
Pre-surgical prostate-specific antigen concentration (ng/mL, mean, SD)	393	6.3 (4.6)
Blood loss during surgery (mL, mean, SD)	358	246.3 (203.3)
Neurovascular bundle preservation (%)	351	
Non-nerve sparing		19.4
Unilateral neurovascular bundle spared		15.4
Bilateral nerve sparing		65.2
Surgical procedure (%)	365	
Minimally-invasive (robotic and laparoscopic)		92.3
Open		7.7
Bladder reconstruction	364	53.0
BPH-related factors		
Prostate size (grams, mean, SD)	288	43.5 (16.6)
IPSS score at baseline (mean, SD)	249	8.6 (6.7)
BPH medication use at baseline (%)	395	13.2
α-blocker use		10.4
5α-reductase inhibitor (and α-blocker) use		2.8
Urinary and sexual function-related factors		
Reported Kegel exercises		
5 weeks post-surgery	358	67.3
12 months post-surgery	332	31.3
ED medication or device use (%)		
Baseline	365	4.8
5 weeks post-surgery	365	30.1
12 months post-surgery	336	18.2

Table 1 (continued)

BPH benign prostatic hyperplasia, *ED* erectile dysfunction, *IPSS* International Prostate Symptom Score, *SD* standard deviation

(22.1% of men at 5 weeks; 50.9% at 12 months), followed by sexual bother (7.3% at 5 weeks; 10.6% at 12 months), and urinary function (9.8% at 12 months, Tables 2 and 3). Lesser proportions of men experienced improvement in incontinence-related bother and sexual function (< 5%). Of note, improvement beyond baseline was observed even as early as 5 weeks post-surgery, particularly for voiding dysfunction-related and sexual bother.

Factors associated with improvement beyond baseline in urinary and sexual outcomes

No significant associations were observed for BPH- or ED-related factors with improved or maintained urinary function or incontinence-related bother after surgery (only evaluable at 12 months, Table 2 and Additional file 1: Table 1). In contrast, each of the individual measures of BPH, as well as the BPH composite measure, were associated with improved voiding dysfunction-related bother at both 5 weeks and 12 months post-surgery (5 weeks: odds ratio [OR] = 3.9, 95% confidence interval [CI]: 2.1–7.2; 12 months: OR = 3.3, 95% CI: 2.0–5.7 for the BPH composite measure). No associations were observed for ED medication or device use at baseline or follow-up.

With respect to sexual outcomes, no significant associations were observed for BPH- or ED-related factors with improved or maintained sexual function. In contrast, the BPH composite measure was associated with improved sexual bother at both 5 weeks (OR = 5.7, 95% CI:1.7–19.3) and 12 months post-surgery (OR = 3.0, 95% CI: 1.2–7.1, Table 3 and Additional file 1: Table 2). Positive associations were also observed for several of the individual measures of BPH, including α-blocker use (OR = 4.4, 95% CI: 1.1–18.0) with improvement in sexual function at 12 months post-surgery, and BPH medication use (OR = 5.4, 95% CI: 2.2–13.0) and α-blocker use (OR = 5.6, 95% CI: 2.2–14.6) with improvement in sexual bother at 5 weeks. Finally, an inverse association was observed for ED medication or device use during follow-up with maintained sexual function (OR = 0.5, 95% CI: 0.3–0.9) and bother (OR = 0.5, 95% CI: 0.3–1.0) compared to impaired function and bother 12 months post-surgery. This is likely due to confounding by indication, whereby men who experienced large declines in sexual function may have been more likely to use ED medications or devices after surgery.

Similar results were observed in sensitivity analyses: (1) adjusting for age, smoking status, living arrangement, and neurovascular bundle preservation; (2) using the lower

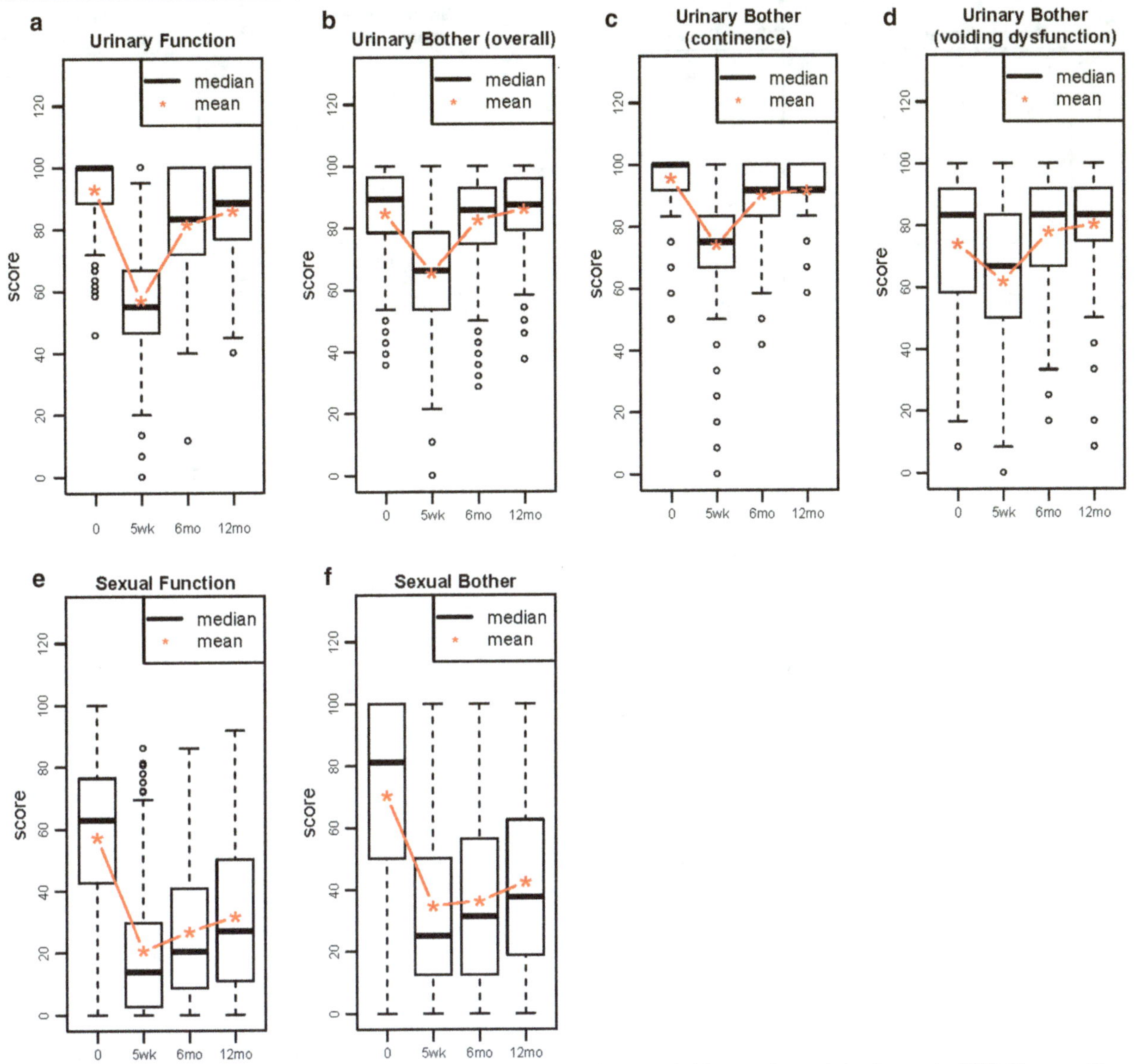

Fig. 1 Changes in Urinary and Sexual Outcomes (mean values) Assessed by the Expanded Prostate Cancer Index Composite (EPIC)-50 among Men in the Prostatectomy, Incontinence and Erectile Function (PIE) Study, between Baseline and 12 Months Post-Radical Prostatectomy

bounds of the EPIC-50 sub-scale-specific MCID ranges; (3) excluding men with high pre-surgical scores in each EPIC-50 sub-scale; (4) restricting to men with complete outcome data at baseline, 5 weeks and 12 months; and (5) examining the 6-month follow-up data (results not shown).

Discussion

Similar to previous studies, our study demonstrated sharp declines in mean urinary and sexual outcomes 5 weeks post-RP, followed by recovery to near, but below, baseline values for urinary incontinence-related outcomes, and to improved, but well below, baseline values for sexual outcomes. However, by examining individual participant trajectories, we also identified several groups of men who experienced improvement beyond their baseline values in each urinary and sexual outcome. Notably, a considerable proportion of men experienced immediate and long-term improvement in voiding dysfunction-related bother, and a small proportion experienced long-term improvement in urinary function (continence) and sexual bother. To our knowledge, improvement in outcomes besides voiding dysfunction has not previously been documented. Additionally, we found that pre-surgical BPH

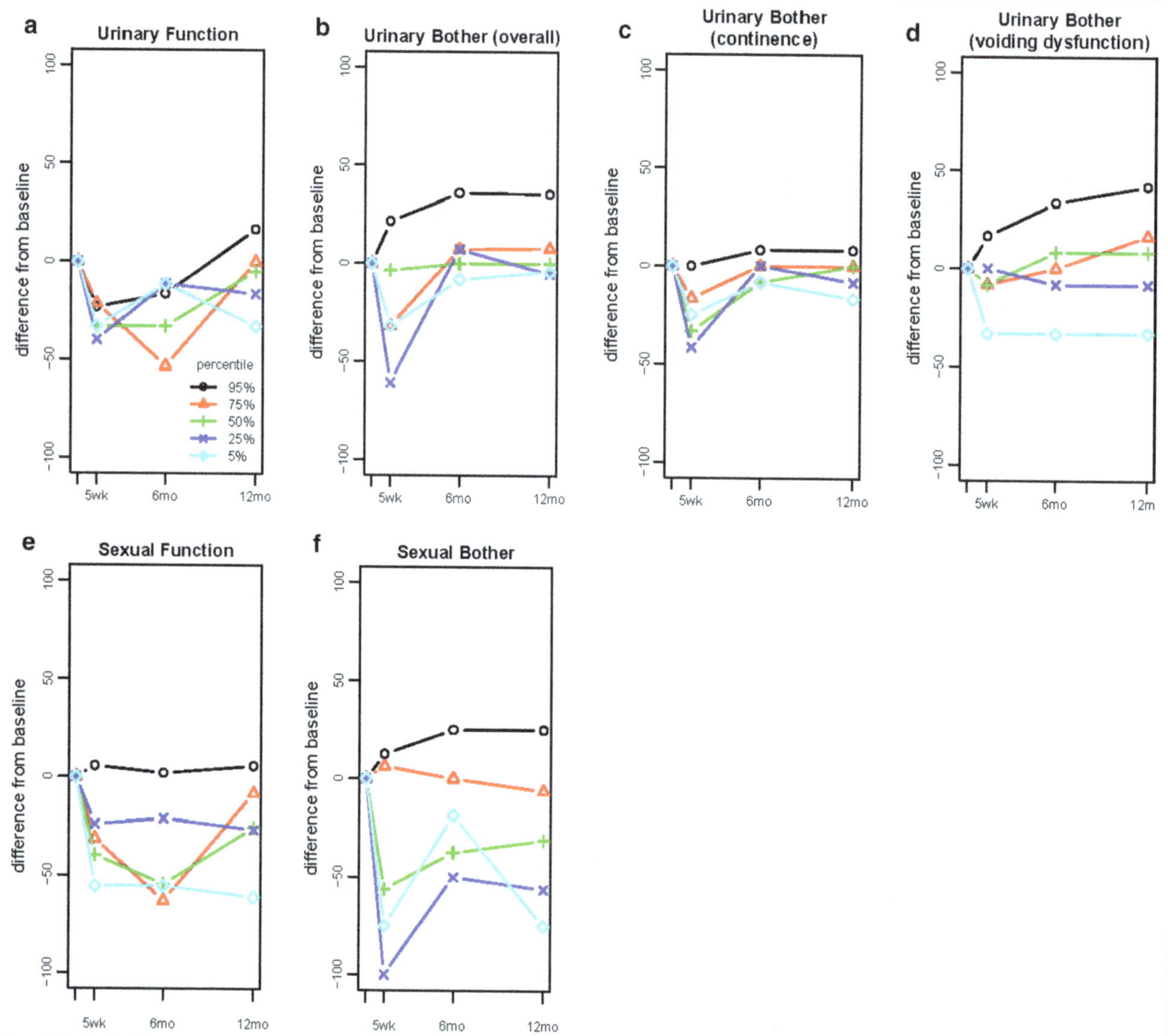

Fig. 2 Individual Trajectories of Urinary and Sexual Outcomes Assessed by the Expanded Prostate Cancer Index Composite (EPIC)-50 among Men in the Prostatectomy, Incontinence and Erectile Function (PIE) Study from Baseline through 12 Months Post-Radical Prostatectomy (The trajectories for five different individuals per domain are presented in each graph. These individuals were selected by subtracting each participant's 12 month follow-up values in each EPIC-50 domain from their baseline values and then by ranking these differences. The outcome trajectories for participants ranked at the 5th, 25th, 50th, 75th, and 95th percentiles of change for each domain are presented to illustrate the range of trajectories experienced by participants. In each domain, participants at the 95th percentile experienced improvement)

was associated with improvement beyond baseline in both voiding dysfunction and sexual bother, strengthening the evidence in national urologic oncology guidelines to recommend surgical treatment for appropriate prostate cancer patients with BPH.

Our finding of clinically meaningful improvement in urinary continence among a small proportion of men treated for prostate cancer by RP was unexpected and differs from most previously published findings [10, 21, 22]. One possible explanation for this finding may be surgical elimination of bladder outlet resistance by RP. Studies of bladder outlet resistance have demonstrated that the bladder detrusor muscle undergoes structural and functional changes, with initial hypertrophy, then compensation, and then decompensation [23–25]. The bladders of men with BPH who undergo RP for prostate cancer may lie anywhere along this spectrum. Men in an initial hypertrophic stage may have some degree of urge-related urinary incontinence, which may be relieved by bladder remodelling following surgical elimination of outlet resistance by RP. Likewise, men in a late decompensated stage may have some degree of stress-related

Table 2 Factors Associated with urinary outcome trajectories assessed by the expanded prostate cancer index composite (EPIC)-50 among men in the prostatectomy, incontinence and erectile dysfunction (PIE) study

	All participants n (%)	BPH-related factors								ED-related factors			
		Prostate size		IPSS score		BPH medication use at baseline		BPH composite measure		ED medication use at baseline		ED medication or device use at follow-up	
		< 40 g	≥ 40 g	< 8	≥ 8	No	Yes	No BPH	Any BPH	No	Yes	No	Yes
Urinary function (continence) 5 weeks post-surgery (n = 377)													
Impaired													
N	346 (91.8)												
OR 95% CI													
Maintained													
N	28 (7.4)												
OR 95% CI													
Improved													
N	3 (0.8)												
OR 95% CI													
Urinary function (continence) 12 months post-surgery (n = 347)													
Impaired													
N	145 (41.8)	57	51	53	46	129	16	63	82	137	8	46	94
OR 95% CI		Reference		Reference		Reference		Reference		Reference		Reference	
Maintained													
N	168 (48.4)	52	71	58	51	148	20	64	104	163	5	59	102
OR 95% CI		1.5 (0.9 to 2.6)		1.0 (0.6 to 1.7)		1.1 (0.5 to 2.2)		1.2 (0.8 to 2.0)		0.5 (0.2 to 1.6)		0.8 (0.5 to 1.4)	
Improved													
N	34 (9.8)	11	17	6	11	28	6	11	23	31	3	13	18
OR 95% CI		1.7 (0.6 to 4.0)		2.1 (0.7 to 6.2)		1.7 (0.6 to 4.8)		1.6 (0.7 to 3.5)		1.7 (0.4 to 6.6)		0.7 (0.3 to 1.5)	
Incontinence-related bother 5 weeks post-surgery (n = 379)													
Impaired													
N	266 (70.3)												
OR 95% CI													
Maintained													
N	110 (29.0)												
OR 95% CI													
Improved													
N	3 (0.8)												
OR 95% CI													

Table 2 (continued)

	All participants n (%)	BPH-related factors								ED-related factors			
		Prostate size		IPSS score		BPH medication use at baseline		BPH composite measure		ED medication use at baseline		ED medication or device use at follow-up	
		< 40 g	≥ 40 g	< 8	≥ 8	No	Yes	No BPH	Any BPH	No	Yes	No	Yes
Incontinence-related bother 12 months post-surgery (n = 348)													
Impaired													
N	53 (15.2)	16	22	25	14	47	6	23	30	50	3	18	33
OR 95% CI		Reference		Reference		Reference		Reference		Reference		Reference	
Maintained													
N	282 (81.0)	103	109	91	87	251	31	113	169	269	13	97	174
OR 95% CI		0.8 (0.4 to 1.5)		1.7 (0.8 to 3.5)		1 (0.4 to 2.4)		1.1 (0.6 to 2.1)		0.8 (0.2 to 2.9)		1.0 (0.5 to 1.8)	
Improved													
N	13 (3.7)	5	7	2	6	9	4	3	10	13	0	6	6
OR 95% CI		1.0 (0.3 to 3.8)		5.4 (1.0 to 30.2)		3.5 (0.8 to 15)		2.6 (0.6 to 10.4)		NE		0.5 (0.2 to 1.9)	
Voiding dysfunction-related bother 5 weeks post-surgery (n = 380)													
Impaired													
N	238 (62.6)	93	89	91	54	212	26	109	129	226	12	126	99
OR 95% CI		Reference		Reference		Reference		Reference		Reference		Reference	
Maintained													
N	58 (15.3)	21	18	23	15	54	4	27	31	55	3	22	33
OR 95% CI		0.9 (0.4 to 1.8)		1.1 (0.5 to 2.3)		0.6 (0.2 to 1.8)		1.0 (0.5 to 1.7)		1.0 (0.3 to 3.8)		1.9 (1.0 to 3.5)	
Improved													
N	84 (22.1)	20	41	14	46	63	21	15	69	80	4	38	40
OR 95% CI		2.1 (1.2 to 3.9)		5.5 (2.8 to 11.0)		2.7 (1.4 to 5.2)		3.9 (2.1 to 7.2)		0.9 (0.3 to 3.0)		1.3 (0.8 to 2.2)	
Voiding dysfunction-related bother 12 months post-surgery (n = 348)													
Impaired													
N	91 (26.1)	38	32	36	20	84	7	49	42	87	4	32	57
OR 95% CI		Reference		Reference		Reference		Reference		Reference		Reference	
Maintained													
N	80 (23.0)	37	26	35	13	75	5	44	36	76	4	22	53
OR 95% CI		0.8 (0.4 to 1.7)		0.7 (0.3 to 1.5)		0.8 (0.2 to 2.6)		1.0 (0.5 to 1.7)		1.1 (0.3 to 4.7)		1.4 (0.7 to 2.6)	
Improved													
N	177 (50.9)	49	80	47	74	148	29	46	131	169	8	67	103

Table 2 (continued)

All participants n (%)	BPH-related factors								ED-related factors			
	Prostate size		IPSS score		BPH medication use at baseline		BPH composite measure		ED medication use at baseline		ED medication or device use at follow-up	
	< 40 g	≥ 40 g	< 8	≥ 8	No	Yes	No BPH	Any BPH	No	Yes	No	Yes
OR 95% CI	1.9 (1.1 to 3.5)		2.8 (1.5 to 5.5)		2.4 (1.0 to 5.6)		3.3 (2.0 to 5.7)		1.0 (0.3 to 3.5)		0.9 (0.5 to 1.5)	

BPH benign prostatic hyperplasia, *CI* confidence interval, *ED* erectile dysfunction, *IPSS* International Prostate Symptom Score, *OR* odds ratio, *NE* not estimable

EPIC-50 measured urinary and sexual outcome trajectories were defined as impaired (negative change greater than the upper bound of minimally important difference), maintained, and improved (positive change greater than the upper bound of minimally important difference). Urinary function, incontinence-related bother: impaired (change < 9); maintained (− 9 ≤ change ≤ 9); improved (change ≥ 9). Voiding dysfunction-related bother: impaired (change < 7); maintained (− 7 ≤ change ≤ 7); improved (change ≥ 7)

Table 3 Factors associated with sexual outcome trajectories assessed by the expanded prostate cancer index composite (EPIC)-50 among men in the prostatectomy, incontinence and erectile dysfunction (PIE) study

	All participants n (%)	BPH-related factors								ED -elated factors			
		Prostate size		IPSS score		BPH medication use at baseline		BPH composite measure		ED medication use at baseline ED medication use at baseline		ED medication or device use at follow-up	
		<40 g	≥40 g	<8	≥8	No	Yes	No BPH	Any BPH	No	Yes	No	Yes
Sexual function 5 weeks post-surgery (n=357)													
Impaired													
N	262 (79.0)												
OR 95% CI													
Maintained													
N	69 (19.3)												
OR 95% CI													
Improved													
N	6 (1.7)												
OR 95% CI													
Sexual function 12 months post-surgery (n=332)													
Impaired													
N	229 (69.0)	76	96	73	73	205	24	91	138	217	12	70	154
OR 95% CI		Reference		Reference		Reference		Reference		Reference		Reference	
Maintained													
N	92 (27.7)	39	28	35	28	80	12	40	52	88	4	40	48
OR 95% CI		0.6 (0.3 to 1.0)		0.8 (0.4 to 1.4)		1.3 (0.6 to 2.7)		0.8 (0.5 to 1.4)		0.8 (0.3 to 2.6)		0.5 (0.3 to 0.9)	
Improved													
N	11 (3.3)	3	6	4	4	8	3	2	9	11	0	2	5
OR 95% CI		1.6 (0.4 to 6.5)		1.0 (0.2 to 4.2)		3.2 (0.8 to 13)		3.0 (0.6 to 14)		NE		1.1 (0.2 to 6.0)	
Sexual bother 5 weeks post-surgery (n=354)													
Impaired													
N	259 (73.2)	94	96	86	77	232	27	110	149	243	16	117	131
OR 95% CI		Reference		Reference		Reference		Reference		Reference		Reference	
Maintained													
N	69 (19.5)	27	27	27	22	61	8	30	39	69	0	36	24
OR 95% CI		1.0 (0.5 to 1.8)		0.9 (0.5 to 1.7)		1.1 (0.5 to 2.6)		1.0 (0.6 to 1.6)		NE		0.6 (0.3 to 1.1)	
Improved													
N	26 (7.3)	6	11	8	11	16	10	3	23	24	2	16	10
OR 95% CI		1.8 (0.6 to 5.1)		1.5 (0.6 to 4.0)		5.4 (2.2 to 13.0)		5.7 (1.7 to 19.3)		1.3 (0.3 to 5.8)		0.6 (0.2 to 1.3)	

Table 3 (continued)

	All participants n (%)	BPH-related factors								ED -elated factors			
		Prostate size		IPSS score		BPH medication use at baseline		BPH composite measure		ED medication use at baseline ED medication use at baseline		ED medication or device use at follow-up	
		< 40 g	≥ 40 g	< 8	≥ 8	No	Yes	No BPH	Any BPH	No	Yes	No	Yes
Sexual bother 12 months post-surgery (n = 329)													
Impaired													
N	229 (69.6)	78	89	81	67	206	23	98	131	216	13	68	157
OR 95% CI		Reference		Reference		Reference		Reference		Reference		Reference	
Maintained													
N	65 (19.8)	28	23	22	19	56	9	28	37	62	3	27	34
OR 95% CI		0.7 (0.4 to 1.4)		1.0 (0.5 to 2.1)		1.4 (0.6 to 3.3)		1.0 (0.6 to 1.7)		0.8 (0.2 to 2.9)		0.5 (0.3 to 1.0)	
Improved													
N	35 (10.6)	8	19	11	15	30	5	7	28	35	0	13	16
OR 95% CI		2.1 (0.9 to 5.0)		1.6 (0.7 to 3.8)		1.5 (0.5 to 4.2)		3.0 (1.2 to 7.1)		NE		0.5 (0.2 to 1.2)	

BPH benign prostatic hyperplasia, *CI* confidence interval, *ED* erectile dysfunction, *IPSS* International Prostate Symptom Score, *OR* odds ratio, *NE* not estimable

EPIC-50 measured urinary and sexual outcome trajectories were defined as impaired (negative change greater than the upper bound of minimally important difference), maintained, and improved (positive change greater than the upper bound of minimally important difference). Sexual function, sexual bother: impaired (change < 12); maintained (-12 ≤ change ≤ 12); improved (change ≥ 12)

urinary incontinence owing to chronic subclinical urinary retention, which may also be relieved by RP.

An additional unexpected observation was our finding that a small proportion of men who underwent RP experienced improvements beyond baseline in sexual outcomes, particularly long-term sexual bother, independent of ED therapy. Although resolution of neuropraxia might explain recovery in these outcomes to baseline levels, we believe it is unlikely to explain improvements beyond baseline. Another possible explanation is improved communication surrounding sexual function. Prostate cancer treatment and its known sexual side effects may be a launching point for men to have an open conversation with their providers and partners about their sexual function. Previous studies have demonstrated that spousal communication is a key factor in healthy sexual function recovery after prostate cancer treatment [26]. For many men, prostate cancer treatment discussions may prompt discussions regarding sexual function that have not been addressed in the past. The mechanisms through which open communication may improve post-RP sexual outcomes might be similar to those in studies of premenopausal women with dyspareunia, which found that open communication between partners was critical for improving sexual function and distress [27].

Another possible explanation for improvement in sexual bother could be relief of sexual bother related to voiding dysfunction post-RP. This hypothesis is supported by growing evidence that BPH and ED may be caused by common biologic mechanisms [28]. As such, improvements in BPH-related symptoms from RP may also result in improvements in sexual outcomes. Alternatively, certain BPH-related medications are known to be associated with decreased sexual function [29]. Therefore, discontinuation of these drugs may contribute to improvement following RP, as was observed for men taking α-blockers pre-RP in our sample. In support of both of these mechanisms, our data demonstrated a higher odds of improved sexual bother associated with the BPH composite index. Finally, it is also possible that RP may relieve sexual pain in men with pre-surgical chronic prostatitis/chronic pelvic pain syndrome, thereby contributing to improvements in sexual bother. Although each of these explanations is speculative, we believe they warrant further study for their possible, eventual guidance for prostate cancer therapeutic decision-making and overall patient counseling.

Strengths of this study include its prospective design, large sample size, frequent follow-up of participants over the one-year study period, and use of validated outcome measures designed specifically for prostate cancer survivors. Additionally, use of the EPIC-50 rather than the shorter EPIC-26 allowed us to gain a more comprehensive understanding of both urinary and sexual function and bother; and our unique statistical analysis allowed us to explore the full range of outcome trajectories rather than just mean outcome levels. However, it is also important to note the limitations of this analysis. Specifically, information on co-existing urological conditions was not collected systematically on all participants, but was only available from participants ' medical records, which may not have had complete information on these conditions. Additionally, data were not collected between 5 weeks and 6 months (e.g., 3 months) to allow us to identify when some outcomes returned to baseline levels.

Conclusions

We observed improvements in urinary and sexual outcomes among non-trivial proportions of men who underwent RP. Although reasons for improvement in urinary function (continence) and sexual bother are unclear, improvement in voiding dysfunction-related bother likely relates to relief of BPH symptoms by RP, as prostatectomy is a known, effective therapy for severe BPH. Therefore, our findings provide additional support for considering baseline BPH symptoms when selecting the best therapy for early-stage prostate cancer.

Supplementary Information

Additional file 1: Supplementary Table 1. Association between Baseline BPH Medication Use with Urinary Outcome Trajectories Assessed by the Expanded Prostate Cancer Index Composite (EPIC)-50 among Men in the Prostatectomy, Incontinence and Erectile Dysfunction (PIE) Study. **Supplementary Table 2**. Association between Baseline BPH Medication Use with Sexual Outcome Trajectories Assessed by the Expanded Prostate Cancer Index Composite (EPIC)-50 among Men in the Prostatectomy, Incontinence and Erectile Dysfunction (PIE) Study.

Acknowledgements

We acknowledge all the participants in this study. A part of the analyses was previously presented at the CanPROS Scientific Conference 2019 and published as an abstract on Current Oncology 2020, 27(1),64–71.

Authors' contributions

All authors contributed to the study conception and design. Material preparation, data collection and analysis were performed by LY, JAL, EH, CP, GAC, RP, KRI, EHK, RLG III, KYW, ASK and SS. The first draft of the manuscript was written by LY and all authors commented on subsequent versions of the manuscript. All authors read and approved the final manuscript.

Author details

[1]Department of Cancer Epidemiology and Prevention Research, Cancer Research and Analytics, Cancer Care Alberta, Alberta Health Services, 5th Floor, Holy Cross Centre, Box ACB, 2210 - 2 St. SW, Calgary, AB T2S 3C3, Canada. [2]Departments of Oncology and Community Health Sciences, University of Calgary, Calgary, Canada. [3]Division of Public Health Sciences, Department of Surgery, Washington University School of Medicine, 600 S. Taylor Ave., 2nd floor, Rm. 208S, Campus Box 8100, St. Louis, MO 63110, USA. [4]Agricultural Statistics Laboratory, University of Arkansas, Fayetteville, USA. [5]Department of Epidemiology, Harvard T.H. Chan School of Public Health, Boston, MA, USA.

[6]Division of Urological Surgery, Department of Surgery, Washington University School of Medicine, St Louis, USA. [7]Department of Urology, Medical University of South Carolina, Charleston, USA. [8]Coeus Health, Chicago, IL, USA. [9]Division of Urology, Department of Surgery, Brigham and Women's Hospital, Boston, USA. [10]Division of Health Behavior Research, Department of Preventive Medicine, Keck School of Medicine of theUniversity of Southern California, 2001 N Soto St., Los Angeles, CA 90032, USA.

References

1. Lin GA, Aaronson DS, Knight SJ, Carroll PR, Dudley RA. Patient decision aids for prostate cancer treatment: a systematic review of the literature. CA Cancer J Clin. 2009;59(6):379–90.
2. Barry MJ. Quality of life and prostate cancer treatment. J Urol. 1999;162(2):407.
3. Sanda MG, Dunn RL, Michalski J, Sandler HM, Northouse L, Hembroff L, Lin X, Greenfield TK, Litwin MS, Saigal CS, et al. Quality of life and satisfaction with outcome among prostate-cancer survivors. N Engl J Med. 2008;358(12):1250–61.
4. McNutt RA. Shared medical decision making: problems, process, progress. JAMA. 2004;292(20):2516–8.
5. Ferrer M, Suarez JF, Guedea F, Fernandez P, Macias V, Marino A, Hervas A, Herruzo I, Ortiz MJ, Villavicencio H, et al. Health-related quality of life 2 years after treatment with radical prostatectomy, prostate brachytherapy, or external beam radiotherapy in patients with clinically localized prostate cancer. Int J Radiat Oncol Biol Phys. 2008;72(2):421–32.
6. Tseng TY, Kuebler HR, Cancel QV, Sun L, Springhart WP, Murphy BC, Albala DM, Dahm P. Prospective health-related quality-of-life assessment in an initial cohort of patients undergoing robotic radical prostatectomy. Urology. 2006;68(5):1061–6.
7. Muramaki M, Miyake H, Behnsawy HM, Furukawa J, Harada K, Fujisawa M. Assessment of postoperative quality of life: comparative study between laparoscopic and minimum incision endoscopic radical prostatectomies. Int J Clin Oncol. 2014;19(6):1092–7.
8. Willis DL, Gonzalgo ML, Brotzman M, Feng Z, Trock B, Su LM. Comparison of outcomes between pure laparoscopic vs robot-assisted laparoscopic radical prostatectomy: a study of comparative effectiveness based upon validated quality of life outcomes. BJU Int. 2012;109(6):898–905.
9. Parker WR, Wang R, He C, Wood DP Jr. Five year expanded prostate cancer index composite-based quality of life outcomes after prostatectomy for localized prostate cancer. BJU Int. 2011;107(4):585–90.
10. Miyake H, Miyazaki A, Furukawa J, Hinata N, Fujisawa M. Prospective assessment of time-dependent changes in quality of life of Japanese patients with prostate cancer following robot-assisted radical prostatectomy. J Robot Surg. 2016;10(3):201–7.
11. Pardo Y, Guedea F, Aguilo F, Fernandez P, Macias V, Marino A, Hervas A, Herruzo I, Ortiz MJ, Ponce de Leon J et al. Quality-of-life impact of primary treatments for localized prostate cancer in patients without hormonal treatment. J Clin Oncol. 2010; 28(31):4687–4696.
12. Jeldres C, Cullen J, Hurwitz LM, Wolff EM, Levie KE, Odem-Davis K, Johnston RB, Pham KN, Rosner IL, Brand TC, et al. Prospective quality-of-life outcomes for low-risk prostate cancer: active surveillance versus radical prostatectomy. Cancer. 2015;121(14):2465–73.
13. Chang P, Regan MM, Ferrer M, Guedea F, Patil D, Wei JT, Hembroff LA, Michalski JM, Saigal CS, Litwin MS et al. Relief of urinary symptom burden after primary prostate cancer treatment. J Urol 2016.
14. Sanda MG, Cadeddu JA, Kirkby E, Chen RC, Crispino T, Fontanarosa J, Freedland SJ, Greene K, Klotz LH, Makarov DV, et al. Clinically Localized Prostate Cancer: AUA/ASTRO/SUO Guideline. Part I: risk stratification, shared decision making, and care options. J Urol. 2018;199(3):683–90.
15. Wei JT, Dunn RL, Litwin MS, Sandler HM, Sanda MG. Development and validation of the expanded prostate cancer index composite (EPIC) for comprehensive assessment of health-related quality of life in men with prostate cancer. Urology. 2000;56(6):899–905.
16. Yang L, Kibel AS, Colditz GA, Pakpahan R, Imm KR, Izadi S, Grubb RL 3rd, Wolin KY, Sutcliffe S. Caution with use of the expanded prostate cancer index composite-50 urinary bother scale: how voiding dysfunction modifies its performance. J Urol. 2017;198(6):1397–403.
17. Skolarus TA, Dunn RL, Sanda MG, Chang P, Greenfield TK, Litwin MS, Wei JT. Minimally important difference for the Expanded Prostate Cancer Index Composite Short Form. Urology. 2015;85(1):101–5.
18. Yang L, Lee J, Kibel AS, Pernar C, Colditz GA, Pakpahan R, Imm KR, Izadi S, Grubb RL III, Wolin KY, et al. One-year urinary and sexual outcome trajectories in prostate cancer patients treated by radical prostatectomy: a prospective study. Curr Oncol. 2020;27(1):e71.
19. Romero FR, Romero AW, Filho TB, Kulysz D, Oliveira FC, Filho RT. The prostate exam. Health Educ J. 2011;71(2):239–50.
20. Barry MJ, Fowler FJ Jr, O'Leary MP, Bruskewitz RC, Holtgrewe HL, Mebust WK, Cockett AT. The American Urological Association symptom index for benign prostatic hyperplasia. The Measurement Committee of the American Urological Association. J Urol. 1992;148(5):1549–64.
21. Punnen S, Cowan JE, Chan JM, Carroll PR, Cooperberg MR. Long-term health-related quality of life after primary treatment for localized prostate cancer: results from the CaPSURE registry. Eur Urol. 2015;68(4):600–8.
22. Levinson AW, Bagga HS, Pavlovich CP, Mettee LZ, Ward NT, Link RE, Su LM. The impact of prostate size on urinary quality of life indexes following laparoscopic radical prostatectomy. J Urol. 2008;179(5):1818–22.
23. Buttyan R, Chen MW, Levin RM. Animal models of bladder outlet obstruction and molecular insights into the basis for the development of bladder dysfunction. Eur Urol. 1997;32(Suppl 1):32–9.
24. Levin RM, Haugaard N, O'Connor L, Buttyan R, Das A, Dixon JS, Gosling JA. Obstructive response of human bladder to BPH vs. rabbit bladder response to partial outlet obstruction: a direct comparison. Neurourol Urodyn. 2000;19(5):609–29.
25. Fusco F, Creta M, De Nunzio C, Iacovelli V, Mangiapia F, Li Marzi V, Finazzi Agro E. Progressive bladder remodeling due to bladder outlet obstruction: a systematic review of morphological and molecular evidences in humans. BMC Urol. 2018;18(1):15.
26. Badr H, Taylor CL. Sexual dysfunction and spousal communication in couples coping with prostate cancer. Psychooncology. 2009;18(7):735–46.
27. Pazmany E, Bergeron S, Verhaeghe J, Van Oudenhove L, Enzlin P. Dyadic sexual communication in pre-menopausal women with self-reported dyspareunia and their partners: associations with sexual function, sexual distress and dyadic adjustment. J Sex Med. 2015;12(2):516–28.
28. Zhao C, Kwan Park J. Phosphodiesterase type 5 inhibitor and erectile dysfunction in lower urinary tract symptoms. Lower Urinary Tract Symptoms. 2012;4(Suppl 1):75–80.
29. Mirone V, Sessa A, Giuliano F, Berges R, Kirby M, Moncada I. Current benign prostatic hyperplasia treatment: impact on sexual function and management of related sexual adverse events. Int J Clin Pract. 2011;65(9):1005–13.

8

The role of mpMRI in qualification of patients with ISUP 1 prostate cancer on biopsy to radical prostatectomy

Łukasz Nyk[1], Omar Tayara[1], Tomasz Ząbkowski[2*], Piotr Kryst[1], Aneta Andrychowicz[3] and Wojciech Malewski[1]

Abstract

Background: To investigate the role of mpMRI and high PIRADS score as independent triggers in the qualification of patients with ISUP 1 prostate cancer on biopsy to radical prostatectomy.

Methods: Between January 2017 and June 2019, 494 laparoscopic radical prostatectomies were performed in our institution, including 203 patients (41.1%) with ISUP 1 cT1c-2c PCa on biopsy. Data regarding biopsy results, digital rectal examination, PSA, mpMRI and postoperative pathological report have been retrospectively analysed.

Results: In 183 cases (90.1%) mpMRI has been performed at least 6 weeks after biopsy. Final pathology revealed ISUP Gleason Grade Group upgrade in 62.6% of cases. PIRADS 5, PIRADS 4 and PIRADS 3 were associated with Gleason Grade Group upgrade in 70.5%, 62.8%, 48.3% of patients on final pathology, respectively. Within PIRADS 5 group, the number of upgraded cases was statistically significant.

Conclusions: PIRADS score correlates with an upgrade on final pathology and may justify shared decision of radical treatment in patients unwilling to repeated biopsies. However, the use of PIRADS 5 score as a sole indicator for prostatectomy may result in nonnegligible overtreatment rate.

Keywords: Active surveillance, Gleason upgrading, Prostate cancer, MpMRI of prostate, PIRADS score

Background

Prostate cancer is diagnosed in 1.1 million men annually [1]. The introduction of prostate specific antigen (PSA) screening attributes to common low risk disease diagnoses [2]. The indolent nature of the majority of cases encourages preservative management of this type of malignancy. Active surveillance (AS) is a recommended approach in low risk prostate cancer and selected cases of intermediate disease [3]. It aims to avoid serious complications of radical treatments such as incontinence or erectile dysfunction. AS studies report high cancer specific survival rates of up to 99% at 15 years [4]. Despite promising outcomes, this management method still raises doubts as to proper selection criteria. There are several AS protocols recommending specific measures to include patients' safely. Most of them are based on PSA and biopsy results as well as digital rectal examination (DRE). In recent years, intriguing diagnostic tool—multiparametric resonance imaging (mpMRI) of the prostate has been developed. The sensitivity in detecting clinically significant cancer regarding the Gleason grade group is 95% [5]. Nevertheless, mpMRI is not recommended in any protocol as selection criterion of AS. Several studies proved that among patients eligible for AS, upstaging and upgrading in postoperative pathology report accounts for up to 47.3% and 59.7% of cases, respectively [6]. The EAU Guidelines recommend mpMRI performance before the confirmatory biopsy within AS management,

*Correspondence: urodent@wp.pl
[2] Department of Urology, Military Institute of Medicine, Warsaw, Poland
Full list of author information is available at the end of the article

which should be repeated at least every 2–3 years [7]. However, multiple repeated biopsies are associated with an increase of inflammation within the prostate and may influence the course of potential prostatectomy procedure and its functional results [8, 9]. Moreover, prostate biopsy itself is not devoid of acute and chronic complications, some of which require hospitalization. Chronic consequences of prostate biopsy may involve even erectile dysfunction [10]. Given the efficacy of mpMRI in detecting clinically significant prostate cancer and disadvantages of repeated prostate biopsies, we hypothesized that some patients with ISUP Gleason Grade Group 1 (GS6) on biopsy and high prostate imaging and report and data system (PIRADS)score on confirmatory biopsy may be skipped and radical treatment can be offered.

This study aimed to investigate the role of mpMRI and high PIRADS score as independent triggers in the qualification of patients with ISUP 1 prostate cancer on biopsy to radical prostatectomy.

Methods

Between January 2017 and June 2019, 494 laparoscopic radical prostatectomies with or without extended lymph node dissection were performed in our institution. Data regarding biopsy results, DRE, PSA, mpMRI, and postoperative pathological report have been prospectively summarized. We identified 203 patients with ISUP Gleason Grade Group 1(ISUP 1) on biopsy. Based on DRE and PSA level, included patients were subdivided into risk groups: low risk group (PSA < 10 ng/mL and cT < 1–2a), intermediate risk group (PSA 10–20 ng/mL or cT2b), and high risk group (PSA > 20 or cT2c) [11]. In 183 cases, mpMRI has been performed at least 6 weeks after biopsy. Every mpMRI have been assessed during qualification appointment and clinical rounds. The assessment was based on MR prostate imaging reporting and data system version 2.0, and proper PIRADS grades from 2 to 5 were ascribed to visible lesions. Within this group, no cases were suspected of extraprostatic extension (EPE) based on DRE. All patients who underwent laparoscopic radical prostatectomies due to ISUP 1 prostate cancer had thorough preoperative discussion about possible risk of overtreatment, complications, and other management options including AS.

All patients signed the informed consent that their medical data might be used in the future as part of retrospective study. The analyzed datasets were anonymised before we used it for the purpose of current study. According to the Act of 6 September 2001 Pharmaceutical Law the study was qualified as noninterventional observation study. Thus, this study did not require approval by Ethics Committee and registration in Central Register of Clinical Studies.

Statistical analysis

Statistical analyses were performed using IBM SPSS Statistics 26.

The χ^2 was used for the categorical and nonparametric continuous variable comparison to check a statistical significance. There were three significance levels determined namely: $p < 0.001$ (***), $p < 0.01$ (**), and $p < 0.05$ (*). This test was applied in the UPGRADE and GLS LPR comparison and showed a statistical significance. Furthermore, a correlation between GLS LPR and MRI PIRADS was analyzed and showed a correlation close to the statistical significance.

The Kruskal–Wallis test was used for the ordinal and measurement variable comparison to check for a statistical significance. There were three significance levels determined as $p < 0.001$ (***), $p < 0.01$ (**), and $p < 0.05$ (*). This test compared a correlation between PSA and GLS LPR as well as PSA and MRI PIRADS and showed statistically significant differences between PSA and GLS LPR variables; however, no statistical significance within PSA and MRI PIRADS variables.

In addition, the Mann-Whitney U test was used for the MRI PIRADS and GLS LPR variable comparison. This test showed a statistical significance between the two groups. Categorical variables were listed using the number, and percentage values; however, nonparametric continuous variables were defined using the median, minimum, and maximum values. The odds ratio (OR) with 95% confidence interval (CI) were reported for each factor.

Results

The analysis involved 183 patients with ISUP 1 on prostate biopsy with preoperative mpMRI. Median PSA was 9.4 ng/mL with a density of 0.20. According to DRE, there was no EPE suspicion in any case. MpMRI of the prostate indicated EPE suspicion in 5.6% of patients. Final pathological report revealed EPE in 13% of cases. According to EAU risk group classification, 88.7% of patients presented low and intermediate risk disease. According to PIRADS classification, PIRADS 5, 4, 3, and 2 lesions occurred in 32.8%, 47%, 16.4%, and 3.8%, respectively (Table 1). Distribution of variables: clinical stage according to DRE and mpMRI as well as corresponding pathological stage are presented in Table 1. Final pathology revealed ISUP Gleason Grade Group upgrade in 62.6% of cases.

ISUP Gleason Grade Group upgrade occurred in 126 of 203 patients (62.1%).

In the low risk group, there was no statistically significant difference in number of upgraded and non-upgraded cases on final pathological result ($p < 0.098$). The intermediate risk group entailed upgrade in 66.7% of cases.

Table 1 Characteristics of the study group

	Number of patients	% of patients
Clinical stage based on DRE		
cT1	40	19.7
cT2a	40	19.7
cT2b	119	58.6
cT2c	4	2
Clinical stage based on MRI		
iT0	7	3.4
iT2a	35	17.2
iT2b	40	19.7
iT2c	86	42.4
iT3a	10	4.9
iT3b	5	2.5
Missing	20	9.9
PIRADS category in MRI		
PIRADS 3	29	15,8
PIRADS 4	86	47
PIRADS 5	61	33,3
BCR risk according to EAU criteria		
Low	29	14.3
Intermediate	151	74.4
High	23	11.3

BCR biochemical recurrence, *DRE* digital rectal examination, *MRI* magnetic resonance imaging

Moreover, there was statistically significant linear correlation between the PSA result and upgrade on final pathological result (Fig. 1).

PIRADS 5, PIRADS 4 and PIRADS 3 were associated with Gleason Grade Group upgrade in 70.5%, 62.8%, 48.3% of patients on final pathology, respectively. Only within PIRADS 5 group, the difference between the number of upgraded and non-upgraded cases was statistically significant ($p < 0.016$) (Table 2, Fig. 2).

Discussion

Management of low risk prostate cancer remains a controversial issue. Concerns about complications of the radical treatment encourage implementation of the conservative approach. Low risk prostate cancer is invariably associated with pathological diagnosis of ISUP Gleason Grade Group 1 (Gleason 6[3+3]) (ISUP 1) on prostate biopsy [12]. ISUP 1 prostate cancer lacks metastatic potential. There was no single lymph node metastasis among more than 14,000 prostate and lymph node specimens after radical treatment with ISUP 1 analyzed by Ross et al. However, cases with even a single microfocus of ISUP 1defined as 5% or less in one biopsy core might be upgraded and have adverse pathological features in up to 22% of patients [13]. Moreover, the large analysis of Surveillance, Epidemiology, and End Results database revealed that 44% of low risk prostate cancer defined as cT1c/2a, ISUP 1, and PSA below 10 ng/mL was upgraded

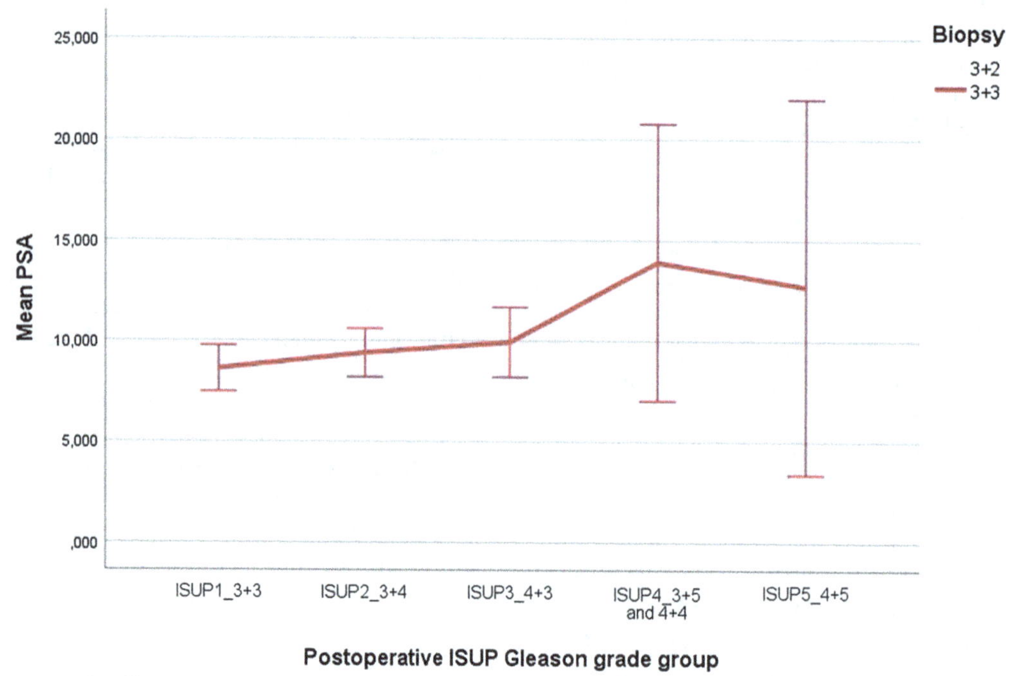

Fig. 1 Postoperative ISUP Gleason grade group with regard to mean PSA

Table 2 Comparison of upgraded or nonupgraded cases within different PIRADS score groups

	Upgrade	Non-upgrade	Total n(%)	*p* value
ISUP1 + PIRADS5	43 (70.5%)	18 (29.5%)	61 (100%)	0.016
ISUP1 + PIRADS4	54 (62.7%)	32 (37%)	86 (100%)	0.062
ISUP1 + PIRADS3	12 (44%)	15 (55%)	27 (100%)	0.086

at final pathological report [14]. Consequently, ISUP Gleason Grade Group 1 detection may indicate disease of metastatic potential in almost half of cases. Nevertheless, current guidelines recommend AS in any case of low risk prostate cancer and selected cases of intermediate risk disease. MpMRI of the prostate emerges as new diagnostic tool that is suggested to be used even before prostate biopsy. It is strongly recommended before second biopsy in case of persistent prostate cancer suspicion and before confirmatory biopsy within the AS protocol [15]. Standardization of mpMRI interpretation was first proposed within the PIRADS in 2012 [16, 17]. This protocol was improved in PIRADS version 2.0, where prostate lesions were scored from 1 to 5, and scores 4 and 5 indicate likely and very likely presence of significant cancer, respectively [18].

In our study, patients with ISUP 1 PCA on prostate biopsy who underwent preoperative mpMRI and subsequent laparoscopic radical prostatectomies were retrospectively analyzed. We assessed the correlation between mpMRI and final pathological results. To the best of our knowledge, upgrade is analyzed for the first time in terms of final pathological result after radical prostatectomy. The detection rate of clinically significant PCA is high and reaches up to 77% and 83% in case of PIRADS 5 score [19, 20].

Therefore, we hypothesized, that patients diagnosed with ISUP 1 prostate cancer and high PIRADS score confirmatory biopsy may be spared due to substantial probability of at least ISUP 2 prostate cancer in the final specimen.

Most modern studies evaluate the safety of avoidance of biopsy in case of negative mpMRI. They compare the mpMRI result with the biopsy specimen and indicate that the use of mpMRI may significantly decrease unnecessary biopsies [21]. Interestingly, in comparison to systematic biopsy, mpMRI fusion confirmatory biopsy resulted in nonsignificant upgrade rates [22].

On the other hand, Verep et al. looked for upgrading predictors by means of comparing the biopsy result and the final specimen. In this study, upgrade occurred in approximately half of all cases. PSA and PSA density were found to be the strongest upgrade predictors. However, no data on the correlation of upgrade with mpMRI score has been included [23].

MpMRI PIRADS 4 and 5 in the study presented by Propilia et al. were associated with the upgrade of ISUP

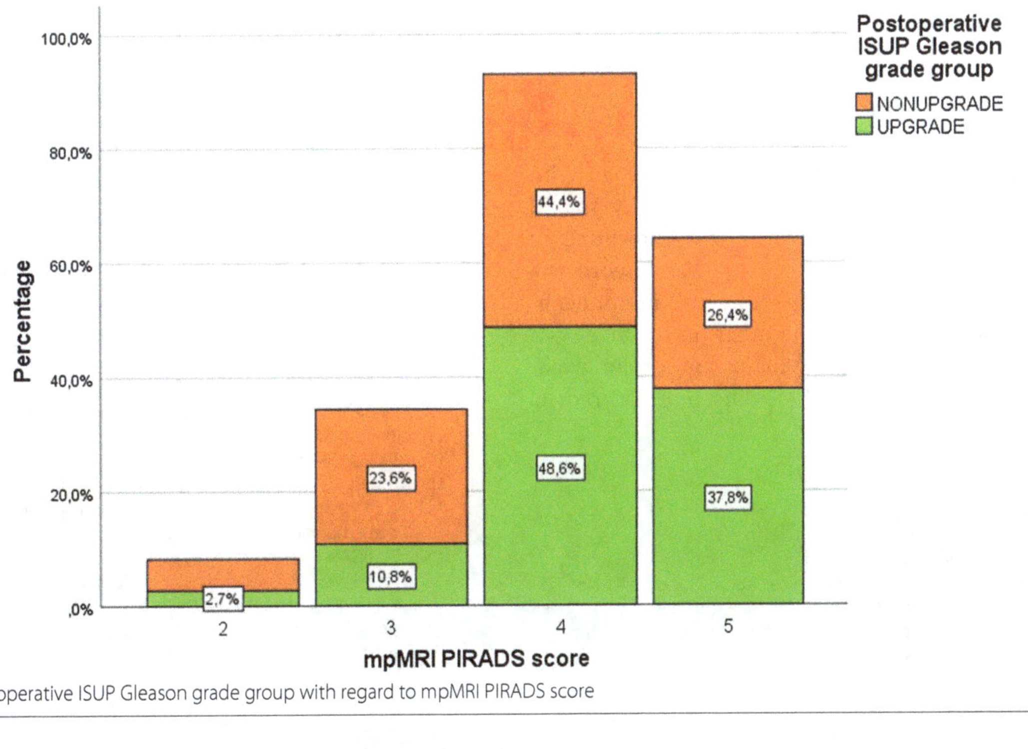

Fig. 2 Postoperative ISUP Gleason grade group with regard to mpMRI PIRADS score

score in 65% of patients who fulfil Epstein criteria of AS (clinical stage T1c, PSA level ≤ 10 ng/mL, GS ≤ 6, PSA-D ≤ 0.15 ng/mL, one or two positive biopsy cores and percentage of core involvement ≤ 50% [24].

In our study, pathological upgrade occurred in 70.5% of patients with biopsy ISUP 1 and PIRADS 5. Similar upgrade occurred within EAU intermediate risk patients. As the risk group stratification was based on DRE and PSA results, these factors in combination with PIRADS score may predict upgrade. Currently, most often deferred treatment is excluded in patients with cT2b < / = disease and PSA above 10 ng/mL [25, 26]. Furthermore, PIRADS 5 and 4scores should be considered in deciding of radical treatment in patients with ISUP Gleason Grade Group 1.

Limitations

We acknowledge several weak points of our study. First of all, its retrospective nature results in selection bias. Clinical stage was assessed by several physicians qualifying the patients for surgery. Therefore, these data may be subjective and heterogeneous. Prostate biopsies were performed in different institutions consequently biopsy protocols and pathological assessment are not uniform. In this group mpMRI has been performed after biopsy. It has been confirmed that use of fusion biopsy decrease the pathological upgrade on final specimen [27]. However, most patients included in our study have been treated in times when recommendation of performing mpMRI before biopsy was not strong according to EAU guidelines.

Conclusions

This study evaluates the correlation between mpMRI, PIRADS score, and ISUP 1 PCA upgrade to significant prostate cancer on final pathology. It correlates with an upgrade on final pathology and may justify shared decision of radical treatment in patients unwilling to repeated biopsies. However, use of PIRADS 5 score as a sole indicator for prostatectomy may result in nonnegligible overtreatment rate. On the other hand, PIRADS 3 and 4 scores should be definite indication for confirmatory biopsy in the course of qualification for radical prostatectomy.

Abbreviations

PSA: Prostate specific antigen; AS: Active surveillance; DRE: Digital rectal examination; mpMRI: Multiparametric resonance imaging; PIRADS: Prostate imaging and report and data system; ISUP: International Society of Urological Pathology; EPE: Extraprostatic extension; GL: Gleason score; LPR: Laparoscopic Prostatectomy; OR: Odds ratio; CI: Confidence interval; PCA: Prostate cancer.

Acknowledgements

Not applicable.

Authors' contributions

LN collected the data, analyzed the data and prepared the manuscript. OT collected the data. TZ analyzed the data and prepared a manuscript. PK analyzed the data and prepared a manuscript. AA prepared a statistical analysis and tables and figures. WM collected the data, analyzed the data and prepared a manuscript. All authors have read and approved the final manuscript.

Author details

[1]Second Department of Urology, Centre of Postgraduate Medical Education, Warsaw, Poland. [2]Department of Urology, Military Institute of Medicine, Warsaw, Poland. [3]Urological Clinic, Warsaw, Poland.

References

1. World Health Organization International Agency for Research on Cancer (IARC). GLOBOCAN 2012: estimated cancer incidence, mortality and prevalence worldwide in 2012. Homepage on the internet; 2012 [cited 2016 Apr 23]. http://globocan.iarc.fr/Pages/fact_sheets_cancer.aspx.
2. Cooperberg MR, Ramakrishna NR, Duff SB, Hughes KE, Sadownik S, Smith JA, et al. Primary treatments for clinically localised prostate cancer: a comprehensive lifetime cost-utility analysis. BJU Int. 2013;111(3):437–50.
3. EAU Guidelines. Edn. Presented at the EAU Annual Congress Amsterdam, 2020. ISBN 978-94-92671-07-3.
4. Klotz L, Vesprini D, Sethukavalan P, Jethava V, Zhang L, Jain S, et al. Long-term follow-up of a large active surveillance cohort of patients with prostate cancer. J Clin Oncol. 2015;33:272–7.
5. Drost FH, Osses DF, Nieboer D, Steyerberg EW, Bangma CH, Roobol MJ, et al. Prostate MRI, with or without MRI-targeted biopsy, and systematic biopsy for detecting prostate cancer. Cochrane Database Syst Rev. 2019;4(4):CD012663.
6. Grasso AA, Cozzi G, Lorenzis DE, Ceruti C, Crivellaro S, Falsaperla M, et al. Multicenter analysis of pathological outcomes of patients eligible for active surveillance according to PRIAS criteria. Minerva Urol Nefrol. 2016;68:237–41.
7. Walton Diaz A, Shakir NA, George AK, Rais-Bahrami S, Turkbey B, Rothwax JT, et al. Use of serial multiparametric magnetic resonance imaging in the management of patients with prostate cancer on active surveillance. Urol Oncol. 2015;33(5):202.e1-202.e7.
8. Olvera-Posada D, Welk B, McClure JA, Winick-Ng J, Izawa JI, Pautler SE. The impact of multiple prostate biopsies on risk for major complications following radical prostatectomy: a population-based cohort study. Urology. 2017;106:125–32.
9. Sooriakumaran P, Calaway A, Sagalovich D, Roy S, Srivastava A, Joneja J, et al. The impact of multiple biopsies on outcomes of nerve-sparing robotic-assisted radical prostatectomy. Int J Impot Res. 2012;24:161–4.
10. Murray KS, Bailey J, Zuk K, Lopez-Corona E, Thrasher JB. A prospective study of erectile function after transrectal ultrasonography-guided prostate biopsy. BJU Int. 2015;116:190–5.
11. Cooperberg MR, Pasta DJ, Elkin EP, Litwin MS, Latini DM, Du Chane J, et al. The University of California, San Francisco Cancer of the Prostate Risk Assessment score: a straightforward and reliable preoperative predictor of disease recurrence after radical prostatectomy. J Urol. 2005;173(6):1938–42.
12. Epstein JI, Zelefsky MJ, Sjoberg DD, Nelson JB, Egevad L, Magi-Galluzzi C, et al. A contemporary prostate cancer grading system: a validated alternative to the Gleason score. Eur Urol. 2016;69(3):428–35.
13. Thong AE, Shikanov S, Katz MH, Gofrit ON, Eggener S, Zagaja GP, et al. A single microfocus (5% or less) of Gleason 6 prostate cancer at biopsy—can we predict adverse pathological outcomes? J Urol. 2008;180(6):2436–40.
14. Dinh KT, Mahal BA, Ziehr DR, Muralidhar V, Chen YW, Viswanathan VB, et al. Incidence and predictors of upgrading and up staging among 10,000 contemporary patients with low risk prostate cancer. J Urol. 2015;194(2):343–9.
15. Kaye DR, Qi J, Morgan TM, Linsell S, Lane BR, Montie JE, et al. Michigan urological surgery improvement collaborative. Association between early confirmatory testing and the adoption of active surveillance for men with favorable-risk prostate cancer. Urology. 2018;118:127–33.

16. Barentsz JO, Richenberg J, Clements R, Choyke P, Verma S, Villeirs G, et al. ESUR prostate MR guidelines 2012. Eur Radiol. 2012;22(4):746–57.
17. Barentsz JO, Weinreb JC, Verma S, Thoeny HC, Tempany CM, Shtern F, et al. Synopsis of the PI-RADS v2 guidelines for multiparametric prostate magnetic resonance imaging and recommendations for use. Eur Urol. 2016;69(1):41–9.
18. American College of Radiology. MR prostate imaging reporting and data system version 2.0. http://www.acr.org/Quality-Safety/Resources/PIRADS/. Accessed 4 Apr 2016.
19. Hofbauer SL, Maxeiner A, Kittner B, Heckmann R, Reimann M, Wiemer L, et al. Validation of prostate imaging reporting and data system version 2 for the detection of prostate cancer. J Urol. 2018;200(4):767–73.
20. Kasivisvanathan V, Rannikko AS, Borghi M, Panebianco V, Mynderse LA, Vaarala MH, et al. MRI-targeted or standard biopsy for prostate-cancer diagnosis. N Engl J Med. 2018;378(19):1767–77.
21. Ahmed HU, El-Shater Bosaily A, Brown LC, Gabe R, Kaplan R, Parmar MK, et al. Diagnostic accuracy of multi-parametric MRI and TRUS biopsy in prostate cancer (PROMIS): a paired validating confirmatory study. Lancet. 2017;389(10071):815–22.
22. Klotz L, Loblaw A, Van Der Kwast T, Fleshner N, Ghai S, Chin J, et al. Active surveillance magnetic resonance imaging study (ASIST): results of a prospective, multicentre, randomized trial. Eur Urol Suppl. 2018;17:e1711–2.
23. Verep S, Erdem S, Ozluk Y, Kilicaslan I, Sanli O, Ozcan F. The pathological upgrading after radical prostatectomy in low-risk prostate cancer patients who are eligible for active surveillance: how safe is it to depend on bioptic pathology? Prostate. 2019;79(13):1523–9.
24. Porpiglia F, Cantiello F, De Luca S, De Pascale A, Manfredi M, Mele F, et al. Multiparametric magnetic resonance imaging and active surveillance: how to better select insignificant prostate cancer? Int J Urol. 2016;23(9):752–7.
25. Thomsen FB, Brasso K, Klotz LH, Røder MA, Berg KD, Iversen P. Active surveillance for clinically localized prostate cancer—a systematic review. J Surg Oncol. 2014;109(8):830–5.
26. Loeb S, Bruinsma SM, Nicholson J, Briganti A, Pickles T, Kakehi Y, et al. Active surveillance for prostate cancer: a systematic review of clinicopathologic variables and biomarkers for risk stratification. Eur Urol. 2015;67(4):619–26.
27. Goel S, Shoag JE, Gross MD, Al Hussein Al Awamlh B, Robinson B, Khani F, et al. Concordance between biopsy and radical prostatectomy pathology in the era of targeted biopsy: a systematic review and meta-analysis. Eur Urol Oncol. 2020;3(1):10–20.

9

Blood transfusion had no influence on the 5-year biochemical recurrence after robot-assisted radical prostatectomy

Jiwon Han[1†], Young-Tae Jeon[1,2†], Jung-Hee Ryu[1,2], Ah-Young Oh[1,2], Hwanik Kim[3], Yu Kyung Bae[1] and Chang-Hoon Koo[1*]

Abstract

Background: Although red blood cells (RBC) transfusion is known to be significantly associated with biochemical recurrence in patients undergoing open prostatectomy, its influence on biochemical recurrence after robot-assisted laparoscopic radical prostatectomy remains unclear. Therefore, this study aimed to validate the effect of RBC transfusion on the 5-year biochemical recurrence in patients undergoing robot-assisted laparoscopic radical prostatectomy.

Methods: This study retrospectively analyzed the medical records of patients who underwent robot-assisted laparoscopic radical prostatectomy at single tertiary academic hospital between October 2007 and December 2014. Univariate and multivariate Cox proportional hazard regression analysis was performed to identify any potential variables associated with 5-year biochemical recurrence.

Results: A total of 1311 patients were included in the final analysis. Of these, 30 patients (2.3%) were transfused with RBC either during robot-assisted laparoscopic radical prostatectomy or during their hospital stay, which corresponded to 5-year biochemical recurrence of 15.7%. Multivariate Cox proportional hazard regression analysis showed that RBC transfusion had no influence on the 5-year biochemical recurrence. Variables including pathologic T stage (Hazard ratio [HR] 3.5, 95% confidence interval [CI] 2.4–5.1 $p < 0.001$), N stage (HR 2.3, 95% CI 1.5–3.7, $p < 0.001$), Gleason score (HR 2.4, 95% CI 1.8–3.2, $p < 0.001$), and surgical margin (HR 2.0, 95% CI 1.5–2.8, $p < 0.001$) were independently associated with the 5-year biochemical recurrence.

Conclusions: RBC transfusion had no significant influence on the 5-year biochemical recurrence in patients undergoing robot-assisted laparoscopic radical prostatectomy.

Keywords: Biochemical recurrence, Red blood cell transfusion, Robot-assisted laparoscopic radical prostatectomy, Prostate cancer

Background

Robot-assisted laparoscopic radical prostatectomy (RARP) is widely used to treat prostate cancer [1]. Advantageously, RARP reduces blood loss, lowers postoperative pain, leads to fewer complications, and promotes better functional outcomes, when compared to conventional approaches [2–4].

*Correspondence: vollock9@gmail.com
†Jiwon Han and Young-Tae Jeon have contributed equally to this work as co first authors.
[1] Department of Anesthesiology and Pain Medicine, Seoul National University Bundang Hospital, Seongnam 13620, Korea
Full list of author information is available at the end of the article

One common benchmark for evaluating treatment efficacy is biochemical recurrence (BCR), which is used as a surrogate marker for prostate cancer and prognostic index for cancer progression, metastasis, and prostate specific mortality [5, 6]. Several studies, as well as a recent meta-analysis, reported that BCR-free survival rates were comparable in patients treated with open radical prostatectomy versus RARP [7, 8]. The 5-year BCR is reported to be 17–19% after open radical prostatectomy [5, 9], and about 14% after RARP [10]. Previous work has identified preoperative prostate specific antigen (PSA), pathologic T stage, surgical margin, as independent predictors of 5-year BCR following open prostatectomy [6]. Moreover, a recent meta-analysis showed that blood transfusion increased the 5-year BCR in patients undergoing open prostatectomy [11]. However, it has not yet been established whether blood transfusion can increase the 5-year BCR in patients undergoing RARP. Therefore, this study aimed to evaluate the effect of blood transfusion on the 5-year BCR in patients undergoing RARP.

Materials and methods

Ethics statement

This retrospective study was approved by the Institutional Review Board of Seoul National University Bundang Hospital (SNUBH; Approval Number: B-2005/615-105). Given the retrospective design, the need for informed consent was waived.

Population

We examined the electronic medical records of patients who were diagnosed with prostate cancer and underwent RARP at SNUBH between October 2007 and December 2014. RARP has been performed in our institution using the da Vinci Surgical System since October 2007. We excluded patients who received radiation therapy or hormonal treatment prior to surgery. Patients whose baseline or postoperative PSA data were missing or incomplete, were also excluded. We also excluded patients whose RARP was converted to open surgery.

Surgical procedures

RARP was conducted by experienced surgeons via transperitoneal approach using the four-armed da Vinci surgical robot system. Patients were placed in lithotomy position. After docking, the following surgical procedures were performed; bladder detachment, endopelvic fascial incision, dissection of dorsal venous complex, bladder neck, vas deference, seminal vesicle, tissue around the prostate, reconstruction and vesicourethral anastomosis [12]. Adjuvant hemostatic agents (mixture of thrombin with gelatin or fibrin) were routinely used by the surgeons. Patients had a Jackson–Pratt drain placed anteriorly to the bladder wall through one of the lateral port sites and secured with a 4-0 nylon stitch. Unless the operation violated oncological guidelines, the neurovascular bundle was spared [13].

Data collection and outcomes

Blood transfusion data were retrieved from electronic medical records of SNUBH and used to evaluate the efficacy of transfusion. Perioperative transfusion was defined as red blood cells (RBC) transfusion either during RARP or within the postoperative hospital stay. RBC was transfused according to the clinical decision of physicians. The demographic (age and body mass index), clinical, and pathological data of patients were collected as covariates. Collected clinical data included American society of anesthesiologists physical status, smoking history, main anesthetic agents, the administration of intraoperative fluid, estimated blood loss during surgery, duration of surgery and anesthesia, and length of hospital stay. Pathologic evaluation of the specimens was consistently performed by urologic pathologists. Pathologic T stage, N stage, margin status, and Gleason score were collected.

BCR was defined as two consecutive serum PSA level of ≥ 0.2 ng/mL. The initial postoperative PSA was evaluated after 6 weeks. Thereafter, PSA was assessed every 3 months for the first year, and every 6 months during the subsequent 4 years.

Statistical analysis

Continuous variables were presented as median with interquartile ranges (IQR), categorical variables were presented as number with percentage. Univariate Cox proportional hazard regression analysis was performed to identify any potential variables associated with the 5-year BCR. Subsequently, variables with a p value < 0.1 in univariate analysis were selected for multivariate Cox proportional hazard regression analysis using forward selection step. In regression analyses, we categorized the pathologic T stage as < pT3 or $\geq$ pT3, and the Gleason score as < 8 or $\geq$ 8. All statistical analyses were performed using SPSS 24. A p value < 0.05 was considered statistically significant.

Results

A total of 1341 patients underwent RARP between October 2007 and December 2014 at SNUBH. Among them, 12 patients were excluded due to a lack of preoperative or postoperative PSA data. An additional 15 patients were excluded for receiving radiation therapy or hormonal treatment prior to surgery. Finally, three additional patients were excluded because they were converted from RARP to the open technique or they received re-operation before discharge. As such, a total of 1311 patients were included in the final analysis (Fig. 1).

Demographic characteristics are summarized in Table 1, and pathologic characteristics are presented in Table 2. Among 1311 patients, 30 patients (2.3%) were transfused with RBCs during RARP or the hospital stay. The median follow-up period after RARP was 102 [IQR 60–146] months, and the 5-year BCR was 15.7% (n = 206). The median time to BCR was 9.8 [IQR 3.4–30.1] months.

Table 3 shows the results of univariate and multivariate Cox proportional regression analysis for the 5-year BCR. In univariate analysis, RBC transfusion was associated with the 5-year BCR (HR 2.159, 95% CI 1.107–4.211, $p = 0.024$). The result also showed the significant association between the number of transfused RBC and 5-year BCR (HR 1.335, 95% CI 1.094–1.631, $p = 0.005$). However, when they were included in the multivariate analysis with preoperative PSA level, pathologic T stage, N stage, gleason score and surgical margin status, both variables were not statistically significant, respectively ($p > 0.05$). Other variables, including preoperative PSA (HR 1.005, 95% CI 1.002–1.009, $p < 0.001$), pathologic T stage ≥ pT3 (HR 3.510, 95% CI 2.426–5.078, $p < 0.001$), N stage (HR 2.337, 95% CI 1.465–3.729, $p < 0.001$), Gleason score ≥ 8 (HR 2.373, 95% CI 1.756–3.207, $p < 0.001$) and positive surgical margin (HR 2.010, 95% CI 1.452–2.782, $p < 0.001$) were found to be independent predictor of 5-year BCR.

Discussion

This study showed that perioperative transfusion was not independent factor for 5-year BCR in patients undergoing RARP. In addition, this study found that pathologic T stage, N stage, Gleason score, and surgical margin were independently associated with an increased 5-year BCR.

Several studies focused on how transfusion causes pro-tumorigenic environment and supported a significant

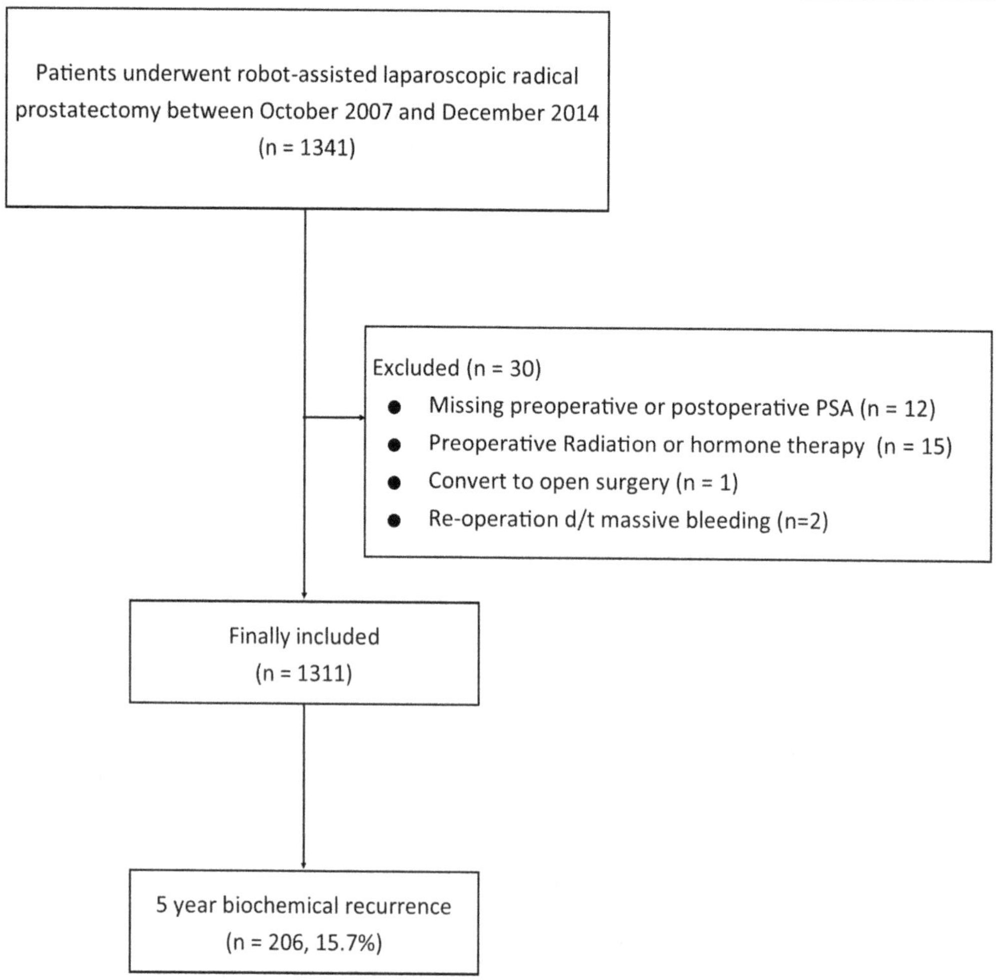

Fig. 1 Flow diagram outlining the inclusion and exclusion criteria with assignment of study cohort

Table 1 Clinical characteristics of included patients (n = 1311)

Variable	
Preoperative variables	
Age, year	66 [61–71]
BMI, kg/m^2	24.6 [22.8–26.2]
ASA physical status, n	
I	436 (33.3%)
II	829 (63.2%)
III	46 (3.5%)
Smoker, n	490 (37.4%)
Preoperative PSA, ng/ml	8.9 [5.6–15.8]
Preoperative Hb, g/dl	14.6 [13.8–15.4]
Preoperative Hct, %	42.8 [40.4–44.9]
Year	
2007-2008	196 (15.0%)
2009-2010	372 (28.4%)
2011-2012	377 (28.8%)
2013-2014	366 (27.9%)
Intraoperative variables	
Main anesthetic agent, n	
Inhalation agent	1217 (92.8%)
Propofol	94 (7.2%)
Fluid administered	
Crystalloid, ml	1204 [900–1651]
Estimated blood loss, ml	200 [100–300]
Duration of surgery, min	200 [175–225]
Duration of anesthesia, min	250 [225–275]
Perioperative transfusion	
Patients who were transfused, n	30 (2.3%)
Number of packed RBC in patients transfused	2 [2–3]
Length of hospital stay, d	11 [9–12]

Values are expressed as median [interquartile range] or number (percentage)

BMI body mass index, *ASA* American society of anesthesiologists, *PSA* prostate-specific antigen, *Hb* hemoglobin, *Hct* hematocrit

Table 2 Pathological characteristics of included patients (n = 1311)

Variable	
Pathologic T stage, n	
pT2	3 (0.2%)
pT2a	109 (8.3%)
pT2c	771 (58.8%)
pT3a	291 (22.2%)
pT3b	129 (9.8%)
pT4	8 (0.6%)
Pathologic N stage, n	
Nx	792 (60.4%)
N0	486 (37.0%)
N1	33 (2.5%)
Gleason score, n	
≤6	116 (8.8%)
7	1025 (78.2%)
8	62 (4.7%)
9	108 (8.2%)
Surgical margin positive, n	393 (30.0%)
1 year BCR	79 (6.0%)
5 year BCR	206 (15.7%)

Values are expressed as median [interquartile range] or number (percentage)

BCR biochemical recurrence

association between transfusion and increased recurrence in patients undergoing surgery for colon, stomach, liver, or bladder cancer [14–17]. There are several pathophysiology to explain the effect of blood transfusion on tumor recurrence in patients undergoing cancer surgery. Surgical manipulation may enable malignant cells to circulate in the bloodstream [18, 19]. Moreover, anesthetics and opioids attenuate host immunity, leading to a permissive tumor environment [20]. Indeed, previous work assessed perioperative changes in the ratio of Th1/Th2 cells period in surgical patients, and observed a shift toward a Th2 immune response, indicative of a significant alteration in the composition of the immune system [21]. Post-surgical immunosuppression may be further aggravated by transfusion as RBCs can also modulate the immune system, a phenomena referred to as transfusion related immunomodulation (TRIM). There are 4 mechanisms for TRIM; (1) suppression of cytotoxic cell and monocyte activity; (2) release of immunosuppressive prostaglandins; (3) inhibition of interleukin-2 production; (4) increased suppressor T-cell activity [22]. Contrary to those studies, we found that transfusion was not associated with increased 5-year BCR in patients undergoing RARP.

There has been some disagreement with regard to whether transfusion may influence on BCR after radical prostatectomy. As mentioned in the introduction, a recent meta-analysis including 8 studies showed that perioperative blood transfusion was associated with decreased overall survival and recurrence-free survival rate following open radical prostatectomy [11]. In contrast to these findings, Boehm et al. analyzed 11,723 patients who were treated with open radical prostatectomy or RARLP and found no correlation between blood transfusion and oncological outcomes [23]. The authors explained this discordance by changes in transfusion standard and reduced immunologic reaction related to transfusion. To the best of our knowledge, this is the first study to evaluate the effect of blood transfusion on BCR in patients undergoing RARP solely.

In the present study, the average patient blood loss was 200 ml, and transfusion rate was 2.3%. These are comparable to previous work which showed that RARP

Table 3 Univariate and Multivariate Cox proportional hazard regression analysis for 5-year biochemical recurrence of prostate cancer

Variable	Univariate analysis		Multivariate analysis	
	HR (95% CI)	*p* value	HR (95% CI)	*p* value
Preoperative variables				
Age, year	1.015 (0.994–1.035)	0.155		
BMI, kg/m2	0.991 (0.951–1.034)	0.678		
ASA physical status				
I	1 (reference)			
II	0.794 (0.597–1.056)	0.112		
III	0.934 (0.451–1.934)	0.854		
Diabetes mellitus	1.321 (0.887–1.968)	0.171		
Hypertension	1.188 (0.887–1.592)	0.248		
Coronary artery disease	1.421 (0.840–2.404)	0.190		
Cerebrovascular accident	1.382 (0.651–2.937)	0.400		
Smoker	0.933 (0.702–1.241)	0.634		
Preoperative PSA, ng/ml	1.015 (1.013–1.018)	**< 0.001***	1.005 (1.002–1.009)	**< 0.001***
Preoperative Hb, g/dl	0.916 (0.826–1.016)	0.098		
Intraoperative variables				
Main anesthetic agent				
Inhalation agent	1 (reference)			
Propofol	0.957 (0.556–1.646)	0.874		
Crystalloid, ml	1.000 (1.000–1.000)	0.968		
Colloid, ml	1.000 (1.000–1.001)	**0.034***		
Estimated blood loss, ml	1.001 (1.000–1.001)	**0.042***		
Perioperative RBC transfusion				
None	1 (reference)			
Transfusion	2.159 (1.107–4.211)	**0.024***		
Number of packed RBC	1.335 (1.094–1.631)	**0.005***		
Pathological variables				
Pathologic T stage				
< pT3	1 (reference)			
≥ pT3	7.197 (5.264–9.839)	**< 0.001***	3.510 (2.426–5.078)	**< 0.001***
Pathologic N stage				
Nx or N0	1 (reference)			
N1	7.080 (4.504–11.129)	**< 0.001***	2.337 (1.465–3.729)	**< 0.001***
Gleason score				
< 8	1 (reference)			
≥ 8	5.478 (4.137–7.254)	**< 0.001***	2.373 (1.756–3.207)	**< 0.001***
Surgical margin positive	4.821 (3.628–6.404)	**< 0.001***	2.010 (1.452–2.782)	**< 0.001***

Statistically significant *p* value (< 0.05) are highlighted in bold

BMI body mass index, *ASA* American society of anesthesiologists, *PSA* prostate-specific antigen, *Hb* hemoglobin

reduced blood loss (188 ml vs. 745 ml) and transfusion rates (16.5% vs. 1.8%) when compared with open prostatectomy [24]. Among the patients who received blood transfusion, the median number of transfused RBC was 2 units. Given that relatively low blood loss and volume, it can be inferred that the volume of transfused RBC was not enough to induce pro-tumor environment or immunomodulation. Difficult surgical conditions such a locally advanced tumor, which is T3 or T4, may increase the risk of transfusion. Therefore, we assessed multicollinearity which means a linear relationship between T stage and transfusion using variance inflation factor. The value of 1.384 suggests that multicollinearity was not a problem in our model.

Consistent with previous work, this study showed that Gleason score, T stage, N stage, and surgical margin, were independent predictors of 5-year BCR. Several large studies with a follow-up more than 5 years have identified predictors of BCR after RARP [10, 25–27]. Despite slightly different definitions of variables among these studies, most studies have reported that Gleason score, pathologic stage, and/or surgical margin were independently associated with 5-year BCR.

It is important to recognize that BCR is not a definitive indicator for the clinical relapse of prostate cancer. However, BCR has been associated with increased mortality [28]. Therefore, physicians should be aware of predictive factors for BCR in prostate cancer patients, and therein stratify high risk patients to prevent clinical progression.

There are several limitations in this study. First, given that relatively small proportion of transfused patient, our findings needed to be interpreted with caution. However, transfusion rate of the present study was similar to the previous study [24]. Second, transfusion was performed in accordance with conventional criteria (Hb 7–8 g/dL or less or Hb 10 g/dL or less if patients has ischemic disease such as coronary atherosclerosis or stroke) but without a predefined protocol. Given that our results are based on a retrospective analysis, further prospective studies are therefore required to validate the association between transfusion and 5-year BCR. Third, the impact of RBC storage was not considered in this study. It has been reported that prolonged RBC storage may have detrimental clinical impacts [29]. However, the small number of patients who were transfused in this study was seemingly insufficient to draw meaningful results from a subgroup analysis based on the duration of RBC storage.

Conclusions

The evidence from this study suggests that blood transfusion was not associated with an increased 5-year BCR in patients undergoing RARP. We hope that our research will be helpful in terms of perioperative blood management in patients undergoing RARP.

Acknowledgements
Not applicable.

Authors' contributions
Conceptualization and Study validation: C-HK; Data Acquisition: JH, Y-TJ, J-HR, A-YO, HK; Data analysis and interpretation: JH, Y-TJ, YKB; Writing original draft: JH, Y-TJ, C-HK; Revising and Editing draft: J-HR, A-YO, YKB, HK; Supervision: C-HK. All authors have agreed both to be personally accountable for the author's own contributions and all aspects of the work. All authors read and approved the final manuscript.

Author details
[1]Department of Anesthesiology and Pain Medicine, Seoul National University Bundang Hospital, Seongnam 13620, Korea. [2]Department of Anesthesiology and Pain Medicine, Seoul National University College of Medicine, Seoul 03080, Korea. [3]Department of Urology, Seoul National University Bundang Hospital, Seongnam 13620, Korea.

References

1. Mottrie A, De Naeyer G, Novara G, Ficarra V. Robotic radical prostatectomy: a critical analysis of the impact on cancer control. Curr Opin Urol. 2011;21(3):179–84.
2. Gandaglia G, Sammon JD, Chang SL, Choueiri TK, Hu JC, Karakiewicz PI, et al. Comparative effectiveness of robot-assisted and open radical prostatectomy in the postdissemination era. J Clin Oncol. 2014;32(14):1419–26.
3. Murphy DG, Kerger M, Crowe H, Peters JS, Costello AJ. Operative details and oncological and functional outcome of robotic-assisted laparoscopic radical prostatectomy: 400 cases with a minimum of 12 months follow-up. Eur Urol. 2009;55(6):1358–66.
4. Novara G, Ficarra V, Mocellin S, Ahlering TE, Carroll PR, Graefen M, et al. Systematic review and meta-analysis of studies reporting oncologic outcome after robot-assisted radical prostatectomy. Eur Urol. 2012;62(3):382–404.
5. Freedland SJ, Humphreys EB, Mangold LA, Eisenberger M, Dorey FJ, Walsh PC, et al. Risk of prostate cancer–specific mortality following biochemical recurrence after radical prostatectomy. JAMA. 2005;294(4):433–9.
6. McCormick BZ, Mahmoud AM, Williams SB, Davis JW. Biochemical recurrence after radical prostatectomy: current status of its use as a treatment endpoint and early management strategies. Indian J Urol. 2019;35(1):6–17.
7. Haese A, Knipper S, Isbarn H, Heinzer H, Tilki D, Salomon G, et al. A comparative study of robot-assisted and open radical prostatectomy in 10,790 men treated by highly trained surgeons for both procedures. BJU Int. 2019;123(6):1031–40.
8. Seo HJ, Lee NR, Son SK, Kim DK, Rha KH, Lee SH. Comparison of robot-assisted radical prostatectomy and open radical prostatectomy outcomes: a systematic review and meta-analysis. Yonsei Med J. 2016;57(5):1165.
9. Han M, Partin AW, Zahurak M, Piantadosi S, Epstein JI, Walsh PC. Biochemical (prostate specific antigen) recurrence probability following radical prostatectomy for clinically localized prostate cancer. J Urol. 2003;169(2):517–23.
10. Liss MA, Lusch A, Morales B, Beheshti N, Skarecky D, Narula N, et al. Robot-assisted radical prostatectomy: 5-year oncological and biochemical outcomes. J Urol. 2012;188(6):2205–10.
11. Pushan Z, Manbiao C, Sulai L, Jun L, Ruidong Z, Hanshen Y. The impact of perioperative blood transfusion on survival and recurrence after radical prostatectomy for prostate cancer: a systematic review and meta-analysis. J Cancer Res Ther. 2018;14(Supplement):S701-S7.
12. Mottrie A, Mazzone E, Wiklund P, Graefen M, Collins JW, De Groote R, Dell'Oglio P, Puliatti S, Gallagher AG. Objective assessment of intraoperative skills for robot-assisted radical prostatectomy (RARP): results from the ERUS Scientific and Educational Working Groups Metrics Initiative. BJU Int. 2021;128(1):103–11.
13. Lee YJ, Jung JW, Lee S, Lee SW, Kim JH, Hong SK, Byun SS, Lee SE, Jeong SJ. Contemporary trends in radical prostatectomy and predictors of recovery of urinary continence in men aged over 70 years: comparisons between cohorts aged over 70 and less than 70 years. Asian J Androl. 2020;22(3):280–6.
14. Amato A, Pescatori M. Perioperative blood transfusions for the recurrence of colorectal cancer. Cochrane Database Syst Rev. 2006;2006(1):CD005033.
15. Linder BJ, Frank I, Cheville JC, Tollefson MK, Thompson RH, Tarrell RF, et al. The impact of perioperative blood transfusion on cancer recurrence and survival following radical cystectomy. Eur Urol. 2013;63(5):839–45.
16. Makino Y, Yamanoi A, Kimoto T, El-Assal ON, Kohno H, Nagasue N. The influence of perioperative blood transfusion on intrahepatic recurrence after curative resection of hepatocellular carcinoma. Am J Gastroenterol. 2000;95(5):1294–300.
17. Squires MH, Kooby DA, Poultsides GA, Weber SM, Bloomston M, Fields RC, et al. Effect of perioperative transfusion on recurrence and survival after gastric cancer resection: a 7-institution analysis of 765 patients from the US gastric cancer collaborative. J Am Coll Surg. 2015;221(3):767–77.
18. Bosch B, Guller U, Schnider A, Maurer R, Harder F, Metzger U, et al. Perioperative detection of disseminated tumour cells is an independ-

ent prognostic factor in patients with colorectal cancer. Br J Surg. 2003;90(7):882–8.

19. Yamaguchi K, Takagi Y, Aoki S, Futamura M, Saji S. Significant detection of circulating cancer cells in the blood by reverse transcriptase-polymerase chain reaction during colorectal cancer resection. Ann Surg. 2000;232(1):58–65.
20. Ash SA, Buggy DJ. Does regional anaesthesia and analgesia or opioid analgesia influence recurrence after primary cancer surgery? An update of available evidence. Best Pract Res Clin Anaesthesiol. 2013;27(4):441–56.
21. Ishikawa M, Nishioka M, Hanaki N, Miyauchi T, Kashiwagi Y, Ioki H, et al. Perioperative immune responses in cancer patients undergoing digestive surgeries. World J Surg Oncol. 2009;7:7.
22. Cata JP, Wang H, Gottumukkala V, Reuben J, Sessler DI. Inflammatory response, immunosuppression, and cancer recurrence after perioperative blood transfusions. Br J Anaesth. 2013;110(5):690–701.
23. Boehm K, Beyer B, Tennstedt P, Schiffmann J, Budaeus L, Haese A et al. No impact of blood transfusion on oncological outcome after radical prostatectomy in patients with prostate cancer. World J Urol. 2015;33(6):801–6.
24. Tewari A, Sooriakumaran P, Bloch DA, Seshadri-Kreaden U, Hebert AE, Wiklund P. Positive surgical margin and perioperative complication rates of primary surgical treatments for prostate cancer: a systematic review and meta-analysis comparing retropubic, laparoscopic, and robotic prostatectomy. Eur Urol. 2012;62(1):1–15.
25. Menon M, Bhandari M, Gupta N, Lane Z, Peabody JO, Rogers CG, et al. Biochemical recurrence following robot-assisted radical prostatectomy: analysis of 1384 patients with a median 5-year follow-up. Eur Urol. 2010;58(6):838–46.
26. Sooriakumaran P, Haendler L, Nyberg T, Gronberg H, Nilsson A, Carlsson S, et al. Biochemical recurrence after robot-assisted radical prostatectomy in a European single-centre cohort with a minimum follow-up time of 5 years. Eur Urol. 2012;62(5):768–74.
27. Suardi N, Ficarra V, Willemsen P, De Wil P, Gallina A, De Naeyer G, et al. Long-term biochemical recurrence rates after robot-assisted radical prostatectomy: analysis of a single-center series of patients with a minimum follow-up of 5 years. Urology. 2012;79(1):133–8.
28. Uchio EM, Aslan M, Wells CK, Calderone J, Concato J. Impact of biochemical recurrence in prostate cancer among US veterans. Arch Intern Med. 2010;170(15):1390–5.
29. Tinmouth A, Fergusson D, Yee IC, Hebert PC, Investigators A, Canadian Critical Care Trials G. Clinical consequences of red cell storage in the critically ill. Transfusion. 2006;46(11):2014–27.

10

Visualization of the renal vein filled with contrast agent may indicate the renal vein injury during percutaneous nephrolithotomy: Two case reports

Xiao-Feng Chen[1,2], Jian-Jun Zhou[3], Jian-Ming Sun[1,2], Guo-Can Cao[3], Yi-Hua Zou[1,2] and Wang-Long Deng[1,2*]

Abstract

Background: Intravenous misplacement of a nephrostomy tube is a rare complication of percutaneous nephrolithotomy (PCNL) or percutaneous nephrostomy. The mechanism of misplacement of a nephrostomy tube into the vascular system is seldom investigated. One type of the possible mechanism is that the puncture needle penetrates a major intrarenal tributary of the renal vein and enters the collecting system. However, the guidewire is located outside the collecting system near the large branches of renal vein or perforates into the renal vein. The dilation is performed and causes a large torn injury. Subsequently, the nephrostomy tube is placed inside the vessel when radiological monitoring is not used. However, there is no imaging evidence and the scene of procedure is not demonstrated. This paper reports two cases of visualization of the renal vein filled with contrast agent during PCNL. The findings may be good evidence to support the step of renal vein injury in patients with intravenous nephrostomy tube misplacement.

Case presentation: We presented two cases with visualization of the renal vein filled with contrast agent during PCNL. In the process of injecting the contrast agent through the puncture needle, we could see the renal vein. Moreover, it was identified that the puncture needle tip was not on the optimal position. The position of puncture needle tip lay outside the collecting system, which was close to the calyceal infundibulum and branches of renal vein.

Conclusions: Visualization of the renal vein filled with contrast agent may be good evidence to verify the renal vein injury in patients with intravenous nephrostomy tube misplacement during PCNL or percutaneous nephrostomy. The suboptimal location of the puncture needle tip and visualization of the renal vein filled with contrast agent indicate the renal vein injury. One type of mechanism of intravenous nephrostomy tube misplacement is as following. Firstly, the guidewire stays outside the collecting system. Subsequently, dilatation directed by the guidewire results in the injury of the vein. Then, the nephrostomy tube migrates into the venous system due to prompt tube inserting and the direction of the sheath and/or the guidewire to the injured vein.

Keywords: Nephrostomy, Percutaneous, Tube, Complication, Intravenous

Background

Intravenous misplacement of a nephrostomy tube is a rare event of percutaneous nephrolithotomy (PCNL) or percutaneous nephrostomy (PCN) [1–6]. Limited literatures have reported the misplacement of a nephrostomy tube in the renal vein, inferior vena cava (IVC) or atrium. The mechanisms of misplacement of a nephrostomy

*Correspondence: 93644294@qq.com
[1] Department of Urology, The First People's Hospital of Chenzhou, 102 Luojiajing, Chenzhou 423000, Hunan, People's Republic of China
Full list of author information is available at the end of the article

tube into the vascular system are also seldom investigated. One type of the possible mechanism is that the puncture needle penetrates a major intrarenal tributary of the renal vein and enters the collecting system. However, the guidewire is located outside the collecting system near the large branches of renal vein or perforates into the renal vein. The dilation is performed and causes a large torn injury. Subsequently, the nephrostomy tube is placed inside the vessel when radiological monitoring is not used [6, 9]. However, there is no imaging evidence and the scene of procedure is not demonstrated.

In the present study, we report two cases of visualization of the renal vein filled with contrast agent during PCNL at our centers. The findings may be good evidence to support the step of renal vein injury in patients with intravenous nephrostomy tube misplacement.

Case presentation

Patient 1 was a 45-year-old man who presented with left flank pain. His medical history indicated that he had renal stone. His physical examination was positive for tenderness upon palpation of his left flank. The initial laboratory evaluation showed normal. The computed tomography (CT) scan of abdomen and pelvis showed left moderate hydronephrosis and an upper ureteral stone was measured at 1.3 cm. Our patient was diagnosed with left upper ureteral stone with moderate hydronephrosis. The procedure of PCNL was carried out. A ureteral catheter was inserted retrogradely into the left pelvic under ureteroscopy. The puncture target calix was the middle posterior calix. The puncture site of the target calyceal fornix was localized under C-arm radiological monitoring using contrast agent injected through ureteral catheter, producing a retrograde pyelography (RP). An 18 gauge, 2 piece entry needle was used. Clear urine was seen when the needle stylet was removed. When we injected the contrast agent into his left collecting system through the puncture needle, we were able to see his left renal vein (Fig. 1). Moreover, we could identify that the location of the puncture needle tip was not optimal, the reason was that the puncture needle tip was located outside the collecting system near the calyceal infundibulum. At the moment, the patient had a hemodynamic stability and the puncture needle was maintained in its original place. Additional lower pole calix puncture was performed under radiological monitoring. Clear urine was also seen when the needle stylet was removed. Injection of contrast agent in his left collecting system through the later puncture needle showed the collecting system, without visualization of the renal vein (Fig. 2). In the process of injecting saline into his left collecting system by ureteral catheter, we were able to see the light red drips through the former puncture needle, and the clear drips through the latter puncture needle. The former puncture needle was pulled out and simultaneous PCNL was performed. An 18 gauge, 2 piece entry needle was advanced into the

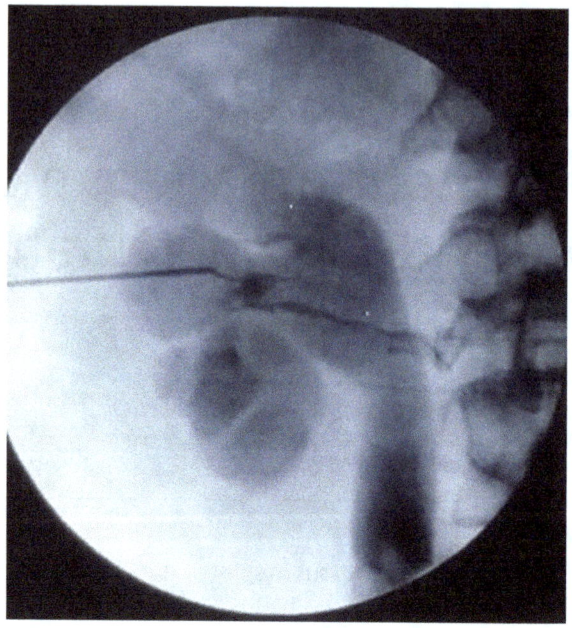

Fig. 1 The radiograph of the kidneys, ureters and bladder revealing the left renal vein, the collecting system, and the suboptimal position of the puncture needle tip

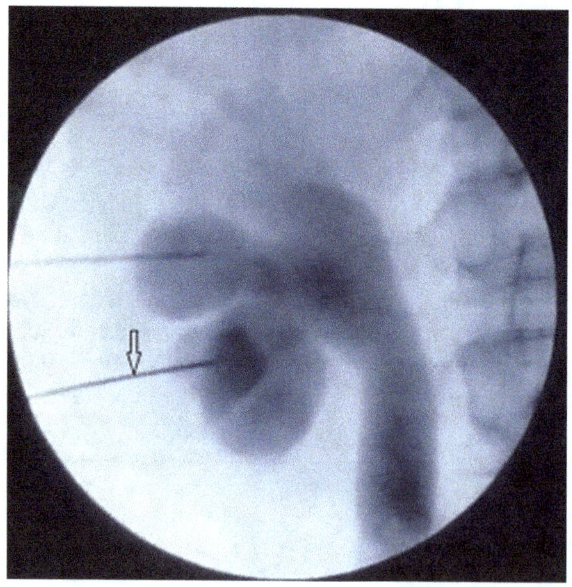

Fig. 2 The radiograph of the kidneys, ureters and bladder revealing the collecting system, without visualization of the renal vein by injection of contrast agent through the latter puncture needle (arrow)

lower pole calix under fluoroscopy guidance. A zebra guidewire was inserted into the collecting system. The tract was dilated with fascial dilators to accommodate an 18 French sheath. The renal calculus was removed uneventfully.

Patient 2 was a 41-year-old woman who presented with left flank pain. Her medical history was unremarkable. White blood cells were detected in the urine. Empirical antibiotics were started. A CT scan of abdomen and pelvis showed the presence of left mild hydronephrosis and renal calculi was measured at 2.2 cm. The patient was diagnosed with renal calculi and mild hydronephrosis. A PCNL procedure protocol was planned. A ureteral catheter was inserted into the left ureter retrogradely. The target calix was the middle posterior calix. The puncture site of the target calyceal fornix was localized under fluoroscopy monitoring using contrast agent injected through ureteral catheter, producing a RP. Clear urine was seen on withdrawal of the stylet. During an injection of contrast agent in her left collecting system through the puncture needle, we were able to visualize her left renal vein filled with contrast agent (Fig. 3). We could also identify that the location of the puncture needle tip was not optimal. The puncture needle tip was near the calyceal infundibulum. The puncture needle was pulled out. A puncture tract passing through the middle posterior caliceal fornix was performed simultaneously and the renal calculi was removed uneventfully. The operative steps were as same as patient 1.

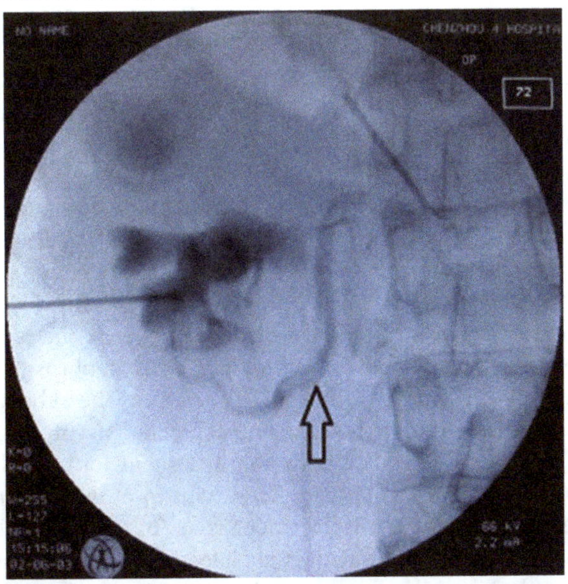

Fig. 3 The radiograph of the kidneys, ureters and bladder revealing the left renal vein (arrow), the inferior calyx, and the suboptimal position of the puncture needle tip

Among our two patients, we saw the renal vein filled with contrast agent during PCNL and identified the location of the puncture needle tip was not optimal. The puncture needle tip was located outside the collecting system near the calyceal infundibulum in the two patients. The visualization of renal vein branches during antegrade pyelography and bloody fluid drips confirmed the puncture needle tips located in a vein vessel or injured a vessel. The following procedures were not carried out. The original operation PCNL was performed successfully by another puncture tract in the two patients. They were discharged uneventfully with the stones cleaned by simultaneous PCNL.

Six articles relevant to the vein injury during PCN or PCNL were selected [3, 5–9]. The data of the six articles were summarized in Table 1. As noted in Table 1, the vein injury in patient undergoing PCN occurred in the initial stage of the operation. The guidewire or catheter perforated and migrated into the vein directly. In patient undergoing PCNL, the vein injury occurred either in the initial stage due to the dilator tearing motion or during the operation due to the fragmentation energy.

Discussion and conclusions

Intravenous tube misplacement is a rare complication of PCNL or PCN with the incidence of 0.02–0.05% [6, 9].

Three types of mechanism of intravenous tube misplacement were mentioned in literatures. The first type of mechanism was described by Chen et al. [6] and Fu et al. [9]. Firstly, the puncture needle passes through a branch of renal vein and its tip enter the collecting system. During inserting the guidewire through the puncture needle, the tip of puncture needle moves outside of the collecting system due to such factors as respiratory movement, narrow space between staghorn calculi and collecting system. The guidewire stays just outside the collecting system near the injured renal vein branch or perforates into the renal vein. If the misplaced improper location of guidewire is not recognized by the surgeon. Dilatation directed by the guidewire results in a torn lesion of the vein. Heavy venous bleeding occurs as soon as the dilator is removed. The nephrostomy tube migrates into the vascular system due to the prompt tube inserting and the direction of the sheath and\or the guidewire to the injured vein.

The second type of mechanism is as Mazzucchi et al. [5] and Wang et al. [7] describes. Firstly, the instruments used during surgery cause a lesion in a large branch of renal vein. Secondly, the sheath directs the nephrostomy tube inside the vascular system. The third mechanism can be observed in catheter placement [3, 8]. Firstly, the

Table 1 Reports of mechanism of intravenous nephrostomy tube misplacement

First author	References	Original operation	Steps: first step	Steps: second step	Steps: third step	Is the guidewire in the vein?	When is the vein torn?
Dias-Filho	[3]	Tuber placement	A vein is perforated by a guidewire	The injured vein is dilated	The catheter is placed inside the vein	Yes	During dilating at the initial stage of operation
Kotb	[8]	Tuber placement	The silicon catheter passes into a major vein after penetrating the renal parenchymal			The guidewire is not used	At the initial stage of operation
Chen	[6]	PCNL	The fascial dilators tear a large vein	The sheath directs the catheter inside the vessels		No	During dilating at the initial stage of operation
Fu	[9]	PCNL	The dilator sheath injures the renal vein	The guidewire perforates into the renal vein and the injured vein is dilatated	The catheter is placed inside the vessels	Yes	During dilating at the initial stage of operation
Mazzucchi	[5]	PCNL	A lesion in a large renal vein branch is caused by the instruments	The sheath directs the catheter inside the vessels		No	During the fragmentation process
Wang	[7]	PCNL	A lesion in a large renal vein branch is caused by the instruments	The sheath directs the catheter inside the vessels		No	During the fragmentation process

nephrostomy tube or the guidewire perforates a major branch of the renal vein. Then, the tube is placed inside the vessel directly, or guided by the guidewire.

Here we provide two patients with the imaging evidence and the scene of procedure demonstration to verify the renal vein injury in the first mechanism. In our patients 1 and 2 the location of the puncture needle tip was not optimal. We are able to visualize the renal vein and collecting system during an injection of contrast agent through the puncture needle. It indicates that the tip of puncture needle has pass through the branch of the renal vein and enters into the collecting system initially. However, during fluoroscopic imaging the tip of puncture needle moves outside of the collecting system. It stays near or inside the branch of the renal vein outside the collecting system. If the guidewire is inserted through the puncture needle, it will just stay outside the calix or perforate into the renal vein. Dilatation directed by the guidewire will result in the injury of the vein. The nephrostomy tube will migrate into the vascular system directed by the dilator sheath and\or the guidewire. To prevent such complication, review of previous imaging, including ultrasound, CT, or magnetic resonance imaging should be performed, to identify valuable anatomic information as to the optimal access entrance before establishing percutaneous access. The ideal entrance point should be along the avascular plane of Brodel in a position that is lateral to the renal calyx, and directed toward the renal pelvis. The puncture tract should pass through the caliceal fornix. After the tip of the needle is confirmed within the collecting system under ultrasound or fluoroscopy guidance. The tip of the needle should be maintained in the initial position with the needle depth no changing. Then, a guidewire is carefully and gently inserted into the renal collecting system. The guidewire should be also confirmed curling in the renal collecting system under ultrasound or fluoroscopy guidance.

In conclusion, visualization of the renal vein filled with contrast agent may be good evidence to verify the renal vein injury in patients with intravenous nephrostomy tube misplacement during PCNL or PCN. The suboptimal location of the puncture needle tip and visualization of the renal vein filled with contrast agent indicate the renal vein injury. One type of mechanism of intravenous nephrostomy tube misplacement is as following. Firstly, the guidewire stays outside the collecting system. Subsequently, dilatation directed by the guidewire results in the injury of the vein. Then, the nephrostomy tube migrates into the venous system due to prompt tube inserting and the direction of the sheath and\or the guidewire to the injured vein.

Abbreviations
CT: Computed tomography; IVC: Inferior vena cava; PCNL: Percutaneous nephrolithotomy; PCN: Percutaneous nephrostomy; RP: Retrograde pyelography.

Acknowledgements
We also thank the two patients for giving us the permission to use the medical information for this publication.

Authors' contributions
XFC drafted the manuscript. WLD was responsible for critical revision of the manuscript. JMS, GCC and YHZ performed the operation. JJZ was responsible for the conception and design of this study, interpretation of the data. All authors read and approved the final manuscript.

Author details
[1]Department of Urology, The First People's Hospital of Chenzhou, 102 Luojiajing, Chenzhou 423000, Hunan, People's Republic of China. [2]Department of Urology, The First Clinical College of Xiangnan University, 102 Luojiajing, Chenzhou 423000, Hunan, People's Republic of China. [3]Department of Urology, The Fourth People's Hospital of Chenzhou, Chenzhou, Hunan, People's Republic of China.

References
1. Mirheydar HS, Palazzi KL, Derweesh IH, Chang DC, Sur RL. Percutaneous nephrolithotomy use is increasing in the United States: an analysis of trends and complications. J Endourol. 2013;27:979–83.
2. Taylor E, Miller J, Chi T, Stoller ML. Complications associated with percutaneous nephrolithotomy. Transl Androl Urol. 2012;1:223–8.
3. Dias-Filho AC, Coaracy GA, Borges W. Right atrial migration of nephrostomy catheter. Int Braz J Urol. 2005;31:470–1.
4. Shaw G, Wah TM, Kellett MJ, Choong SK. Management of renal vein perforation during a challenging percutaneous nephrolithotomy. J Endourol. 2005;19:722–3.
5. Mazzucchi E, Mitre A, Brito A, Arap M, Murta C, Srougi M. Intravenous misplacement of the nephrostomy catheter following percutaneous nephrostolithotomy: two case reports. Clinics (Sao Paulo). 2009;64:69–70.
6. Chen XF, Chen SQ, Xu LY, Gong Y, Chen ZF, Zheng SB. Intravenous misplacement of nephrostomy tube following percutaneous nephrolithotomy: three new cases and review of seven cases in the literature. Int Braz J Urol. 2014;40:690–6.
7. Wang C, Chen S, Tang F, Shen B. Metachronous renal vein and artery injure after percutaneous nephrostolithotomy. BMC Urol. 2013;13:1–5.
8. Kotb AF, Elabbady A, Mohamed KR, Atta MA. Percutaneous silicon catheter insertion into the inferior vena cava, following percutaneous nephrostomy exchange. Can Urol Assoc J. 2013;7:e505–7.
9. Fu W, Yang Z, Xie Z, Yan H. Intravenous misplacement of the nephrostomy catheter following percutaneous nephrostolithotomy: two case reports and literature review. BMC Urol. 2017;17:43.

11

A 3D printing personalized percutaneous puncture guide access plate for percutaneous nephrolithotomy

Gao Keyu[1†], Li Shuaishuai[2†], Ashok Raj[2†], Li Shuofeng[1], Liu Shuai[3], Zhang Yuan[4], Zhu Haitao[1] and Wang Junqi[1*]

Abstract

Objective: CT-Urography combined with 3D printing technology, digital design, construction of individualized PCNL puncture guides, and preliminary analyze their efficacy, safety puncture positioning for PCNL.

Methods: Twenty-two patients with renal calculi were randomly selected at the affiliated Hospital of Xuzhou Medical University during 2017–2018. We randomly divided the patients into two groups: in 10 experimental groups, we used our 3D printing personalized percutaneous puncture guide access plate for PCNL, and in the control group, 12 patients with standard USG guide PCNL. The accuracy of puncture position, puncture time, and intraoperative blood loss was compared.

Results: In the experimental group, 10 patients with 3D printing personalized percutaneous puncture guide access plate. The puncture needle was accessed through the guide plate and verified by the color Doppler. The single puncture, needle position, and depth success rate were 100.00% (10/10). The angles were consistent with the preoperative design. In the control group, 12 patients via USG guided PCNL success rate was 75.00% (9/12). The puncture time and amount of hemorrhage was (7.78 ± 0.94) min and (49.31 ± 6.43) mL, and (9.04 ± 1.09) min and (60.08 ± 12.18) mL, respectively. The above data of the two groups were statistically significant ($P < 0.05$).

Conclusion: 3D printing personalized percutaneous nephrolithotomy guide plate for PCNL can improve PCNL renal puncture channel positioning accuracy, shorten puncture time, reduce intraoperative blood loss, bleeding-related complications and provide a new method for PCNL renal puncture positioning, which is worthy of further clinical exploration.

Keywords: Percutaneous nephrolithotomy (PCNL), 3D Printing technology, Puncture, Guide plate

Introduction

Percutaneous nephrolithotomy (PCNL) is still the mainstream treatment for complex renal calculi. However, the complications such as bleeding, Infection, and residual stones during and after PCNL operation are the main burden needed more attention. Among them, bleeding is the most common complication, and the cause of bleeding is mainly the poor selection of renal puncture site and damage to renal vessels· The establishment of the best skin-to-target renal puncture channel is a critical factor for successful operation. At present, the main preferable clinical methods of stone localization are X-ray (fluoroscopy) and Ultrasound [1, 2]. Fluoroscopy is a two-dimensional imagining system that lacks the stereoscopic sense of kidney tissue and stone location, with a low success rate of puncture and radiation damage [3]. Ultrasound can position calculi in multiple layers and effectively

*Correspondence: 389747002@qq.com
†Gao Keyu, Li Shuaishuai and Ashok Raj contributed equally to the work.
[1] Department of Urology, The Affiliated Hospital of Xuzhou Medical University, Xuzhou 221000, China
Full list of author information is available at the end of the article

improve the accuracy of positioning. However, its low resolution and high requirements on ultrasonic technology of the surgeons limit its clinical application to a certain extent. 3D printing technology is a new technology developed in recent years. Using 3D printing technology to make personalized guide plates for different surgeries has been more and more applied in orthopedics and stomatology [4, 5]. However, this technology is still in the preliminary exploration stage in urology. The 3D printing plate can be implemented to avoid the damage of renal vascular puncture in the process of renal puncture localization and improve the accuracy of puncture localization. Through the 3D reconstruction model, doctors, patients, and their families can more clearly understand the stone localization, making the communication between doctors and patients more comfortable and has guiding significance for the planning of clinical surgery plans. In the experimental group, 10 patients who planned to undergo PCNL in the Affiliated Hospital of Xuzhou Medical University from 2017 to 2018 were selected. Using Computed Tomography Urography (CTU), combined with 3D printing technology and digital design, the individualized percutaneous nephrolithotomy guide plate was developed. The feasibility of its application in PCNL puncture localization was preliminarily discussed.

Materials and methods

General information

From 2017 to 2018, in the Affiliated Hospital of Xuzhou Medical University, a total of 22 patients with kidney stones were randomly selected for our study. All patients have signed informed consent forms. The experimental group (n = 10) had five males and five females. According to the stone side, there were 4 cases on the left side and 6 cases on the right side. According to the type of calculi, there were 5 cases of staghorn calculus, 2 cases of single calculi, and 3 cases of multiple calculi. Among them, lumbar pain and discomfort were found in 6 cases, an asymptomatic physical examination was found in 2 cases, gross hematuria in 2 cases. Two patients had a history of hypertension, and 4 patients had undergone extracorporeal shock wave lithotripsy (ESWL). The mean age was 48.60 ± 9.69 (28–62) years old. The control group (n = 12) had 7 males and 5 males. According to the stone side, there were 5 cases on the left side and 7 cases on the right side. According to the type of calculi, there were 4 staghorn calculi, 5 single calculi, and 3 multiple calculi. 7 cases complained of lumbar pain and discomfort, 3 were found asymptomatic on physical examination, and 2 were found gross hematuria. ESWL was performed in 5 patients. The mean age was 45.33 ± 8.52 (22–58) years old. There was no statistically significant difference in age, sex, stone side, stone type, and stone associated symptoms between the two groups ($P > 0.05$) (Table 1). Inclusion criteria: 1. All patients were diagnosed as renal calculi by CTU before surgery; 2. Surgical indications are consistent with PCNL [6]; 3. There was no significant disease of cardiopulmonary and other vital organ dysfunction; 4. Preoperative urine culture was negative, no urinary tract infection or Infection had been controlled; 5. No obvious bleeding tendency, normal liver and kidney function; 6. Invertebrate deformity and unable to prone patients; 7. communicate with patients and their families about the PCNL combined with 3D technology, digital design, and development of personalized percutaneous nephrolithotomy guide plate, obtain the consent of patients and their families, and sign the informed consent surgery.

A construction of 3D printing individualized percutaneous nephroscopy guides plate

All 10 patients in the experimental group were placed in the supine position. CTU examination (256-slice spiral CT Philips) was performed with 5 mm thickness and 1.25 mm reconstruction. During a plain scan, the gray values of ribs and stones were higher than those of surrounding soft tissues, and the gray values of ureters, pelvis, and calyx were higher than those of renal artery, renal vein, aorta, and renal cortex; during arterial phase, the gray values of ureters, pelvis, and calyx were higher than those of renal artery, renal vein. During the excretion period, the gray value of the pelvis, calyx, and ureter can be increased because of the contrast agent to distinguish it from other soft tissues. The Dicom image file obtained by CT scan is used as initial data. Then, the Dicom file is imported into Mimics 17.0 software (Materialise Company of Belgium); according to the corresponding threshold segmentation and regional growth functions, kidney and pelvic calculi are established. 3-D reconstruction models of ribs and skin are saved in STL format.

Table 1 General information of two groups of patients

Patients profile	Experience group (n = 10)	Control group (n = 12)	*P*
Age: (years)	48.60 ± 9.69	45.33 ± 8.52	0.410
Stone side: (L/R)	4/6	5/7	0.937
Gender: (M/L)	5/5	7/5	0.696
Stone types: (staghorn/solitary/multiple occurrences (e.g.)	5/2/3	4/5/3	0.542
Complaint: (lumbar pain/discomfort/naked hematuria)	6/2/2	7/3/2	0.953

Then STL was imported into 3-Matic software, and the skin was smoothed with the guide plate. L1 and L2 were fixed points, and the lower edge of twelve or eleven ribs of the posterior axillary line were puncture points. Draw the surface surrounded by the positioning point, cut the surface appropriately, make the middle hollow, leave space for the color Doppler ultrasound probe, simulate the needle insertion cylinder to increase to 5 mm, use "Boolean subtraction" to determine the inner diameter of the needle insertion channel (1.5 mm), and generate the digital model of the guide. PLA material is used to print on the 3D printer (Raise 3D N2, Suzhou Wuchuang 3D Technology Co., Ltd.); after printing, the guiding device is used for reserve during operation after plasma sterilization (Fig. 1). Each guide plate costs about 500 USD. We also built the spinal model according to CTU, then designed the guide plate according to the position of the spinal model L1 and L2, and determined the point position of L1 and L2 on the guide plate. Before surgery, the patient was placed in a left decubitus position, and the patient grasped his hands over his knees to bend the spine. The surgeon found the bone marks on L1 and L2 body surfaces by hand touch and marked them on the body surface with a marker pen, respectively. During the operation, the position of the L1 and L2 guide plate was aligned with the marked on body surface to determine the position of the guide plate. During surgery, the guide plate is positioned with L1 and L2 markers aligned with L1 and L2 markers on the body surface.

Position and surgical methods

Under general anesthesia, all 22 patients were placed in a prone position. Then, the surgical area was disinfected and draped. In the experimental group, we wear virtual reality glasses and can observe the 3D model established before the operation, better assisting the surgical puncture. During the operation, the patients' breathing is maintained by the ventilator. During the puncture, we will suspend the operation of the ventilator (within 1 min) or reduce the tidal volume of the ventilator to control the impact of breathing activities on the puncture. The X area in Figure E in Fig. 1 is reserved for the ultrasonic probe to monitor the depth and angle of the puncture needle in real-time. If any deviation, it can be

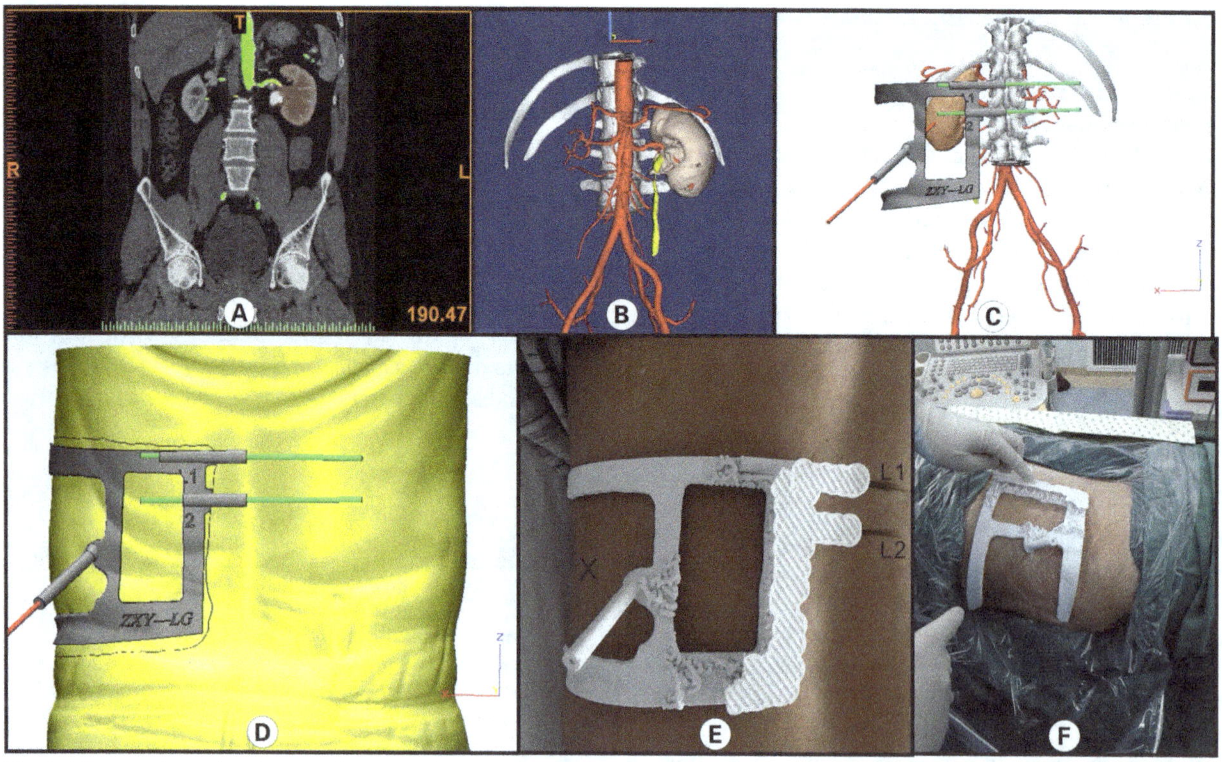

Fig. 1 A Construction and application of a 3-D printing personalized percutaneous nephroscope puncture guide for a patient with left-sided kidney stones shown above. **A** CTU examination shows arterial phase and left kidney stone; **B** three-dimensional reconstruction of the kidney, renal vessels, and kidney stones was achieved by software through CTU images; **C** reconstructing the puncture location point according to the model, the angle, and depth of puncture, avoiding the main vessels; **D** designing the puncture guide plate that fits the skin; **E** 3D printed percutaneous nephroscope puncture guide plate was fixed on the patient skin. **F** The percutaneous puncture localized in patients with percutaneous nephroscope puncture guides by 3-D printing. (**Figure Legend** This figure is our own, drawn by Gao Keyu[1*], Li Shuaishuai[2*], and Ashok Raj[*])

adjusted in real-time After that, the sterilized puncture guide plate was fixed on the patient body. The assistant holds the puncture guide plate to prevent displacement. Then, the puncture needle was inserted through a puncture hole, and the angular position and accuracy of the puncture needle were assessed under USG. In the control group, a Puncture needle was inserted under the direct guidance of USG to locate a stone in the renal pelvis. Then, the PCNL procedure was performed in both groups.

The accuracy of puncture (success rate of single needle puncture)

Intraoperative blood loss (intraoperative blood loss = Hb concentration in the sample of flushing fluid * volume of flushing fluid/preoperative Hb concentration [7]. Combined with intraoperative estimation), puncture time (puncture start to find the calyces where the stones are successfully located) were recorded.

Statistical data analyzed by SPSS 20.0 software

The mean of measurement data (± standard deviation, *t* test, counting data (%), and Fisher exact test for statistical analysis. There was a significant difference in $P<0.05$.

Results

Before the operation, all ten patients were successfully designed and printed with a 3D percutaneous nephrolithotomy guide plate in the experimental group. The direction, depth, and angle of puncture were consistent with the design in the solid computer model. In all ten patients, the intraoperative puncture guide plate fitted to the patients' body skin, and the puncture needle under the guidance of the guide plate and verified by Ultrasound, the success of one puncture was 100.00% (10/10). In the control group, the success rate of one puncture was 75.00% (9/12), and there was no statistical significance between the two groups ($P>0.05$). In both experimental and control groups, the puncture time and intraoperative blood losses were (7.78 ± 0.94/9.04 ± 1.09) min and (49.31 ± 6.43/60.08 ± 12.18) mL, respectively; there was a significant difference between the two groups ($P<0.05$, Table 2).

Discussion

PCNL is an effective treatment for complicated kidney stones [8]. Previous studies have reported that PCNL stone clearance rate and surgical risk are closely related to the choice of the renal puncture site, and the establishment of the correct renal puncture channel is the premise to complete lithotripsy and reduce the incidence of complications such as intraoperative and postoperative massive hemorrhage, liver and pleural injury, and intestinal injury [9]. Therefore, the successful establishment of the renal puncture pathway is the main factor and difficulty of PCNL. We have researched and produced 3D printed guide plates to solve puncture positioning problems and increase puncture positioning accuracy and safety. The traditional methods of assisted renal puncture positioning mainly include X-ray or Ultrasound. Ultrasound and X-ray have their advantages and disadvantages. The X-ray can detect the whole process of a puncture in real-time and determine the residual stones after lithotripsy.

However, there is radiation damage to patients and surgeons, and the vertical depth of the stones is not feasible, and multiple puncture positioning may be required for patients with mild hydronephrosis [10, 11]. Ultrasound can distinguish the location of renal calculi and the thickness of surrounding renal parenchyma without radiation damage, thus improving the success rate of puncture and reducing the bleeding-related complications. However, Ultrasound requires the high ultrasonic skill of the surgeon and a long learning period, and it is not as straightforward as X-ray for stone imaging [12].

In this study, we found that the 3D percutaneous nephrolithotomy guide plate was made and applied to locate the kidney before puncture and guide the direction and angle of the puncture needle during puncture to reach the optimal renal calyx where the calculi were located, which could increase the accuracy of kidney puncture and simplify the puncture process and improve

Table 2 Comparison of puncture time, intraoperative bleeding, and puncture success of the first attempt between two groups

Parameter	Puncture time (min)	Blood loss (mL)	Successful puncture rate in the first attempt (%)
Experimental group	7.78 ± 0.94	49.31 ± 6.43	100.00 (10)
Control group	9.04 ± 1.09	60.08 ± 12.18	75.00 (9)
T	2.913	2.652	
P	0.010	0.017	0.221*

* Fisher Precise test

the puncture accuracy. Moreover, the 3D reconstruction model can enable patients and their families to a more precise understanding of the location of stones, specific surgical methods, and possible surgical risks compared with other imaging assistance techniques: which has a guiding significance for the planning of clinical, surgical plans, improve patients' trust in doctors, and makes the doctor-patient relationship more harmonious.

In this study, we designed an individualized percutaneous nephrolithotomy guide plate with 3D printing. L1 and L2 were selected as a bone landmark, and the puncture guide plate was reconstructed according to the scanning data of CTU in the plain scan period, arterial phase, and excretion period combined with PLA material. The thickness of the guide plate base is designed to be about 1 mm. The angle and depth of the puncture hole of the guide plate were selected according to the three-dimensional reconstructed renal vascular structure, the relatively large safety gap was selected, and the internal diameter of the puncture hole is designed to be 1.5 mm according to the type of the puncture needle. The excess internal diameter of the puncture hole would increase the puncture needle's instability and may cause the puncture angle deviation. The shape of the whole guide plate is designed as a long strip according to the bony marks and puncture points. The hollow design is adopted in part without support, which can save costs and leave space for the color ultrasound probe to monitor the puncture progress in real-time and assist positioning during puncture. We use PLA material because it has the characteristics of heat resistance, impact resistance, low cost, and low pollution, which can reduce the possibility of deformation of the guide plate in the progress of sterilization and disinfection. Under ultrasound-assisted verification during the operation, all the ten patients succeeded in one needle puncture (100.00%) under the guidance of a percutaneous nephroscope puncture guide plate. The positioning of the entry point, the depth, and the puncture angle were consistent with the preoperative design. Compared with the control group (75.00%), the accuracy of puncture location was significantly increased in the experimental group, and shortened the puncture time, and reduced the amount of intraoperative bleeding.

In the localization of renal puncture in PCNL surgery, we need to pay attention to uncontrollable factors such as (1) change in body position: the patients in the supine CT scan and prone position during surgery. (2) bony marker localization deviation. (3) respiratory activity. (4) intestinal or other intraperitoneal organ interference can reduce puncture accuracy and even lead to puncture failure. In order to minimize these uncontrollable factors, we will take the following measures in the future: (1) Preoperative CT scan position consistent with intraoperative position remain prone position and should be given abdominal augmentation according to PCNL position requirements, select the same hardness and flat operation beds because of the change of subtle body position will cause stones and surrounding tissue structure difference. (2) Before CT-urography, we can place two metal patches on the patients' body surface, design the puncture guide model according to the position of the two metal patches, and then keep the metal patches on the patients. During surgery, the marking points of the metal patch on the puncture guide plate are directly aligned with the metal patches on the patients' body surface, making the localization more accurate.

Although the above measures were taken to minimize the influence of uncontrollable factors, we believed that because preoperative intestinal preparation, intraoperative abdominal elevation, respiration, and other factors of the patient could not be consistent with preoperative conditions, there might be some deviation between the intraoperative renal position of the patient and the preoperative CTU, which could affect the puncture accuracy. In the past, 3D printing technology has been extensively used in orthopedics and maxillofacial surgery because of its bony structure, relative position is fixed, but percutaneous renal puncture for breathing is very demanding, mild kidney movement can affect puncture. Even if intraoperative breathing pause is used, the relative kidney position at this time cannot be guaranteed to be the same as that at preoperative CT examination. We preserve ample space for the ultrasonic probe under the puncture guide plate. During the puncture process, we can fine-tune the puncture angle in real-time and correct the puncture accuracy according to the images provided by the Ultrasound, which solves the above problems. However, the puncture template is already finalized and constructed; the puncture angle and position cannot be adjusted too much during the surgery. In the following improvement, we will connect the puncture channel and the base of the puncture template in the way of the ball joint, which is believed to solve this problem more perfectly. The error between clinical positioning of template and computer simulation can be reduced as much as possible through the above methods. In this paper, the 3D puncture guide plate relies on CTU, and CTU is related to patients' renal function. If patients' renal function is inferior, it may affect the CTU imaging, which is a limitation. We can consider combining various imaging techniques to establish a 3D model in context improvements, such as magnetic resonance urography. It should be emphasized that in the development of the model, we did not use ultrasound technology but only used Ultrasound to detect the position of the puncture needle for fine-tuning during the operation. The kidney is located behind the peritoneum. Considering the intestinal tract and other abdominal organs, we selected the puncture point below the 12th rib or around the 11th intercostal rib in the posterior axillary line. Then, the puncture access was determined in combination with the CTU scan results, and the position of the puncture needle was monitored in real-time by Ultrasound, which will minimize damage to the abdominal organs. At the same time, in the improved experiment, the patients' CTU examination position was taken as prone as possible to restore the operation. In addition, the puncture channel adopts a spherical joint, which can also avoid the injury of abdominal organs. As for the intraoperative placement of the guide plate, we had determined the bone marks on the patients' body surface before surgery and marked them with a marker pen. Therefore, we only needed to align the guide plate's L1 and L2 marker points with the body surface markers during the operation, and then the assistant helped to press the guide plate. The whole process does not take much time. With the development of 3D technology, we believe that these aspects will not impose restrictions on the clinical application of 3D printing technology in the urology department. In addition, another limitation of this paper is that the sample size is too small, which may affect our statistical result. Therefore, in the following work, we still need more samples to verify our conclusion.

Conclusion

In summary, the 3D printing puncture guide provides a new method for PCNL puncture with high accuracy and safety compared with traditional color ultrasound puncture. This paper is a preliminary exploration of the application of 3D printing technology in a clinical puncture in urology. It is believed that with the maturation and development of 3D printing technology, it will be more prevalent in urology in the future.

Acknowledgements
None.

Authors' contributions
GK: Data Collection, Manuscript Writing, Data Analysis. LS: Data Collection, Manuscript Writing, Data Analysis. AR: Data Collection, Manuscript Writing, Data Analysis. LS: Data Collection. LS: Data Collection. ZY: Data Collection. ZH: Manuscript Writing. WJ: Manuscript Writing. All authors read and approved the final manuscript.

Author details
[1]Department of Urology, The Affiliated Hospital of Xuzhou Medical University, Xuzhou 221000, China. [2]Xuzhou Medical University, Xuzhou 221000, China. [3]Xuzhou Central Hospital, Xuzhou 221000, China. [4]Xuzhou Children's Hospital, Xuzhou 221000, China.

References

1. Lojanapiwat B. The ideal puncture approach for PCNL: fluoroscopy, ultrasound or endoscopy? Indian J Urol IJU J Urol Soc India. 2013;29(3):208.
2. Ullah A, Khan MK, Rahman AU, Naeem M, Khan S, Rehman R. Total ultrasound guided percutaneous nephrolithotomy: a novel technique. Gomal J Med Sci. 2013; 11(2).
3. Chu C, Masic S, Usawachintachit M, Hu W, Yang W, Stoller M, et al. Ultrasound-guided renal access for percutaneous nephrolithotomy: a description of three novel ultrasound-guided needle techniques. J Endourol. 2016;30(2):153–8.
4. Eltorai AE, Nguyen E, Daniels AHJO. Three-dimensional printing in orthopedic surgery. Orthopedics. 2015;38(11):684–7.
5. Dawood A, Marti BM, Sauret-Jackson V, Darwood A. 3D printing in dentistry. Br Dent J. 2015;219(11):521.
6. Assimos DG. Re: EAU guidelines on interventional treatment for urolithiasis. J Urol. 2016;195(3):659.
7. Kukreja R, Desai M, Patel S, Bapat S, Desai M. First prize: factors affecting blood loss during percutaneous nephrolithotomy: prospective Study. J Endourol. 2004;18(8):715–22.
8. Bird VG, Fallon B, Winfield H. Practice patterns in the treatment of large renal stones. J Endourol. 2003;17(6):355–63.
9. Bader MJ, Gratzke C, Seitz M, Sharma R, Stief CG, Desai M. The, "all-seeing needle": initial results of an optical puncture system confirming access in percutaneous nephrolithotomy. Eur Urol. 2011;59(6):1054–9.
10. Osman M, Wendt-Nordahl G, Heger K, Michel MS, Alken P, Knoll T. Percutaneous nephrolithotomy with ultrasonography-guided renal access: experience from over 300 cases. BJU Int. 2005;96(6):875–8.
11. Zegel H, Pollack H, Banner M, Goldberg B, Arger P, Mulhern C, et al. Percutaneous nephrostomy: comparison of sonographic and fluoroscopic guidance. Am J Roentgenol. 1981;137(5):925–7.
12. Wang K, Zhang P, Xu X, Fan M. Ultrasonographic versus fluoroscopic access for percutaneous nephrolithotomy: a meta-analysis. Urol Int. 2015;95(1):15–25.

12

Risk factor analysis of intravesical recurrence after retroperitoneoscopic nephroureterectomy for upper tract urothelial carcinoma

Masato Yanagi[1*], Tsutomu Hamasaki[2], Jun Akatsuka[1], Yuki Endo[1], Hayato Takeda[1] and Yukihiro Kondo[1]

Abstract

Background: One of the major concerns of patients with upper tract urothelial carcinoma (UTUC) treated with nephroureterectomy is intravesical recurrence (IVR). The purpose of the present study was to investigate the predictive risk factors for IVR after retroperitoneoscopic nephroureterectomy (RNU) for UTUC.

Methods: Clinicopathological and surgical information were collected from the medical records of 73 patients treated with RNU for non-metastatic UTUC, without a history of or concomitant bladder cancer. The association between IVR after RNU and clinicopathological and surgery-related factors, including preoperative urine cytology and pneumoretroperitoneum time, was analyzed using the Fisher exact test.

Results: During the median follow-up time of 39.1 months, 18 (24.7%) patients had subsequent IVR after RNU. The 1- and 3-year IVR-free survival rates were 85.9% and 76.5%, respectively. The Fisher exact test revealed that prolonged pneumoretroperitoneum time of ≥ 210 min was a risk factor for IVR in 1 year after RNU ($p = 0.0358$) and positive urine cytology was a risk factor for IVR in 3 years after RNU ($p = 0.0352$).

Conclusions: In UTUC, the occurrences of IVR in 1 and 3 years after RNU are highly probable when the pneumoretroperitoneum time is prolonged (≥ 210 min) and in patients with positive urine cytology, respectively. Strict follow-up after RNU is more probable recommended for these patients.

Keywords: Upper urinary tract, Urothelial carcinoma, Retroperitoneoscopic nephroureterectomy, Pneumoretroperitoneum time, Intravesical recurrence, Urine cytology

Background

Upper tract urothelial carcinoma (UTUC) is a relatively uncommon condition and accounts for 5–10% of all urothelial malignancies [1]. Nephroureterectomy (NU) with excision of the bladder cuff is the gold standard treatment for non-metastatic UTUC. However, intravesical recurrence (IVR) after NU for UTUC frequently occurs, with an incidence rate of approximately 22–47% [1–4]. Several studies have investigated the risk factors of IVR after NU for UTUC. Reportedly, the risk factors for IVR after NU for UTUC include positive preoperative urine cytology, preoperative diagnostic ureteroscopic biopsy for UTUC, surgery-related factors, such as laparoscopic surgery or endoscopic approach of the bladder cuff excision, lymphovascular invasion (LVI), and concomitant carcinoma in situ (CIS) [4–8].

Recently, laparoscopic NU (LNU) and retroperitoneoscopic NU (RNU) are being performed globally for UTUC. However, there have been discussions about whether LNU and RNU increase the risk of postoperative IVR compared to open NU, and a consensus is yet to be reached [9–13]. On the other hand, few studies have

*Correspondence: area-i@nms.ac.jp
[1] Department of Urology, Nippon Medical School Hospital, 1-1-5, Sendagi, Bunkyo-ku, Tokyo 113-8603, Japan
Full list of author information is available at the end of the article

investigated the risk factors of IVR after LNU and RNU, including surgery-related factors.

The purpose of the present study was to investigate the association between IVR after RNU for UTUC and clinicopathological and surgical factors, including preoperative urine cytology, urinary bladder tumor antigen (BTA), urinary nuclear mitotic apparatus protein (NMP22), and pneumoretroperitoneum time.

Methods

Patient selection

We retrospectively identified 102 patients treated with RNU for non-metastatic UTUC at Nippon Medical School Hospital between 2012 and 2020. UTUC was diagnosed using computed tomography (CT), magnetic resonance imaging (MRI), and urine cytology. A diagnostic ureteroscopic biopsy was performed when required. All patients underwent preoperative cystoscopy. Of the 102 patients, 29 patients with a history of bladder cancer or concomitant bladder cancer were excluded from our study. Finally, 73 patients were included in the study.

Clinicopathological data

From the medical records, we collected clinicopathological and surgical information of the patients, including age, sex, laterality and location of the main tumor, presence or absence of hydronephrosis, preoperative urine cytology, preoperative urinary BTA level, preoperative urinary NMP22 level, necessity of diagnostic ureteroscopic biopsy, pneumoretroperitoneum time, total operating time, multifocality of the tumor, tumor size, pathological characteristics, necessity of adjuvant systemic chemotherapy (ASC), and oncological outcomes. Tumors were staged according to the 2002 American Joint Committee of Cancer tumor-node-metastasis classification and were graded according to the 2004 World Health Organization classification [14].

Surgical procedure

While performing RNU, retroperitoneoscopic procedures were performed in the kidney position, with 8 mmHg CO_2 gas pressure in all cases. The CO_2 gas pressure was increased temporally when necessary. The maximum pressure of the CO_2 gas was 12 mmHg. In the retroperitoneoscopic procedure, we clamped the ureter after ligation of the renal arteries. In all patients, a small iliac incision (Gibson incision) or lower abdominal midline incision was made to retrieve the kidney and ureter and to perform bladder cuff resection with sufficient surgical margin using the extravesical approach. In our institution, we have performed RNU in patients with non-metastatic localized or locally advanced UTUC (cTa-3N0M0). Lymphadenectomy was not performed in this study.

Adjuvant therapy and follow-up

Adjuvant intravesical therapy is not administered at our institution. Four courses of ASC, such as the gemcitabine/cisplatin regimen or gemcitabine/carboplatin regimen, were administered to select pT2–4 patients. Of these patients, those with an estimated glomerular filtration rate (eGFR) of < 30 ml/min/1.73 m^2 received ASC with the gemcitabine/carboplatin regimen, and the other patients received ASC with the gemcitabine/cisplatin regimen. After RNU, all patients were generally followed-up using blood tests, urine analysis, urine cytology, cystoscopy, and CT scan every three months for two years, and every six months thereafter. We defined IVR as a pathologically diagnosed bladder cancer after RNU. We also defined progression disease as radiologically diagnosed local or distance recurrence.

Endpoint of the present study

The primary endpoint of the present study was to investigate the association between IVR after RNU for UTUC and clinicopathological and surgical factors, including preoperative factors of urine cytology, urinary BTA, urinary NMP22, and pneumoretroperitoneum time.

Statistical analysis

Statistical analyses were performed using JMP® 13 (SAS Institute Inc., Cary, NC, USA). The value of statistical significance was set at $p < 0.05$. The categorical variables were compared using the Fisher exact test and continuous variables using the t-test or the Mann–Whitney U test, depending on the results of the one-sample Kolmogorov–Smirnov test. Survival curves were constructed using the Kaplan–Meier method. To determine the risk factors for IVR in 1 and 3 years after RNU, the Fisher exact test was performed. In the analyses of IVR and progression 1 year after RNU, no IVR and progression cases without 1 year or >1 year of follow-up were excluded. In the analyses of IVR and progression 3 years after RNU, no IVR and progression cases without 3 years or >3 years of follow-up were excluded. The cut-off value of the pneumoretroperitoneum time of RNU was 210 min, which was defined as the maximum pneumoretroperitoneum time in the technical certification test of RNU by the Japanese Society of Endourology [15].

Results

Table 1 demonstrates the characteristics of 73 patients treated with RNU for UTUC. Surgical margins of the bladder cuff were negative in all patients.

Table 1 Characteristics of patients treated with RNU for upper urinary tract carcinoma

Preoperative factors		**n = 73 (%)**
Age (years)	Median (IQR 25–75)	74 (67–79)
Gender	Male/female	56 (76.7)/17 (23.3)
Laterality	Right/left	37 (50.7)/36 (49.3)
Location of main tumor	Ureter/renal pelvis	33 (45.2)/40 (54.8)
Hydronephrosis	Yes/no	24 (32.9)/49 (67.1)
Urine cytology	Positive/negative	32 (43.8)/41 (56.2)
Urinary BTA	Positive/negative	29 (39.7)/44 (60.3)
Urinary NMP22	Positive/negative	36 (49.3)/37 (50.7)
Diagnostic ureteroscopic biopsy	Yes/no	24 (32.9)/49 (67.1)
Intraoperative and postoperative factors		
Pneumoretroperitoneum time (min)	Median (IQR 25–75)	202 (170–268)
	≥210/<210	32 (43.8)/41 (56.2)
Total operating time (min)	median (IQR 25–75)	352 (302–402)
	≥360/<360	32 (43.8)/41 (56.2)
Multifocality	multiple/ single	11 (15.1)/62 (84.9)
Tumor size (cm)	≥3/<3	40 (54.8)/33 (43.8)
Pathological T stage	≤1/2/≥3	30 (41.1)/18 (24.7)/25 (34.2)
Grade	1, 2/3	37 (50.7)/36 (49.3)
LVI	Positive/negative	18 (24.7)/55 (75.3)
INF	a/b, c	21 (28.8)/52 (71.2)
ASC	Yes/ no	23 (31.5)/50 (68.5)

IQR interquartile range, *BTA* bladder tumor antigen, *NMP22* nuclear mitotic apparatus protein, *LVI* lymphovascular invasion, *INF* infiltrative growth, *ASC* adjuvant systemic chemotherapy

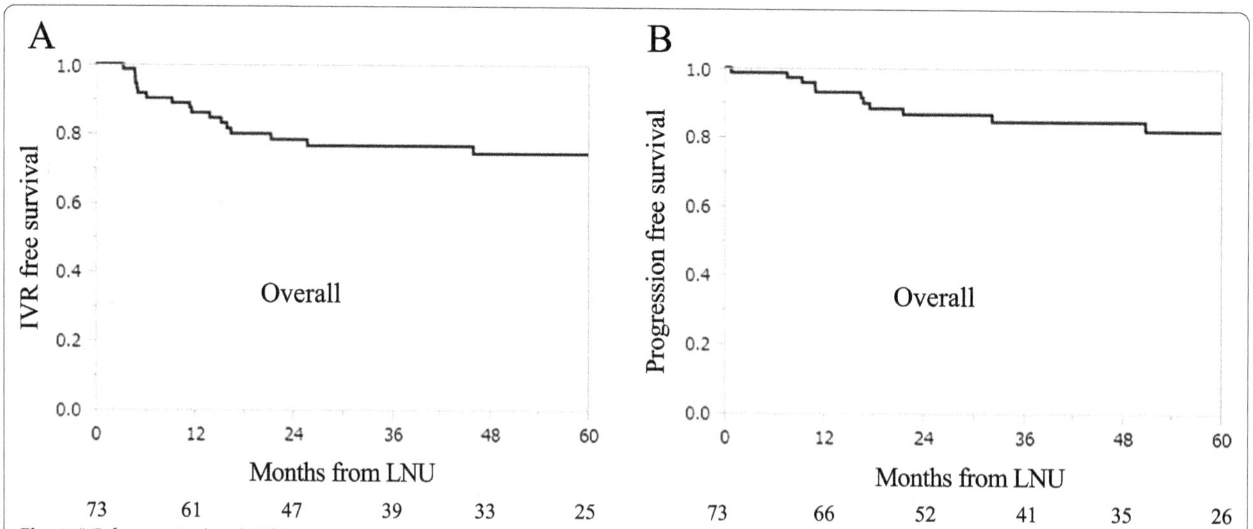

Fig. 1 IVR-free survival and PFS in 73 patients. **A** Kaplan–Meier curves of IVR-free survival in 73 patients. **B** Kaplan–Meier curves of PFS in 73 patients

During the median follow-up of 39.1 months after RNU, 18 (24.7%) patients had IVR. The 1-year and 3-year IVR-free survival rates were 85.9% and 76.5%, respectively (Fig. 1A). The histological type of bladder cancer in 18 patients was urothelial carcinoma. Table 2 demonstrates the multifocality and location of IVR tumors. In 50% of these bladder cancers, the grade was lower than that of the initial UTUC diagnosis. In the other 50% of bladder cancer cases, the grade was the same grade as that of the initial UTUC. None of

Table 2 Multifocality and location of intravesical recurrence tumors

	n = 18 (%)
Multifocality	
Single	14 (77.8)
Multiple	4 (22.2)
Tumor location	
Scar site	11 (61.1)
Bladder neck	5 (27.8)
Lateral wall	4 (22.2)
Dome	1 (5.5)
Posterior wall	1 (5.5)

the bladder cancers had a higher grade than the initial UTUC diagnosis.

The Fisher exact test revealed that prolonged pneumoretroperitoneum time of ≥210 min was a risk factor for IVR in 1 year after RNU ($p=0.0358$) (Table 3) and positive urine cytology was a risk factor for IVR in 3 years after RNU ($p=0.0352$) (Table 4).

Table 5 demonstrates two group analyses based on the pneumoretroperitoneum time of 210 min to investigate the presence of bias. No significant difference between these two groups was noted.

Of the 73 cases, 15 (20.5%) were positive for urine cytology, NMP22, and BTA, and 18 (24.7%) were positive for two of these three.

During the median follow-up of 41.9 months after LNU, 12 (16.4%) patients had a metastatic recurrence. The 1-year and 3-year progression-free survival (PFS) rates were 92.9% and 84.5%, respectively (Fig. 1B). The Fisher exact test revealed that pathological T ≥ 3 was a risk factor for progression in 1 year after RNU (p = 0.0439) (Table 6), and pathological T ≥ 3 ($p=0.0007$), Grade 3 ($p=0.0145$), LNI ($p=0.0073$), and ASC ($p=0.0088$) were the risk factors for progression in 3 years after RNU (Table 7).

Discussion

LNU is the mainstream surgery for UTUC and RNU is not popularly performed [8, 16, 17]. Therefore, most studies are focused on LNU. Here, we focused on RNU. This is the first report investigating the risk factors, including the pneumoretroperitoneum time, for IVR after RNU.

In this study, prolonged pneumoretroperitoneum time of ≥210 min was a risk factor for IVR in 1 year after RNU, with 8 mmHg CO_2 gas pressure (Table 3). In a previous study, Shigeta et al. reported that prolonged pneumoperitoneum time of LNU for UTUC was an independent risk factor for IVR [8]. They performed LNU (62.8%) and RNU (37.2%) for their cohort. The results of the present and the previous studies suggested that CO_2 gas pressure time impact on IVR. Shigeta et al. analyzed a cohort similar to this study that excluded patients with a history of bladder cancer or concomitant bladder cancer; the IVR rate was 47.3% during the median follow-up of 31.1 months postoperatively. They performed LNU or RNU with 10 mmHg CO_2 gas pressure and the median pneumoperitoneum or pneumoretroperitoneum time was 150 min; meanwhile, the median pneumoretroperitoneum time of the present study was 202 min, which was significantly longer than that of their study. However, in the present study, the IVR rate after RNU was 24.7% during the median follow-up of 39.1 months postoperatively, which was significantly lower than that of the study by Shigeta et al. When the two studies were compared, the differences were observed in CO_2 gas pressure and surgical procedure. It was suggested that a low CO_2 gas pressure of 8 mmHg and/or RNU in the present study might have influenced the low IVR rates. Further studies with large cohorts comparing different CO_2 gas pressures are needed to investigate the impact of CO_2 gas pressure on IVR postoperatively. Moreover, we only analyzed RNU in this study; therefore, it remains unclear whether the results of this study apply to LNU, because the pressure on the ureter during surgery might be different between RNU and LNU. Further studies comparing RNU and LNU are required.

This study was a retrospective study without a pilot study. The study began in February 2021, and the results were disclosed to all urologists at our institution in April 2021. Therefore, there was no bias of knowledge in the study results. We also analyzed the factors related to prolonged pneumoretroperitoneum time. However, any factors related to prolonged pneumoretroperitoneum time were not present (Table 5).

Recent molecular genetic studies have suggested that intraluminal seeding is one of the main mechanisms of IVR after NU [18–20]. It was also reported that continuous intravesical irrigation with distilled water or physiological saline solution during LNU decreased the rate of IVR incidence [16]. They concluded that continuous intravesical irrigation might eliminate cancer cells floating in the bladder during surgery before they become engrafted on the mucous membrane of the bladder. This result suggests that IVR after NU occurs due to intraluminal seeding. Recent studies demonstrated that prolonged CO_2 gas pressure time and diagnostic ureteroscopic biopsy are independent factors of IVR after NU [5, 8]. Based on these results of past studies, long-term CO_2 gas pressure to the tumor and direct destruction of the tumor by diagnostic ureteroscopic biopsy might

Table 3 Risk factor analysis of IVR in 1 year after RNU

Variables		No IVR n = 60 (%)	IVR n = 10 (%)	*p*-value
Age (years)	≥ 70	42 (70.0)	5 (50.0)	0.2790
Gender	Male	45 (75.0)	8 (80.0)	1.0000
Laterality	Right	32 (53.3)	4 (40.0)	0.5079
Location of main tumor	Ureter	25 (41.7)	6 (60.0)	0.3203
Hydronephrosis	Yes	19 (31.7)	3 (30.0)	1.0000
Urine cytology	Positive	24 (40.0)	7 (70.0)	0.0956
Urinary BTA	Positive	22 (36.7)	6 (60.0)	0.1833
Urinary NMP22	Positive	28 (46.7)	5 (50.0)	1.0000
Diagnostic ureteroscopic biopsy	Yes	18 (30.0)	5 (50.0)	0.2790
Multifocality	Multiple	6 (10.0)	3 (30.0)	0.1120
Tumor size (cm)	≥ 3	29 (48.3)	3 (30.0)	0.3263
Pathological T stage	≥ 3	19 (31.7)	5 (50.0)	0.2945
Grade	3	29 (48.3)	5 (50.0)	1.0000
LVI	Positive	15 (25.0)	2 (20.0)	1.0000
INF	b, c	41 (68.3)	9 (90.0)	0.2618
Pneumoretroperitoneum time (min)	≥ 210	24 (40.0)	8 (80.0)	0.0358*
Total operating time (min)	≥ 360	25 (41.7)	6 (60.0)	0.3203
ASC	Yes	19 (31.7)	4 (40.0)	0.7192

IVR intravesical recurrence, *BTA* bladder tumor antigen, *NMP22* nuclear mitotic apparatus protein, *LVI* lymphovascular invasion, *INF* infiltrative growth, *ASC* adjuvant systemic chemotherapy

*$p < 0.05$

Table 4 Risk factor analysis of IVR in 3 years after RNU

Variables		No IVR n = 38 (%)	IVR n = 16 (%)	*p*-value
Age (years)	≥ 70	26 (68.4)	7 (43.8)	0.1280
Gender	Male	29 (76.3)	12 (75.0)	1.0000
Laterality	Right	18 (47.3)	7 (43.8)	1.0000
Location of main tumor	Ureter	18 (47.3)	8 (50.0)	1.0000
Hydronephrosis	Yes	11 (28.9)	6 (37.5)	0.5402
Urine cytology	Positive	15 (39.5)	12 (75.0)	0.0352*
Urinary BTA	Positive	15 (39.5)	9 (56.3)	0.3695
Urinary NMP22	Positive	17 (44.7)	8 (50.0)	0.7718
Diagnostic ureteroscopic biopsy	Yes	12 (31.6)	8 (50.0)	0.2301
Multifocality	Multiple	3 (7.9)	3 (18.8)	0.3461
Tumor size (cm)	≥ 3	16 (42.1)	7 (43.8)	1.0000
Pathological T stage	≥ 3	11 (28.9)	6 (37.5)	0.5402
Grade	3	16 (42.1)	9 (56.3)	0.3836
LVI	Positive	7 (18.4)	5 (31.3)	0.3090
INF	b, c	27 (71.1)	13 (81.3)	0.5155
Pneumoretroperitoneum time (min)	≥ 210	16 (42.1)	11 (68.8)	0.1350
Total operating time (min)	≥ 360	16 (42.1)	10 (62.5)	0.2358
ASC	Yes	13 (34.2)	5 (31.3)	1.0000

IVR intravesical recurrence, *BTA* bladder tumor antigen, *NMP22* nuclear mitotic apparatus protein, *LVI* lymphovascular invasion, *INF* infiltrative growth; ASC, adjuvant systemic chemotherapy

*$p < 0.05$

Table 5 The characteristics of patients according to pneumoretroperitoneum time

Variables		PT < 210 min n = 41 (%)	PT ≥ 210 min n = 32 (%)	*p*-value
Age (years)	Median (IQR 25–75)	75 (67–80)	74 (67–78)	0.4168
Gender	Male	32 (78.0)	24 (75.0)	0.7865
Laterality	Right	18 (43.9)	19 (59.4)	0.2405
Location of main tumor	Ureter	19 (46.3)	14 (43.8)	1.0000
Hydronephrosis	Yes	15 (36.6)	9 (28.1)	0.4655
Urine cytology	Positive	15 (36.6)	17 (53.1)	0.2345
Urinary BTA	Positive	12 (29.3)	17 (53.1)	0.1496
Urinary NMP22	Positive	20 (48.8)	16 (50.0)	1.0000
Diagnostic ureteroscopic biopsy	Yes	15 (36.6)	9 (28.1)	0.4655
Multifocality	Multiple	6 (14.6)	5 (15.6)	1.0000
Tumor size (cm)	≥ 3	19 (46.3)	14 (43.8)	1.0000
Pathological T stage	≥ 3	15 (36.6)	10 (31.3)	0.8041
Grade	3	22 (53.7)	14 (43.8)	0.4818
LVI	Positive	10 (24.3)	8 (25.0)	1.0000
INF	b, c	30 (73.2)	22 (68.8)	0.7958
ASC	Yes	13 (31.7)	10 (31.3)	1.0000

PT pneumoretroperitoneum time, *IQR* interquartile range, *BTA* bladder tumor antigen, *NMP22* nuclear mitotic apparatus protein, *LVI* lymphovascular invasion, *INF* infiltrative growth, *ASC* adjuvant systemic chemotherapy

Table 6 Risk factor analysis of progression in 1 year after RNU

Variables		No progression n = 65 (%)	Progression n = 5 (%)	*p*-value
Age (years)	≥ 70	42 (64.6)	5 (100.0)	0.1639
Gender	Male	48 (73.8)	5 (100.0)	0.3255
Laterality	Right	33 (50.8)	3 (60.0)	1.0000
Location of main tumor	Ureter	28 (43.1)	3 (60.0)	0.6489
Hydronephrosis	Yes	20 (30.8)	2 (40.0)	0.6463
Urine cytology	Positive	31 (47.7)	0 (0.0)	0.0616
Urinary BTA	Positive	27 (41.5)	1 (20.0)	0.6415
Urinary NMP22	Positive	32 (49.2)	1 (20.0)	0.3608
Diagnostic ureteroscopic biopsy	Yes	21 (32.3)	2 (40.0)	1.0000
Multifocality	Multiple	9 (13.8)	0 (0.0)	1.0000
Tumor size (cm)	≥ 3	28 (43.1)	4 (80.0)	0.1710
Pathological T stage	≥ 3	20 (30.8)	4 (80.0)	0.0439*
Grade	3	30 (46.2)	4 (80.0)	0.1921
LVI	Positive	15 (23.1)	2 (40.0)	0.5887
INF	b, c	45 (69.2)	5 (100.0)	0.3117
Pneumoretroperitoneum time (min)	≥ 210	30 (46.2)	2 (40.0)	1.0000
Total operating time (min)	≥ 360	29 (44.6)	2 (40.0)	1.0000
ASC	Yes	20 (30.8)	3 (60.0)	0.3221

BTA bladder tumor antigen, *NMP22* nuclear mitotic apparatus protein, *LVI* lymphovascular invasion, *INF* infiltrative growth, *ASC* adjuvant systemic chemotherapy

*$p < 0.05$

contribute to intraluminal seeding. In the present study, the grade of bladder cancer with IVR was not higher than that of initial UTUC. It has also been suggested that IVR tumors are caused by intraluminal seeding from UTUC.

Table 7 Risk factor analysis of progression in 3 years after RNU

Variables		No progression n = 40 (%)	Progression n = 10 (%)	*p*-value
Age (years)	≥70	24 (60.0)	7 (70.0)	0.7222
Gender	Male	29 (72.5)	8 (80.0)	1.0000
Laterality	Right	17 (42.5)	6 (60.0)	0.4804
Location of main tumor	Ureter	19 (47.5)	6 (60.0)	0.7252
Hydronephrosis	Yes	12 (30.0)	3 (30.0)	1.0000
Urine cytology	Positive	19 (47.5)	5 (50.0)	1.0000
Urinary BTA	Positive	18 (45.0)	3 (30.0)	0.4880
Urinary NMP22	Positive	18 (45.0)	5 (50.0)	1.0000
Diagnostic ureteroscopic biopsy	Yes	12 (30.0)	3 (30.0)	1.0000
Multifocality	Multiple	4 (10.0)	0 (0.0)	0.5710
Tumor size (cm)	≥3	14 (35.0)	8 (80.0)	0.0836
Pathological T stage	≥3	8 (20.0)	8 (80.0)	0.0007*
Grade	3	22 (55.0)	9 (90.0)	0.0145*
LVI	Positive	6 (15.0)	6 (60.0)	0.0073*
INF	b, c	28 (70.0)	10 (100.0)	0.0920
Pneumoretroperitoneum time (min)	≥210	20 (50.0)	5 (50.0)	1.0000
Total operating time (min)	≥360	19 (47.5)	5 (50.0)	1.0000
ASC	Yes	12 (30.0)	8 (80.0)	0.0088*

BTA bladder tumor antigen, *NMP22* nuclear mitotic apparatus protein, *LVI* lymphovascular invasion, *INF* infiltrative growth, *ASC* adjuvant systemic chemotherapy

*$p < 0.05$

The BTA test detects the human complement factor H-related protein secreted in the urine. While the NMP22 test detects the protein level of the nuclear mitotic apparatus. Positive urinary BTA and NMP22 have been reported as predictors of the presence of bladder cancer and UTUC, along with positive urine cytology [21–24]. In the present study, the risk factor for IVR 3 years after RNU was not positive urinary BTA or urinary NMP22, but positive urine cytology (Table 4). Additionally, only 20.5% of patients had all three positive urine cytology, urinary BTA, and urinary NMP22. There is not much overlap between urine cytology, urinary BTA, and urinary NMP22. Urinary BTA and NMP22 are considered unsuitable for predicting IVR after RNU because the values of urinary BTA and NMP22 generally have a positive correlation with tumor volume; however, urinary BTA and NMP22 do not directly detect cancer cells.

Physical injury to the bladder is associated with increased adherence of tumor cells to the urothelium [25]. In NU, the bladder cuff and ureteral orifice are resected, while a urethral catheter is maintained in the bladder during and several days after NU. Physical injury to the urothelium, such as bladder cuff resection and stimulation of the bladder mucosa with a ureteral catheter, might support the growth of tumor cells in the urothelium [26]. In the present study, 11 (61.1%) and 5 (27.8%) patients had IVR tumors located at scar site and bladder neck, which could have been stimulated by the urethral catheter (Table 2). Hence, this result is consistent with the that of the previous study [26].

Recently, two prospective randomized trials have demonstrated that a single early intravesical chemotherapy cycle using mitomycin C or pirarubicin after NU decreased the risk of IVR [27, 28]. However, the type of patients that will benefit from this treatment remains unclear. In this study, prolonged pneumoretroperitoneum time of ≥210 min was a risk factor for IVR in 1 year after RNU and positive urine cytology was a risk factor for IVR in 3 years after RNU. From our results, we strongly recommend that patients with pneumoperitoneum time of ≥210 min and/or with positive urine cytology should receive a single early intravesical chemotherapy after RNU with 8 mmHg CO_2 gas pressure.

In this study, pathological findings of UTUC were the risk factors for progression after RNU, not pneumoretroperitoneum time (Tables 6, 7). Therefore, when the pneumoretroperitoneum time of RNU is prolonged, an attending physician can perform a follow-up imaging after RNU at normal intervals.

The present study has several limitations. UTUC is a relatively uncommon condition. We excluded patients with a history of bladder cancer or concomitant bladder cancer, because the purpose of the present study was to investigate the risk factors for IVR after RUN for UTUC. In addition, this study was conducted in a single institution; therefore, the cohort in this study was small. Since the study was a retrospective analysis, there might be a selection bias for the surgeons. In this study, 13 surgeons performed the RUN procedure. However, three experienced surgeons who had performed more than 100 laparoscopic surgeries performed or supervised all of the RUN procedures. In addition, the rate of IVR incidence in our study was lower than that reported in previous studies. Based on these facts, we believe that the participation of inexperienced surgeons in RUN had little impact on the IVR rate in the present study. To reduce these limitations, prospective studies with larger cohorts from several institutions are required. Currently, lymphadenectomy is recommended for pathological T ≥ 2 UTUC. However, lymphadenectomy was not performed in this study. The reasons are that there are several discrepancies between the clinical T stage and the pathological T stage, and there are technical issues with retroperitoneoscopic lymphadenectomy. The lack of lymphadenectomy in this study might impact on PFS. In our institution, we performed open NU and lymphadenectomy only in cases suspected of visible lymph node metastasis on CT. There is an urgent need to improve the accuracy of diagnostic imaging for staging and lymphadenectomy for clinical T ≥ 2 UTUC. Finally, the risks of IVR logically related to the time from infusing CO_2 gas pressure to the clipping of the ureter. However, we were only able to collect the data on clipping time of the ureter for some patients using their operation and intraoperative nursing records. Therefore, it was difficult to analyze association between IVR after RNU and the time from infusing CO_2 gas pressure to the clipping of the ureter. Further studies analyzing the association between IVR after RNU and the time from infusing CO_2 gas pressure to the clipping of the ureter are required.

Conclusions

In UTUC, the occurrence of IVR in 1 year after RNU is highly probable when the pneumoretroperitoneum time is prolonged (≥ 210 min) and the occurrence of IVR in 3 years after RNU is highly probable in patients with positive urine cytology. Strict follow-up after RNU is more probable recommended for these patients.

Abbreviations

ASC: Adjuvant systemic chemotherapy; BTA: Bladder tumor antigen; CIS: Carcinoma in situ; CT: Computed tomography; eGFR: Estimated glomerular filtration rate; INF: Infiltrative growth; IVR: Intravesical recurrence; LNU: Laparoscopic nephroureterectomy; LVI: Lymphovascular invasion; NMP22: Nuclear mitotic apparatus protein 22; NU: Nephroureterectomy; PFS: Progression-free survival; RNU: Retroperitoneoscopic nephroureterectomy; UTUC: Upper tract urothelial carcinoma.

Acknowledgements

The authors thank Editage for editing English of our manuscript.

Authors' contributions

Conception and Design: MY Collection of data: MY and YE Data analysis: MY. Manuscript writing: All authors. All authors read and approved the final manuscript.

Author details

[1]Department of Urology, Nippon Medical School Hospital, 1-1-5, Sendagi, Bunkyo-ku, Tokyo 113-8603, Japan. [2]Department of Urology, Nippon Medical School Musashikosugi Hospital, 1-396, Kosugityo, Nakahara-ku, Kawasaki city, Kanagawa 211-8533, Japan.

References

1. Rouprêt M, Babjuk M, Burger M, Capoun O, Cohen D, Compérat EM, et al. European association of urology guidelines on upper urinary tract urothelial carcinoma: 2020 update. Eur Urol. 2021;79:62–79.
2. Tanaka N, Kikuchi E, Kanao K, Matsumoto K, Shirotake S, Kobayashi H, et al. The predictive value of positive urine cytology for outcomes following radical nephroureterectomy in patients with primary upper tract urothelial carcinoma: a multi-institutional study. Urol Oncol. 2014;32(48):e19-26.
3. Hirano D, Okada Y, Nagane Y, Satoh K, Mochida J, Yamanaka Y, et al. Intravesical recurrence after surgical management of urothelial carcinoma of the upper urinary tract. Urol Int. 2012;89:71–7.
4. Liu W, Wang Z, Liu S, Yao Y, Liu Y, Zhang G. Preoperative positive voided urine cytology predicts poor clinical outcomes in patients with upper tract urothelial carcinoma undergoing nephroureterectomy. BMC Cancer. 2020;20:1113.
5. Sharma V, Miest TS, Juvet TS, Toussi A, Packiam V, Chamie K, et al. The impact of upper tract urothelial carcinoma diagnostic modality on intravesical recurrence after radical nephroureterectomy: a single institution series and updated meta-analysis. J Urol. 2021. https://doi.org/10.1097/JU.0000000000001834.
6. Xylinas E, Colin P, Audenet F, Phe V, Cormier L, Cussenot O, et al. Intravesical recurrence after radical nephroureterectomy for upper tract urothelial carcinomas: predictors and impact on subsequent oncological outcomes from a national multicenter study. World J Urol. 2013;31:61–8.
7. Xylinas E, Rink M, Cha EK, Clozel T, Lee RK, Fajkovic H, et al. Upper Tract Urothelial Carcinoma Collaboration. Impact of distal ureter management on oncologic outcomes following radical nephroureterectomy for upper tract urothelial carcinoma. Eur Urol. 2014;65:210–7.
8. Shigeta K, Kikuchi E, Hagiwara M, Ando T, Mizuno R, Miyajima A, et al. Prolonged pneumoperitoneum time is an independent risk factor for intravesical recurrence after laparoscopic radical nephroureterectomy in upper tract urothelial carcinoma. Surg Oncol. 2017;26:73–9.
9. Shigeta K, Kikuchi E, Abe T, Hagiwara M, Ogihara K, Anno T, et al. Long-term oncologic outcomes of laparoscopic versus open radical nephroureterectomy for patients with T3N0M0 upper tract urothelial carcinoma: a multicenter cohort study with adjustment by propensity score matching. Ann Surg Oncol. 2019;26:3774–81.
10. Kim SH, Song MK, Kim JK, Hong B, Kang SH, Ku JH, et al. Laparoscopy versus open nephroureterectomy in prognostic outcome of patients with advanced upper tract urothelial cancer: a retrospective, multicentre, propensity-score matching analysis. Cancer Res Treat. 2019;51:963–72.
11. Piszczek R, Nowak Ł, Krajewski W, Chorbińska J, Poletajew S, Moschini M, et al. Oncological outcomes of laparoscopic versus open nephroureterectomy for the treatment of upper tract urothelial carcinoma: an updated meta-analysis. World J Surg Oncol. 2021;19:129.
12. Ni S, Tao W, Chen Q, Liu L, Jiang H, Hu H, et al. Laparoscopic versus open nephroureterectomy for the treatment of upper urinary tract urothelial carcinoma: a systematic review and cumulative analysis of comparative studies. Eur Urol. 2012;61:1142–53.
13. Seisen T, Granger B, Colin P, Léon P, Utard G, Renard-Penna R, et al. A systematic review and meta-analysis of clinicopathologic factors linked to intravesical recurrence after radical nephroureterectomy to treat upper tract urothelial carcinoma. Eur Urol. 2015;67:1122–33.
14. Soukup V, Čapoun O, Cohen D, Hernández V, Babjuk M, Burger M, et al. Prognostic performance and reproducibility of the 1973 and 2004/2016 World Health Organization Grading Classification Systems in Non-muscle-invasive Bladder Cancer: a European Association of Urology

non-muscle invasive bladder cancer guidelines panel systematic review. Eur Urol. 2017;72:801–13.
15. Yanagi M, Kimura G, Sekine T, Takeda H, Akatsuka J, Endo Y, et al. Factors associated with prolonged retroperitoneal laparoscopic radical nephrectomy performed by non-expert surgeons. J Nippon Med Sch. 2021;88:109–12.
16. Yamamoto S, Sakamoto S, Imamura Y, Sazuka T, Nakamura K, Inoue T, et al. Intravesical irrigation might prevent bladder recurrence in patients undergoing radical nephroureterectomy for upper urinary tract urothelial carcinoma. Int J Urol. 2019;26:791–6.
17. Zou L, Zhang L, Zhang H, Jiang H, Ding Q. Comparison of post-operative intravesical recurrence and oncological outcomes after open versus laparoscopic nephroureterectomy for upper urinary tract urothelial carcinoma. World J Urol. 2014;32:565–70.
18. Hafner C, Knuechel R, Stoehr R, Hartmann A. Clonality of multifocal urothelial carcinomas: 10 years of molecular genetic studies. Int J Cancer. 2002;101:1–6.
19. Hafner C, Knuechel R, Zanardo L, Dietmaier W, Blaszyk H, Cheville J, et al. Evidence for oligoclonality and tumor spread by intraluminal seeding in multifocal urothelial carcinomas of the upper and lower urinary tract. Oncogene. 2001;20:4910–5.
20. Miyake H, Hara I, Kamidono S, Eto H. Multifocal transitional cell carcinoma of the bladder and upper urinary tract: molecular screening of clonal origin by characterizing CD44 alternative splicing patterns. J Urol. 2004;172:1127–9.
21. Babjuk M, Soukup V, Pesl M, Kostírová M, Drncová E, Smolová H, et al. Urinary cytology and quantitative BTA and UBC tests in surveillance of patients with pTapT1 bladder urothelial carcinoma. Urology. 2008;71:718–22.
22. Walsh IK, Keane PF, Ishak LM, Flessland KA. The BTA stat test: a tumor marker for the detection of upper tract transitional cell carcinoma. Urology. 2001;58:532–5.
23. Kumar A, Kumar R, Gupta NP. Comparison of NMP22 BladderChek test and urine cytology for the detection of recurrent bladder cancer. Jpn J Clin Oncol. 2006;36:172–5.
24. Jovanovic M, Soldatovic I, Janjic A, Vuksanovic A, Dzamic Z, Acimovic M, et al. Diagnostic value of the nuclear matrix protein 22 test and urine cytology in upper tract urothelial tumors. Urol Int. 2011;87:134–7.
25. See WA, Chapman PH. Heparin prevention of tumor cell adherence and implantation on injured urothelial surfaces. J Urol. 1987;138:182–6.
26. Ito A, Shintaku I, Satoh M, Ioritani N, Tochigi T, Numata I, et al. Intravesical seeding of upper urinary tract urothelial carcinoma cells during nephroureterectomy: an exploratory analysis from the THPMG trial. Jpn J Clin Oncol. 2013;43:1139–44.
27. Ito A, Shintaku I, Satoh M, Ioritani N, Aizawa M, Tochigi T, et al. Prospective randomized phase II trial of a single early intravesical instillation of pirarubicin (THP) in the prevention of bladder recurrence after nephroureterectomy for upper urinary tract urothelial carcinoma: the THP Monotherapy Study Group Trial. J Clin Oncol. 2013;31:1422–7.
28. O'Brien T, Ray E, Singh R, Coker B, Beard R; British Association of Urological Surgeons Section of Oncology. Prevention of bladder tumours after nephroureterectomy for primary upper urinary tract urothelial carcinoma: a prospective, multicentre, randomised clinical trial of a single postoperative intravesical dose of mitomycin C (the ODMIT-C Trial). Eur Urol. 2011;60:703–10.

13

Three-port approach *vs* standard laparoscopic radical cystectomy with an ileal conduit: A single-centre retrospective study

Zhouting Tuo†, Ying Zhang†, Jinyou Wang, Huan Zhou, Youlu Lu, Xin Wang, Chao Yang, Dexin Yu and Liangkuan Bi*

Abstract

Background: This study aimed to evaluate the effect of the three-port approach and conventional five-port laparoscopic radical cystectomy (LRC) with an ileal conduit.

Methods: Eighty-four patients, who were diagnosed with high-risk non-muscle-invasive and muscle-invasive bladder carcinoma and underwent LRC with an ileal conduit between January 2018 and April 2020, were retrospectively evaluated. Thirty and fifty-four patients respectively underwent the three-port approach and five-port LRC. Clinical characteristics, pathological data, perioperative outcomes, and follow-up data were analysed.

Results: There were no differences in perioperatively surgical outcome, including pathology type, prostate adenocarcinoma incidence, tumour staging, and postoperative creatinine levels between the two groups. The operative time (271.3 ± 24.03 vs. 279.57 ± 48.47 min, $P = 0.299$), estimated blood loss (65 vs. 90 mL, $P = 0.352$), time to passage of flatus (8 vs. 10 days, $P = 0.084$), and duration of hospitalisation post-surgery (11 vs. 12 days, $P = 0.922$) were no clear difference between both groups. Compared with the five-port group, the three-port LRC group was related to lower inpatient costs (12 453 vs. 14 134 \$, $P = 0.021$). Our follow-up results indicated that the rate of postoperative complications, 90-day mortality, and the oncological outcome did not show meaningful differences between these two groups.

Conclusions: Three-port LRC with an ileal conduit is technically safe and feasible for the treatment of bladder cancer. On comparing the three-port LRC with the five-port LRC, our technique does not increase the rate of short-term and long-term complications and tumour recurrence, but the treatment costs of the former were reduced.

Keywords: Three-port, Laparoscopic radical cystectomy, Bladder cancer, Ileal conduit

Background

Radical cystectomy (RC) and urinary diversion remain standard procedures for high-risk non-muscle-invasive and muscle-invasive bladder carcinoma [1]. However, RC is one of the most challenging urologic surgeries because of its postoperative complications and high mortality. Nevertheless, treatment of bladder cancer currently achieves satisfactory therapeutic results through open radical cystectomy (ORC), laparoscopic radical cystectomy (LRC), and robot-assisted radical cystectomy (RARC) [2, 3].

The number of surgeons performing RARC has gradually increased since its first reported use [4]. There is evidence that RARC has the advantages of reducing the complication rate and enhancing postoperative recovery,

*Correspondence: biliangkuan118@yeah.net
†Tuo Zhouting, Ying Zhang, and Jinyou Wang contributed equally to this work and are considered to be co-first authors
Department of Urology, The Second Affiliated Hospital of Anhui Medical University, NO. 678 Furong Road, Hefei 230032, China

and its therapeutic effect is equivalent to that of ORC [3, 5, 6]. Although many bladder cancer patients undergo RARC, the treatment costs remain high [7]. Urologists face this problem in many developing countries. Especially in China, robotic systems only exist in large medical centres, thus limiting RARC availability. Similar situations exist in other developing countries [8]; therefore, traditional LRC is still the mainstay of treatment for bladder cancer.

Traditional LRC usually requires five or four ports and has been popular because of its low cost and satisfactory postoperative outcomes [9]. However, a higher number of ports leads to the requirement of more surgeons and increases the possibility of port site-related complications. With the accumulation of surgical experience using laparoscopy, we devised a modified three-port technique for minimising the number of ports, which could be performed by a single surgeon and one scope assistant [10]. The initial results showed that our modified method was feasible and repeatable. In this investigation, we compared the clinical data of patients who underwent the three-port approach and conventional five-port LRC with an ileal conduit, including surgical, oncological, and postoperative outcomes.

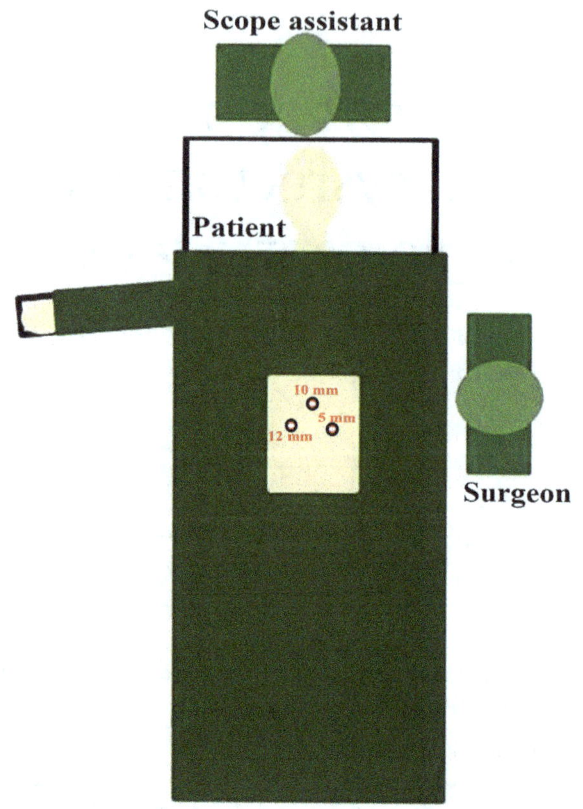

Fig. 1 Schematic diagram of three-port LRC. The surgeon stood on the left side of the patient and scope assistant towards client's head, without another first assistant

Methods

Patients

Patients treated with three-port approach LRC and ileal conduit urinary diversion at our centre from January 2018 to April 2020 were reviewed and included in our study. Their clinical data were identified from the central database. Patients with severe obesity (body mass index [BMI] $\geq$ 35 kg/m^2), distant metastases, poor renal function, severe liver insufficiency, active enteritis, and positive urethral margins were excluded. For comparison with these patients, other patients who underwent conventional five-port LRC and ileal conduit surgery at our centre during the same period were reviewed and matched to the study group by demographic characteristics (e.g. age, sex, BMI, and clinical tumour stage).

Surgical technique

The three-port LRC technique was described in detail in our previous report [10]. In other words, the surgeon stood on the left side of the patient and a scope assistant was oriented toward the client's head, without the need for another first assistant (Fig. 1). The three-port approach was introduced: the first port (10-mm) was placed 2 cm above the umbilicus for the observation hole, followed by a hypogastric 12-mm port at the right lateral rectus line, 3–4 cm below the umbilicus for the main operation hole, and a 5-mm port for the assisted operation hole was placed at the left lateral rectus line, 5–7 cm below the umbilicus (Fig. 2a). Our surgical protocol mainly consists of five steps, with the approximate sequence as follows: dissociation of the ureter, dissociation of bladder and prostate ligaments, removal of the bladder and prostate, pelvic lymph node dissection (PLND), and extracorporeal construction of the ileal conduit. Our specific lateral three-layer approach was used to expose the vital pelvic anatomy, including the external iliac vessel layer, internal iliac vessel layer, and ureter layer. After completing RC and lymphatic dissection, pelvic re-peritonealisation was completed using Hem-o-lok clips (Teleflex Medical, Wayne, PA, USA). A conventional ileal conduit was constructed extracorporeally with a small midline incision. The ureters were implanted using a non-refluxing split-cuff nipple technique, which included a 0.5-cm longitudinal incision in the distal ureter, and the ureteral wall was turned back on itself to construct a nipple. Two F6 single-J stents were placed in the ureter to allow removal approximately 4 weeks postoperatively. The ureters were anastomosed to the ileal conduit in an end-to-side fashion with ureteral stents and secured with 4–0 absorbable suture. The ileal conduit was then placed into the peritoneal cavity, and the distal end of the

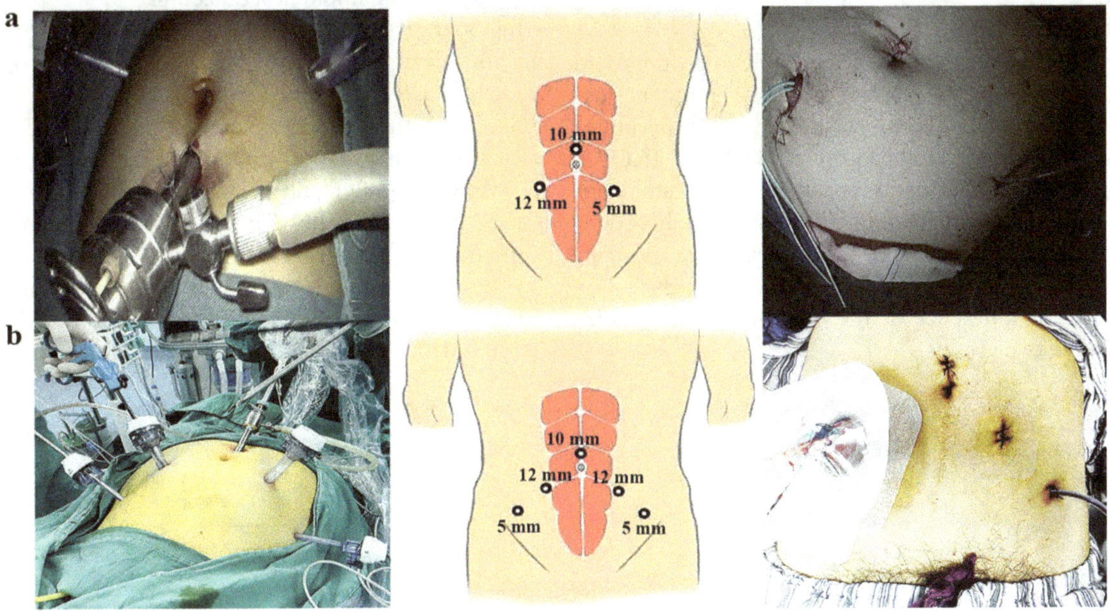

Fig. 2 Position of the trocars and incisions for three-port LRC and five-port LRC. **a** Port placement and operative incision of three-port LRC with an ileal conduit; **b** Port placement and operative incision of five-port LRC with an ileal conduit

ileal segment was anastomosed to the skin in a nipple-to-stoma fashion.

Conventional five-port LRC with an ileal conduit was performed in accordance with a previously described methom [9], including PLND, RC, and the use of a conventional ileal conduit. Five port placements were done in all patients (Fig. 2b). Pelvic re-peritonealisation and non-reflux techniques were used in the five-port group. All patients received standard postoperative care at our institution. All patients are encouraged to have early ambulation after surgery according to the principles of enhanced recovery after surgery (ERAS) [11] and gradually return to a regular diet after intestinal function recovery.

Follow-up evaluation

All patients were followed-up in accordance with the institutional protocol. Follow-up data were obtained through teleconsultations, and outpatient services. Patients were evaluated at 1, 3, 6, and 12 months during the first year after surgery, and then semi-annually. Routine blood tests, renal function tests, urinary ultrasonography, or computed tomography were performed at every outpatient follow-up. The last follow-up time was August 2020.

Data collection

All surgeries were completed by the same team. The data of patients were collected retrospectively, including demographic characteristics (e.g. age, sex, BMI, American Society of Anesthesiology [ASA] score, previous abdominal surgery, previous transurethral resection of bladder tumour [TURBT], smoking status, diabetes mellitus, hypertension, preoperative hydronephrosis, previous chemotherapy, and preoperative creatinine), operative and oncologic outcomes, and follow-up examination results. Complications that occurred within 90 days after surgery were defined as short-term complications, while those that developed 3 months after surgery were defined as long-term complications. Short-term complications (>90 days) were categorised based on the Clavien-Dindo classification [12].

Statistical analysis

All analyses were performed using SPSS 23.0 (IBM, Armonk, NY, USA). Results for continuous variables are expressed as mean ± standard deviations (SD) or median and interquartile range (IQR), and results for categorical variables are reported as the number of cases and percentages. To compare the differences between the two groups, continuous variables were assessed using Student's t-test or the Mann–Whitney *U* test, and categorical variables were evaluated using the Chi-square test or Fisher's exact test. All P values were two-sided, with $P < 0.05$ indicating statistical significance.

Results

Patient characteristics

The demographic characteristics of the two groups were shown in Table 1. We observed a more frequent history of previous abdominal surgery in the experimental group than in the control group (33.33% vs. 16.67%), although the difference was not statistically significant ($P=0.080$). Thirteen patients had preoperative hydronephrosis (20.00% vs. 12.96% in the experimental and control groups, respectively, $P=0.399$). Therefore, there was no significant difference in the baseline characteristics between the two groups.

Operative and pathological outcomes

The operative and pathological outcomes of patients in both groups are presented in Table 2. The operative time (271.30 ± 24.03 vs. 279.57 ± 48.47 min, $P=0.299$) (Fig. 3a), estimated blood loss (65 vs. 90 mL, $P=0.352$) (Fig. 3b), time to passage of flatus (8 vs. 10 days, $P=0.084$) (Fig. 3c), and hospital stay after operation (11 vs. 12 days, $P=0.922$) (Fig. 3d, e) were not significantly different between the two groups. Compared with the five-port group, the treatment cost was significantly lower in the three-port LRC group (12 453 vs. 14 134 $, $P=0.021$). All cases had negative surgical margins, and

Table 1 Demographic characteristics of 84 bladder cancer patients

Variable	Total cases	Three-port LRC (n = 30)	Five-port LRC (n = 54)	P value
Age, [years, mean ± SD]	69.31 ± 9.36	70.84 ± 9.89	68.44 ± 9.03	0.258
Gender, [cases (%)]				0.093
Male	64 (76.2)	26 (86.50)	38 (70.40)	
Female	20 (23.8)	4 (13.50)	16 (29.60)	
Smoking status, [cases (%)]				0.090
Yes	40 (47.62)	18 (60.00)	22 (40.74)	
No	44 (52.38)	12 (40.00)	32 (59..26)	
Diabetes mellitus, [cases (%)]				1.00
Yes	14 (16.67)	5 (16.67)	9 (16.67)	
No	70 (83.33)	25 (83.33)	45 (83.33)	
Hypertension, [cases (%)]				0.461
Yes	32 (38.10)	13 (43.33)	19 (35.19)	
No	52 (61.90)	17 (56.67)	35 (64.81)	
Previous abdominal surgery*, [cases (%)]				0.080
Yes	19 (22.62)	10 (33.33)	9 (16.67)	
No	65 (77.38)	20 (66.67)	45 (83.33)	
Previous TURBT, [cases (%)]				0.973
Yes	31 (36.90)	11 (36.67)	20 (37.04)	
No	53 (63.10)	19 (63.33)	34 (62.96)	
Previous chemotherapy, [cases (%)]				0.398
Yes	26 (30.95)	11 (36.67)	15 (27.78)	
No	58 (59.05)	19 (63.33)	39 (72.22)	
BMI, [kg/m2,mean ± SD]	22.77 ± 3.03	22.36 ± 3.04	23.00 ± 3.03	0.359
ASA score, [cases (%)]				0.471
≤2	60 (71.43)	20 (66.67)	40 (74.07)	
>2	24 (28.57)	10 (33.33)	14 (25.93)	
Preoperative hydronephrosis,[cases (%)]				0.399
Yes	13 (15.48)	6 (20.00)	7 (12.96)	
No	71 (84.52)	24 (80.00)	47 (87.04)	
Clinical tumour stage, [cases (%)]				0.609
≤T1	28 (33.33)	8 (26.67)	20 (37.04)	
T2	32 (38.10)	13 (43.33)	19 (35.18)	
T3-4	24 (28.57)	9 (30.00)	15 (27.78)	
Preoperative creatinine, [umol/L, median (range)]	80 (49.00–143.50)	84 (39.00–143.50)	78 (44.00–135.00)	0.307

* History of abdominal surgery includes appendectomy, hernia operation, intestinal surgery and cesarean section

Table 2 Operative and pathologic outcomes of 84 bladder cancer patients

Variable	Total cases	Three-port LRC (n = 30)	Five-port LRC (n = 54)	*P* value
Operative time, [min,mean ± SD]	276.62 ± 41.45	271.30 ± 24.03	279.57 ± 48.47	0.299
EBL, [mL,median (range)]	80 (30–300)	65 (40–300)	90 (30–300)	0.352
Pathology type, [cases (%)]				0.177
Transitional cell carcinoma	83 (98.81)	29 (96.67)	54 (100)	
Squamous cell carcinoma	1 (1.19)	1 (3.33)	0	
Incidental prostate adenocarcinoma,[cases(%)]	5 (5.95)	3 (10.00)	2 (3.70)	0.243
Pathologic T stage, [cases (%)]				0.166
1	30 (35.71)	6 (20.00)	24 (44.44)	
2	32(38.10)	14 (46.66)	18 (33.33)	
3	18 (21.43)	8 (26.67)	10 (18.52)	
4	4 (4.76)	2 (6.67)	2 (3.71)	
Pathologic N stage, [cases (%)]				0.563
0	75 (89.29)	26 (86.67)	49 (90.74)	
≥ 1	9 (10.71)	4 (13.33)	5 (9.26)	
Time to out-of-bed activity, [d, median (range)]	2 (1–4)	2 (1–4)	2 (1–4)	0.436
Time to passage of flatus, [d, median (range)]	3(2–5)	3(2–5)	3(2–5)	0.084
Time to regular diet, [d, median (range)]	5(4–13)	5(4–13)	6(4–12)	0.065
Time to pelvic drain removal, [d, median (range)]	9(5–18)	8(5–17)	10(5–18)	0.084
Hospital stay after operation, [d, median (range)]	11.5(7–28)	11(8–22)	12(7–28)	0.922
Median treatment cost [$, median (range)]*	13 474 (8 411–24 683)	12 453 (8 411–20 326)	14 134 (8 794–24 683)	0.021

* Treatment costs were converted to 2021 dollars

patients with postoperative pathological results above T2b were administered adjuvant chemotherapy. Transitional cell carcinoma was the predominant type, seen in 83 (98.81%) cases, and squamous cell carcinoma was noted in the remaining cases (1.19%). In general, the surgical and pathological results did not show meaningful differences between these two groups, including pathology type, incidental prostate adenocarcinoma, tumour staging, and postoperative creatinine level (all $P > 0.05$). In addition, the results were similar in both groups in terms of postoperative recovery, such as time to ambulation after surgery, time to passage of flatus, time to regular diet, time to pelvic drain removal, and hospital stay after the operation (all $P > 0.05$).

Postoperative outcomes

The postoperative outcomes of these patients are shown in Table 3. Short-term complications were observed in 28 (33.33%) of 84 patients. Major complications (> grade III) were observed in three (10.00%) cases in the experimental group and in two (3.70%) in the control group ($P = 0.174$). In addition, two (6.67%) patients in the experimental group and one (1.85%) patient in the control group required reoperation due to severe bowel obstruction. However, our results indicated that the rate of short-term complications (43.33% vs. 27.78%, $P = 0.274$) and 90-day mortality (3.33% vs. 1.85%, $P = 0.67$) did not show meaningful differences between groups.

Long-term outcomes

The median follow-up time was 17.5 months (range, 2–29 months) in the three-port group and 19 (range, 2–31) months in the five-port group ($P = 0.433$). Between 4–14 months after surgery, there were two (6.67%) cases of tumour recurrence in the three-port group and two (3.70%) cases in the five-port group ($P = 0.541$); they were undergoing chemoradiotherapy in the oncology department. At one month post-surgery, there were 16 (53.33%) cases of hydronephrosis in the three-port group and 27 (50.00%) cases in the five-port group. Twelve months after surgery, the three-port group had one (3.33%) case of severe hydronephrosis. In the five-port group, two (3.70%) patients with ureteroileal anastomotic stricture were diagnosed at 12 and 16 months after surgery, ipsilaterally in one patient and bilaterally in the other patient. One patient (1.85%) had a parastomal hernia at 10 months after surgery. These patients were kept under close surveillance, and the complications gradually resolved with surgical intervention.

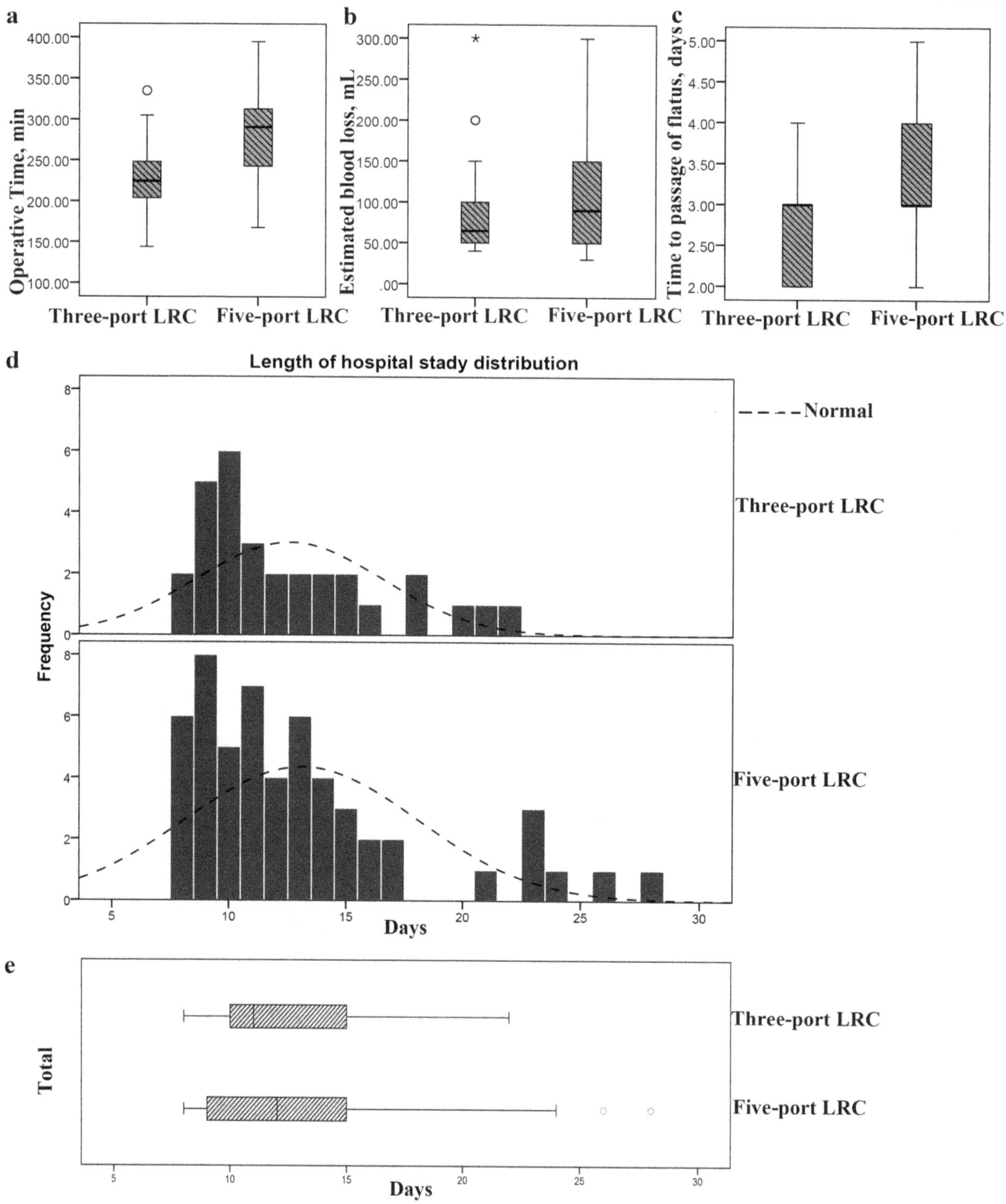

Fig. 3 Comparison of perioperative results for three-port LRC and five-port LRC. **a** Comparison of operative time; **b** Comparison of estimated blood loss; **c** Comparison of time to passage of flatus; **d, e** Comparison of hospital stay after operation

Discussion

This study aimed to compare the clinical outcomes between the three-port approach and conventional five-port LRC for bladder cancer. Our results confirmed the feasibility of three-port LRC with an ileal conduit in treating invasive bladder cancer, with similar

Table 3 Postoperative outcomes of 84 bladder cancer patients

Variable	Total cases	Three-port LRC (n = 30)	Five-port LRC (n = 54)	*P* value
Febrile urinary tract infection, [cases (%)]	11 (13.10)	6 (20.00)	5 (9.26)	0.162
Wound infection, [cases (%)]	5 (5.95)	2 (6.67)	3 (5.56)	0.837
Vein thrombosis, [cases (%)]	2 (2.38)	1 (3.33)	1 (1.85)	0.670
Bowel obstruction, [cases (%)]	6 (7.14)	2 (6.67)	4 (7.40)	0.899
Wound dehiscence, [cases (%)]	2 (2.38)	1 (3.33)	1 (1.85)	0.670
Sepsis, [cases (%)]	2 (2.38)	1 (3.33)	1 (1.85)	0.670
Reoperation, [cases (%)]	3 (3.57)	2 (6.67)	1 (1.85)	0.255
Clavien-Dindo classification (< 90d), [cases (%)]				0.274
I–II	23 (27.38)	10 (33.33)	13 (24.07)	
≥ III	5 (5.95)	3 (10.00)	2 (3.70)	
90-Days mortality, [cases (%)]	2 (2.38)	1 (3.33)	1 (1.85)	0.670

perioperative outcomes and complication rates as the standard five-port LRC, but the treatment costs of the former were significantly less.

ORC is the primary surgical modality for muscular-invasive bladder cancer or high-risk non-muscular-invasive bladder cancer, with a perioperative complication rate of up to 60% due to the complexity of the procedure [13]. With the rapid development of minimally invasive technology, RARC and LRC have become important procedures for bladder cancer management, having been carried out in several medical centres [2]. Numerous studies have demonstrated the advantages of these procedures in reducing the rate of complications and accelerating postoperative recovery, and their safety and tumour therapeutic efficacy are similar to those of ORC [5, 13, 14]. Therefore, they have been used as one of the first-line surgical treatments of bladder cancer in some developed countries. Nevertheless, the complex operation of the robotic system extends the operation time, and the huge costs are not negligible. Morii et al. [15] found that RARC is more expensive than LRC and ORC. In contrast, LRC is widely accepted because of its lower cost and satisfactory efficacy, especially in developing countries such as China. This might not change for a long time. Therefore, traditional LRC remains vital in these countries and has become more prevalent with the increasing incidence of bladder cancer. In fact, owing to the financial cost of RARC [16], standard LRCs are still used in some large medical centres.

For a variety of reasons, urologists in our centre mainly perform LRC with different urinary diversions. Common trocar placement mostly involve the four-port or five-port method in conventional LRC, which is mainly performed by three or four urologists. Although LRC has become quite popular, some limitations have yet to be overcome, such as complex operation, the unfamiliar coordination of the surgeon and assistant, parietal pain, and high operating costs [2, 3, 15]. Recently, reduced port surgery has become increasingly popular for LRC. Single-port and two-port LRC have been reported as minimally invasive methods with potential advantages in port site-related complications, improved cosmesis, and fewer surgical incisions [17, 18]. Moreover, the operation was completed by a urologist and a scope assistant by performing a few incisions. However, these methods have several disadvantages compared with conventional laparoscopic surgery, including long operation time, difficulty in patients with obesity or narrow pelvic space, and a steep learning curve. To overcome the above limitations and the lack of effective coordination due to the operator's and assistant's unfamiliarity with the four-port or five-port LRC, we also attempted to reduce the ports in LRC based on previous surgical experience and performed the three-port procedures for bladder cancer. Our initial goal was to simplify the procedure, make the incision ideal, and facilitate patient recovery [10]. In contrast, the three-port procedure is not substantially different from the single-port and two-port methods and is not restricted by the first assistant compared with the conventional five-port procedure.

Although most of the recent single-centre reports are experiences with RARC and LRC, the availability and cost of technology are major concerns [3, 5, 6]. In our view, three-port LRC has the advantage of an acceptable minimally invasive incision and low cost. Our results show that three-port LRC is not significantly different from standard LRC in oncological results and operative time, but the treatment costs of the former are significantly less. Although inpatient costs are associated with multiple factors, such as the commodity price and health insurance policies, the reduction in the number of surgeons and instruments can avail economic benefits.

Laparoscopic surgery has become quite popular in urology and has potential advantages in precision surgery and tumour control [19]. We also note further modifications of traditional laparoscopic techniques, including the use of the three-port method, in prostate cancer patients. Xu et al. [20] believe that the three-port method has more advantages than traditional laparoscopic radical prostatectomy, including surgical results and postoperative complications. The main benefits of the three-port approach include: (1) fewer surgical incisions and low treatment costs, (2) overcomes the influence of assistants and main equipment, and (3) potential advantages of triangulation. Similarly, our three-port method, which is based on the traditional five-port LRC, overcomes the limitations of the first assistant and the main surgical equipment, which poses significant disadvantages when implementing a five-port technique. Urologists can use left-handed instruments to separate the surrounding tissues and expand the surgical field even for patients with obesity, narrow pelvic organ space, and factors leading to difficulty in exposure. Triangulation is an important basic principle of laparoscopic surgery, which can avoid the formation of narrow spaces and reduce the surgeon's fatigue. The triangular trocar distribution is consistent with the ergonomic principle, which is also in line with the surgeon's habit of laparoscopic surgery. Combined with other urologists' experience in Table 4, we observed that three-port LRC may have an advantage in shortening operative time. It is worth noting that with the reduction in the number of trocars, the three-port approach requires more experience and ability for surgeons. However, our method is difficult to be used by beginners. Therefore, this is recommended for surgeons with extensive experience in laparoscopic surgery.

The Bricker ileal conduit remains the classic and standardized procedure for urinary diversion following RC, widely used by urologists due to its relatively simple procedure and low postoperative complication rate [26]. In our study, all patients underwent a Bricker ileal conduit to reduce the impact of different urinary diversions on postoperative outcomes. Our follow-up results showed that there were no significant differences between the two groups, including short-term and long-term complications. Thus, these results indicate that the three-port LRC with an ileal conduit is feasible for the treatment of bladder cancer. It is important to note that anastomotic techniques may affect the rate of postoperative complications after an ileal conduit, and controversies surrounding refluxing or nonrefluxing anastomotic techniques remain. Nonrefluxing techniques have a higher rate of strictures than the refluxing technique, but the latter has harmful effects on renal function because of potential urinary infection [27, 28]. However, some researchers believe that these techniques have no significant effect on long-term outcomes [29]. In this study, our team performed a split-cuff ureteric nipple to avoid urine reflux according to previous experiences. Our clinical data showed that the rate of postoperative hydronephrosis in the control group was higher than that in the study group, but the difference was not statistically significant. The hydronephrosis in the two groups, which may be related to inflammatory oedema at the anastomotic site, gradually resolved with time after surgery. It is important to protect renal function after an ileal conduit because upper urinary tract obstruction from a stricture is a major cause of renal damage [30]. In our follow-up, these patients had no overtly impaired renal function, and only two patients in the control developed strictures.

Table 4 A synopsis of published series on the surgical treatment of bladder cancer

Reference	Treatment	Case(n)	OT(min)	EBL (ml)	Hospital stay after operation (days)	Complications (%)	PSM (%)
Huang et al. [21]	Single-port LRC with orthotopic ileal neobladder	8	399	154	15	37.50	NA
Ma et al. [18]	Single-port LRC with ileal conduit	5	208.02[a] /135[b]	270	19.5	20.00	0
Angulo et al. [17]	Two-port LRC with urinary diversion	30	330	347.5	10	40.00	0.067
Abraham et al. [22]	Conventional LRC with ileal conduit	20	419	653	9.4	70.00	0
Khan et al. [23]	Conventional LRC with urinary diversion	58	316	480.7	16.1	27.00	0.04
Kim et al. [24]	Conventional LRC with urinary diversion	22	524	400	12	NA	0
Su et al. [25]	Conventional LRC with urinary diversion	126	315	200	10	58.73	0.023

[a] Extirpative operative time; [b]ileal conduit operative time

However, the occurrence of late postoperative strictures requires further investigation.

This study has several limitations that need to be addressed. First, as this was a small-sample retrospective study, randomised controlled trials were not performed and a contemporary historical cohort was used as a control group for comparison. Second, the follow-up time of this study was relatively short, which can fail to determine all complications of the technique, especially long-term complications. Further studies are needed to confirm the clinical relevance of these findings.

Conclusions

In our study, we observed that the perioperative outcomes and complications did not show any significant difference between the three-port LRC with an ileal conduit and a conventional five-port LRC with an ileal conduit, but the treatment costs of the former were reduced. These preliminary data suggest that our three-port LRC may be a viable alternative LRC method. However, further large-sample prospective randomised controlled trials are required to confirm the benefits and long-term effects of the three-port approach.

Abbreviations

LRC: Laparoscopic radical cystectomy; RC: Radical cystectomy; ORC: Open radical cystectomy; LRC: Laparoscopic radical cystectomy; RARC: Robot-assisted radical cystectomy; BMI: Body mass index; PLND: Pelvic lymph node dissection; SD: Standard deviations; IQR: Interquartile range; ASA: American society of anesthesiology; TURBT: Transurethral resection of bladder tumour; ERAS: Enhanced recovery after surgery; OT: Operative time; EBL: Estimated blood loss; PSM: Positive surgical margin; NA: Not available.

Acknowledgements

We would like to thank Editage for English language editing.

Authors' contributions

Each author has participated sufficiently in the work and takes public responsibility for appropriate portions of the content. The authors have agreed to be accountable for all aspects of the work and ensure that questions related to the accuracy or integrity of any part of the work are appropriately investigated and resolved. TZ, ZY and WJ carried out the interpretation of data and drafted the manuscript. ZH, LY and WX participated in the collection of data and data analysis. Literature research was conducted by YC and YD. BL conceived and designed the study. All authors read and approved the final manuscript.

References

1. Ng CK, Kauffman EC, Lee MM, Otto BJ, Portnoff A, Ehrlich JR, Schwartz MJ, Wang GJ, Scherr DS. A comparison of postoperative complications in open versus robotic cystectomy. Eur Urol. 2010;57(2):274–81.
2. Bochner BH, Dalbagni G, Marzouk KH, Sjoberg DD, Lee J, Donat SM, Coleman JA, Vickers A, Herr HW, Laudone VP. Randomized trial comparing open radical cystectomy and robot-assisted laparoscopic radical cystectomy: oncologic outcomes. Eur Urol. 2018;74(4):465–71.
3. Snow-Lisy DC, Campbell SC, Gill IS, Hernandez AV, Fergany A, Kaouk J, Haber GP. Robotic and laparoscopic radical cystectomy for bladder cancer: long-term oncologic outcomes. Eur Urol. 2014;65(1):193–200.
4. Menon M, Hemal AK, Tewari A, Shrivastava A, Shoma AM, El-Tabey NA, Shaaban A, Abol-Enein H, Ghoneim MA. Nerve-sparing robot-assisted radical cystoprostatectomy and urinary diversion. BJU Int. 2003;92(3):232–6.
5. Parekh DJ, Messer J, Fitzgerald J, Ercole B, Svatek R. Perioperative outcomes and oncologic efficacy from a pilot prospective randomized clinical trial of open versus robotic assisted radical cystectomy. J Urol. 2013;189(2):474–9.
6. Martin AD, Nunez RN, Castle EP. Robot-assisted radical cystectomy versus open radical cystectomy: a complete cost analysis. Urology. 2011;77(3):621–5.
7. Yu HY, Hevelone ND, Lipsitz SR, Kowalczyk KJ, Nguyen PL, Choueiri TK, Kibel AS, Hu JC. Comparative analysis of outcomes and costs following open radical cystectomy versus robot-assisted laparoscopic radical cystectomy: results from the US Nationwide Inpatient Sample. Eur Urol. 2012;61(6):1239–44.
8. Sundram M. Asian robotic experience. Urol Oncol. 2010;28(6):677–81.
9. Gao ZL, Fan J, Zhao JJ, Xia SJ, Shi L, Men CP, Wang H, Wang L, Yang DD, Sun DK, et al. Laparoscopic radical cystectomy with extracorporeal ileal conduit urinary diversion for treatment of Chinese bladder cancer patients. Urol Int. 2007;79(3):204–9.
10. Wang X, Lu Y, Tuo Z, Bi L: Our initial experience with the three layers with three-port approach for laparoscopic radical cystectomy. Videosurgery and Other Miniinvasive Techniques/Wideochirurgia i inne techniki małoinwazyjne 2021.
11. Daneshmand S, Ahmadi H, Schuckman AK, Mitra AP, Cai J, Miranda G, Djaladat H. Enhanced recovery protocol after radical cystectomy for bladder cancer. J Urol. 2014;192(1):50–5.
12. Dindo D, Demartines N, Clavien PA. Classification of surgical complications: a new proposal with evaluation in a cohort of 6336 patients and results of a survey. Ann Surg. 2004;240(2):205–13.
13. Kiss B, Burkhard FC, Thalmann GN. Open radical cystectomy: still the gold standard for muscle invasive bladder cancer. World J Urol. 2016;34(1):33–9.
14. Cohen SA, Mirheydar HS, Parsons JK, Palazzi KL, Liss MA, Chang DC, Kane CJ, Kader AK. Minimally invasive cystectomy is associated with improved perioperative patient safety outcomes compared with open cystectomy in a national cohort. Urology. 2014;84(2):314–9.
15. Morii Y, Osawa T, Suzuki T, Shinohara N, Harabayashi T, Ishikawa T, Tanikawa T, Yamashina H, Ogasawara K. Cost comparison between open radical cystectomy, laparoscopic radical cystectomy, and robot-assisted radical cystectomy for patients with bladder cancer: a systematic review of segmental costs. BMC Urol. 2019;19(1):110.
16. Novara G, Catto JW, Wilson T, Annerstedt M, Chan K, Murphy DG, Motttrie A, Peabody JO, Skinner EC, Wiklund PN, et al. Systematic review and cumulative analysis of perioperative outcomes and complications after robot-assisted radical cystectomy. Eur Urol. 2015;67(3):376–401.
17. Angulo JC, García-Tello A, Mateo E, Gimbernat H, Redondo C, Andrés G. Two-port approach compared to standard laparoscopic radical cystectomy. J Endourol. 2015;29(9):1030–7.
18. Ma LL, Bi H, Hou XF, Huang Y, Wang GL, Zhao L, Zhang SD. Laparoendoscopic single-site radical cystectomy and urinary diversion: initial experience in China using a homemade single-port device. J Endourol. 2012;26(4):355–9.
19. Lin T, Fan X, Zhang C, Xu K, Liu H, Zhang J, Jiang C, Huang H, Han J, Yao Y et al. A prospective randomised controlled trial of laparoscopic vs open radical cystectomy for bladder cancer: perioperative and oncologic outcomes with 5-year follow-upT Lin et al. Br J Cancer 2014, 110(4):842–849.
20. Xu B, Peng YJ, Ma GZ, Zhang Q. A novel "three-port" trocar placement technique for laparoscopic radical prostatectomy. World J Surg Oncol. 2020;18(1):279.
21. Huang J, Lin TZ, Xu KW, Han JL, Ye F, Huang H, Jiang C, Zhang CX, Yao YS, Xie WL, et al. Application of modified single port laparoscopic radical cystoprostatectomy and orthotopic ileal neobladder. Zhonghua Yi Xue Za Zhi. 2010;90(22):1542–6.
22. Abraham JB, Young JL, Box GN, Lee HJ, Deane LA, Ornstein DK. Comparative analysis of laparoscopic and robot-assisted radical cystectomy with ileal conduit urinary diversion. J Endourol. 2007;21(12):1473–80.

23. Khan MS, Challacombe B, Elhage O, Rimington P, Coker B, Murphy D, Grieve A, Dasgupta P. A dual-centre, cohort comparison of open, laparoscopic and robotic-assisted radical cystectomy. Int J Clin Pract. 2012;66(7):656–62.
24. Kim TH, Sung HH, Jeon HG, Seo SI, Jeon SS, Lee HM, Choi HY, Jeong BC. Oncological outcomes in patients treated with radical cystectomy for bladder cancer: comparison between open, laparoscopic, and robot-assisted approaches. J Endourol. 2016;30(7):783–91.
25. Su S, Gu L, Ma X, Li H, Wang B, Shi T, Zhang X. Comparison of laparoscopic and robot-assisted radical cystectomy for bladder cancer: perioperative and oncologic outcomes. Clin Genitourin Cancer. 2019;17(5):e1048–53.
26. Siddiqui KM, Izawa JI. Ileal conduit: standard urinary diversion for elderly patients undergoing radical cystectomy. World J Urol. 2016;34(1):19–24.
27. Richards KA, Cohn JA, Large MC, Bales GT, Smith ND, Steinberg GD. The effect of length of ureteral resection on benign ureterointestinal stricture rate in ileal conduit or ileal neobladder urinary diversion following radical cystectomy. Urol Oncol. 2015;33(2):61–5.
28. Pantuck AJ, Han KR, Perrotti M, Weiss RE, Cummings KB. Ureteroenteric anastomosis in continent urinary diversion: long-term results and complications of direct versus nonrefluxing techniques. J Urol. 2000;163(2):450–5.
29. Harraz AM, Mosbah A, Abdel-Latif M, El-Assmy A, Gad H, Shaaban AA. Impact of the type of ureteroileal anastomosis on renal function measured by diuretic scintigraphy: long-term results of a prospective randomized study. BJU Int. 2014;114(2):202–9.
30. Jin XD, Roethlisberger S, Burkhard FC, Birkhaeuser F, Thoeny HC, Studer UE. Long-term renal function after urinary diversion by ileal conduit or orthotopic ileal bladder substitution. Eur Urol. 2012;61(3):491–7.

14

Robotic adrenalectomy in the pediatric population: initial experience case series from a tertiary center

Anirban P. Mitra[1*], Evalynn Vasquez[1,2], Paul Kokorowski[1,2] and Andy Y. Chang[1,2]

Abstract

Background: Laparoscopic resection is the most well described minimally-invasive approach for adrenalectomy. While it allows for improved cosmesis, faster recovery and decreased length of hospital stay compared with the open approach, instrument articulation limitations can hamper surgical dexterity in pediatric patients. Use of robotic assistance can greatly enhance operative field visualization and instrument control, and is in the early stages of adoption in academic centers for pediatric populations.

Case presentation: We present a single-institution series of pediatric adrenalectomy cases. The da Vinci Xi surgical system was used to perform adrenalectomies on three consecutive patients (ages, 2–13 years) at our center. Final pathology revealed ganglioneuroblastoma (n = 2) and pheochromocytoma (n = 1). Median operating time was 244 min (range, 244–265 min); median blood loss was estimated at 100 ml (range, 15–175 ml). Specimens were delivered intact and all margins were negative. Median post-operative hospital stay was 2 days (range, 1–6 days). All patients remain disease-free at median follow-up of 19 months (range, 12–30 months).

Conclusion: Our experience continues to evolve, and suggests that robotic surgery is safe, feasible and oncologically effective for resection of adrenal masses in well-selected pediatric patients.

Keywords: Minimally-invasive surgery, Robotics, Pediatrics, Adrenal mass, Neuroblastoma, Pheochromocytoma, Case report

Background

While no randomized trials have evaluated the efficacy of open versus minimally-invasive surgery for treatment of solid abdominal tumors in pediatric populations, the minimally-invasive approach to adrenalectomy is a feasible alternative in well-selected patients [1, 2]. It offers the advantages of improved exposure, reduced soft tissue dissection, improved cosmesis, decreased morbidity and post-operative pain allowing for early feeding, faster return to activity, and decreased length of stay. In adults, it has been associated with decreased blood loss and need for transfusion [3]. Laparoscopic adrenalectomy is the most extensively described minimally-invasive approach, but can be technically challenging due to the small intra-abdominal spaces of pediatric patients, as well as limited instrument dexterity [4].

Use of robotic assistance allows the added advantages of magnified three-dimensional view and articulating instruments with increased range of motion, tremor control, which facilitate precise dissection and hemostasis. Robotic surgery has also been suggested to further reduce duration of hospital stay and blood loss compared to laparoscopic adrenalectomy [5]. However, the body of literature on robotic adrenalectomy for pediatric patients has been sparse, with only two cases reported thus far

*Correspondence: apmitra@gmail.com
[1] Institute of Urology, University of Southern California, Los Angeles, CA, USA
Full list of author information is available at the end of the article

[6, 7]. We present our technique and initial institutional experience with pediatric adrenalectomies performed using the da Vinci Xi system (Intuitive Surgical, Sunnyvale, CA).

Case presentation

Case 1

A 2-year-old female had previously undergone a robot-assisted adrenal-sparing left upper pole partial nephrectomy at 14 months of age for recurrent febrile urinary tract infections and a poorly functioning renal moiety with ectopic ureter. Postoperative ultrasound showed a new 2.5 cm right adrenal mass, which was confirmed on MRI. Metabolic activity was confirmed by MIBG study (Fig. 1a, b). 24-h urine metanephrines, homovanillate and vanillylmandelate, and corresponding plasma chemistry levels were within normal limits.

Under general anesthesia, the patient was positioned in left lateral decubitus. An 8 mm robotic camera port was introduced at the umbilicus using the Hasson technique [8]. Following low-pressure insufflation, the camera was introduced and visceral injuries were ruled out. Three additional 8 mm robotic ports and a 5 mm assistant port were then placed (Fig. 1c). After docking the da Vinci Xi robot, the hepatic flexure of the right colon was minimally mobilized to aid in visualization of the right adrenal gland. After identifying the right suprarenal vein and adrenal gland, dissection was carried cephalad under the liver. Combination of monopolar and bipolar cautery was used to obtain hemostasis. A tough dissection plane between the medial aspect of the adrenal

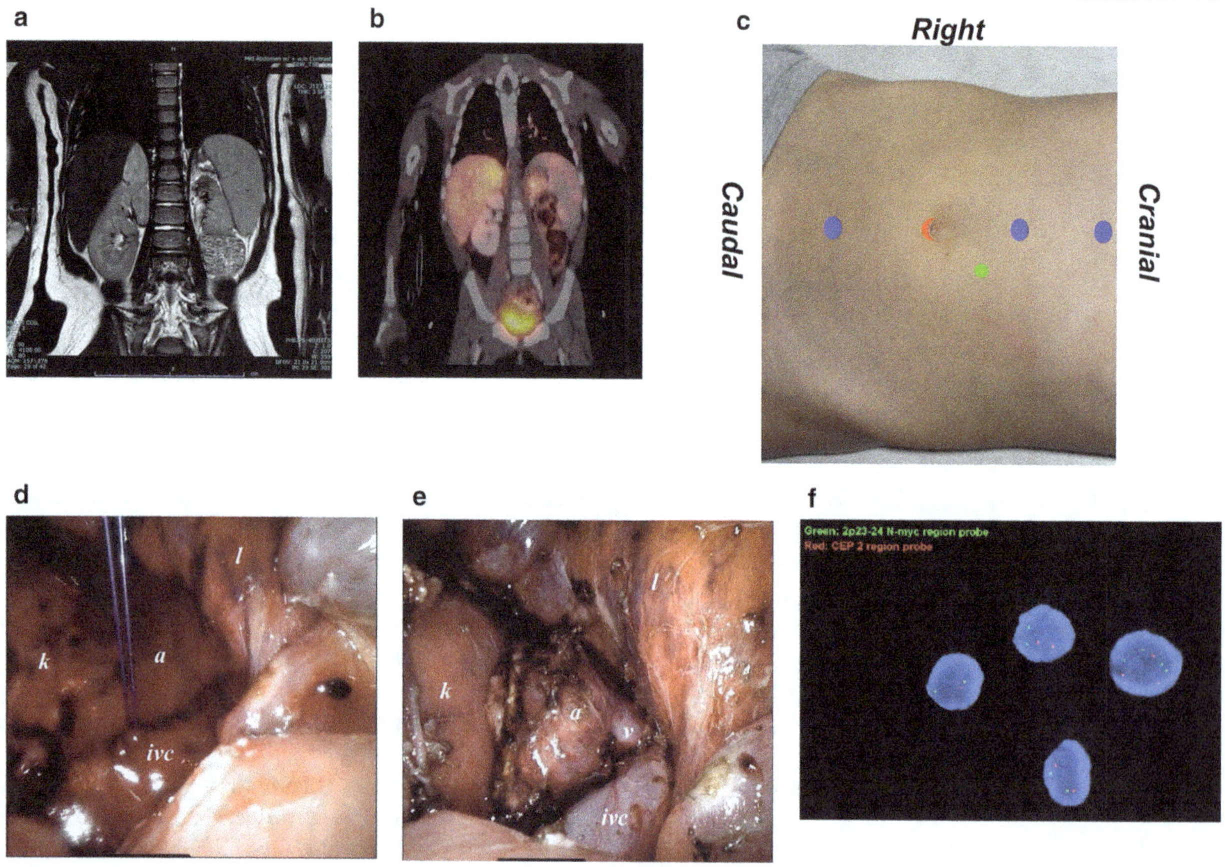

Fig. 1 **a** MRI for *Case 1* showing a 2.1 cm × 1.7 cm × 2.5 cm T2 hyperintense, heterogeneously enhancing lobulated structure replacing the right adrenal gland without gross evidence of local invasion and local or distant adenopathy. **b** MIBG study showing activity in the right adrenal gland without any abnormal foci of uptake elsewhere. **c** Location of ports. After placement of an 8 mm periumbilical robotic camera port (red), additional 8 mm midline robotic ports were placed in the suprapubic and subxiphoid regions, and midway between xiphoid and umbilicus (blue) in a straight line. A 5 mm laparoscopic assistant port with insufflation was placed over the right abdominal wall (*green*). Representative intraoperative screen captures for *Case 1* showing **d** primary repair of a small cavotomy with figure-of-eight 4–0 polypropylene suture, and **e** surgical anatomy of the dissected right adrenal gland (*a*) in relation to the right suprarenal vein (*v*), inferior vena cava (*ivc*), right kidney (*k*) and liver (*l*). **f** FISH of the final tumor specimen did not demonstrate *MYCN* amplification

gland and the inferior vena cava resulted in creation of a small inadvertent cavotomy that was rapidly repaired primarily with figure-of-eight 4–0 polypropylene suture (Fig. 1d). The right adrenal gland was mobilized (Fig. 1e). The adrenal vein was suture-ligated with 4–0 polypropylene suture before transection. Hemostasis was confirmed and the kidney was well perfused throughout. Specimen was delivered intact through the umbilical port incision using an EndoCatch specimen pouch (Covidien, Minneapolis, MN). Estimated blood loss was 175 ml; 125 ml packed red blood cells, 1000 ml crystalloids and 60 ml colloids were transfused intraoperatively. Operative time was 244 min.

Patient had an uneventful hospital course with good in-house pain control and was discharged on post-operative day two. Final pathological evaluation of the 7.1 gm specimen revealed nodular ganglioneuroblastoma that was negative for c-Myc by immunohistochemistry. FISH did not show *MYCN* amplification (Fig. 1e). Surgical margins were negative. No lymphovascular invasion was noted. Patient is being followed with serial MRI, MIBG scan, and urine catecholamines. She remains disease-free at 30 months of post-operative follow-up.

Case 2

A 13-year-old male was noted to be intermittently tachycardic and hypertensive during hospitalization for a pneumonia episode, and found to have a 6 cm right adrenal mass on MRI (Fig. 2). Patient's father has von Hippel-Lindau disease and had undergone bilateral adrenalectomy for pheochromocytoma and bilateral nephrectomy for renal cell carcinoma. A pathogenic *VHL* mutation (c.583C > T, p.Q195X) was found in the patient, which was same as the father. 24-h urine norepinephrine level was elevated.

Three weeks after initiating alpha-adrenergic blockade, patient underwent robotic right adrenalectomy. Patient and robotic port positioning were the same as in *Case 1*. Dissection was performed in the plane between the inferior vena cava and the right adrenal gland, and the latter was also released from the right upper renal pole and liver. After freeing the adrenal gland circumferentially without complication, it was delivered intact by extending the suprapubic port incision using an EndoCatch pouch. Estimated blood loss was 100 ml; 2500 ml crystalloids and 750 ml colloids were transfused intraoperatively. Operative time was 244 min.

Patient's postoperative stay was prolonged due to a generalized morbilliform eruption attributed to a previously unknown allergy to clindamycin. This gradually resolved after administration of systemic corticosteroids and stopping the offending drug, and he was discharged on post-operative day six. Pathological evaluation of the 48.5 gm specimen was consistent with pheochromocytoma. No capsular or vascular invasion was seen. Surgical margins were negative. Patient is being monitored with serial ultrasound and MRI. He remains disease-free at 19 months of post-operative follow-up.

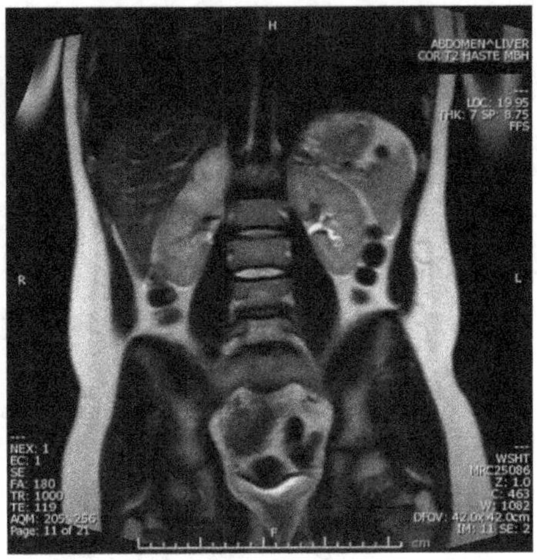

Fig. 2 MRI for *Case 2* showing a 6.0 cm × 3.6 cm × 3.2 cm solid enhancing structure in the right adrenal gland region suggestive of a pheochromocytoma

Case 3

Renal ultrasound for workup of microscopic hematuria in a 4-year-old male showed an incidental mass in the area of the right kidney. A subsequent CT scan showed a 6.4 cm heterogeneous mass replacing the right adrenal gland, which was MIBG-avid (Fig. 3a–c). CT chest and bone scan were negative for metastatic disease. 24-h urine homovanillate and vanillylmandelate were elevated.

The patient underwent robotic right adrenalectomy as described in *Case 1*. Dissection was carried over the inferior vena cava, and small vessels feeding into the mass were controlled with bipolar electrocautery before transection. A prominent lymph node overlying the vena cava was also excised. Specimen was delivered through a mini Pfannenstiel incision along the suprapubic port. Estimated blood loss was 15 ml; 500 ml crystalloids were transfused intraoperatively. Operative time was 265 min.

Patient had an uneventful hospital course and was discharged on post-operative day one. Pathological diagnosis of the 57 gm specimen was intermixed type, Schwannian stroma-rich ganglioneuroblastoma with negative surgical margins. Immunohistochemistry was negative for c-Myc and n-Myc. FISH did not show *MYCN* amplification (Fig. 3d). No malignancy was identified in the resected lymph node. Patient is being followed with serial MRI, MIBG scan, and urine catecholamines.

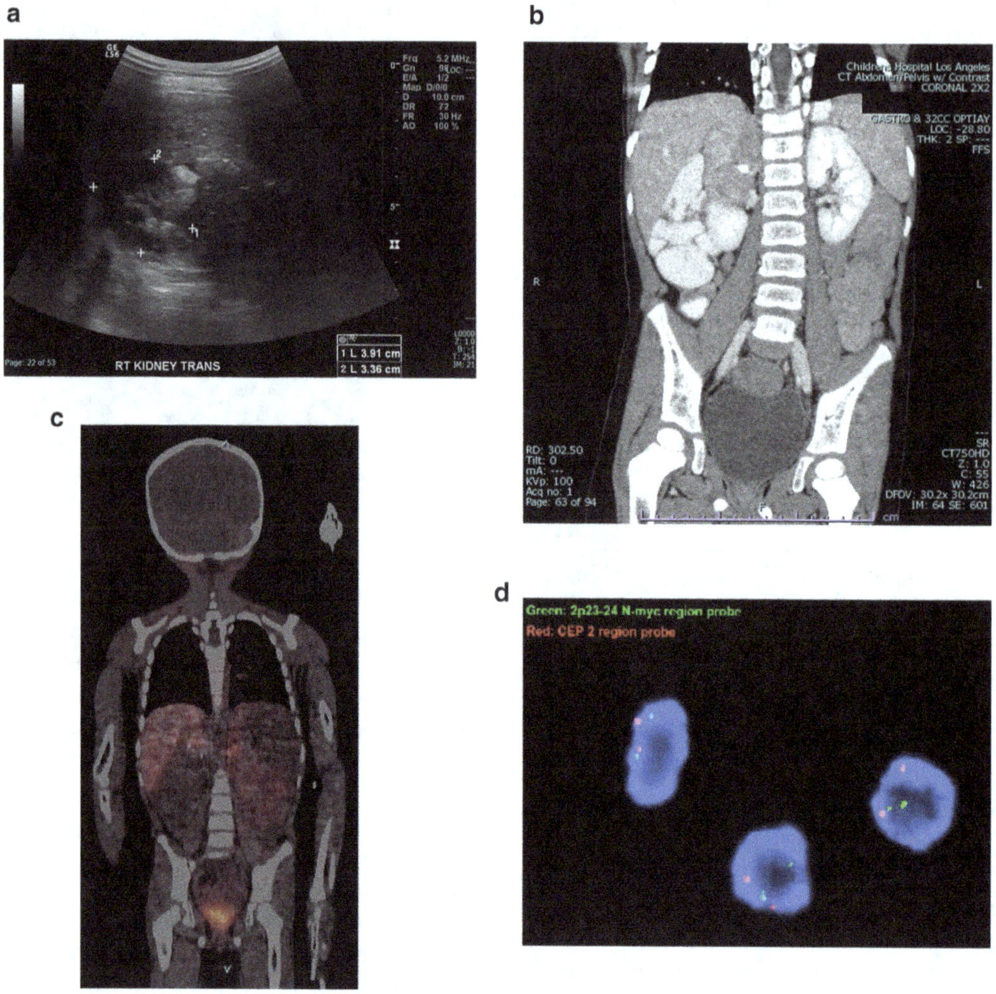

Fig. 3 **a** Renal ultrasound for *Case 3* showing a heterogeneous complex mass in the area of the right kidney. **b** CT scan of abdomen and pelvis showing a 6.4 cm × 4.2 cm × 3.4 cm heterogeneous calcified mass replacing the right adrenal gland concerning for neuroblastoma. No regional or distant lymphadenopathy was noted. **c** MIBG study showing activity in the right adrenal gland without evidence of avid metastatic disease. **d** FISH of the final tumor did not demonstrate *MYCN* amplification

He remains disease-free at 12 months of post-operative follow-up.

Discussion and conclusions

We herein report on the initial experience with robotic pediatric adrenalectomy from our institution. All cases followed a standardized surgical approach independent of suspected adrenal pathology, and none required open conversion. All specimens were resected and delivered intact (median weight, 48.5 g; range, 7.1–57 g), and all surgical margins were negative.

We demonstrate that robotic adrenalectomy is feasible in a wide range of ages and body habitus in the pediatric population. While use of robotic assistance has been described in two pediatric adrenalectomy cases previously [6, 7], this is the first reported series using the da Vinci Xi robot. This provides additional advantages over prior generation robots including improved patient arm clearance, versatility of camera placement into any port, ability to place arms along a single line thereby avoiding clashing, and guided docking and targeting [9].

Median operative time was 244 min (range, 244–265 min), and reflects our initial learning curve in performing this complex surgery at a tertiary center with more than 50% trainee participation in each case. As with most complex robotic procedures, we do anticipate that operative time will continue to improve as our experience matures. However, one is cautioned by findings from the adult population that indicate significantly longer operating time in patients who underwent robotic adrenalectomy when compared with those undergoing laparoscopic resection [10]. Median estimated blood loss was 100 ml (range, 15–175 ml). Injury to surrounding vasculature is a known complication during adrenalectomy; *Case 1* also demonstrates ability of the da Vinci Xi system for rapid control and primary repair of such injuries due to precise articulation of the robotic instruments.

While median post-operative hospital stay for this series was 2 days, one patient had a protracted recovery due to an unexpected drug reaction (range, 1–6 days). Typical postoperative recovery, however, appears to be similar or better to prior reports for minimally-invasive adrenalectomies [4, 6, 7]. At a median post-operative follow-up of 19 months (range, 12–30 months), all patients remain disease-free. Our series represents the longest reported follow-up for pediatric patients undergoing robotic adrenalectomy. There were no mortality and local recurrence or metastases, and biochemical and hormonal parameters have remained within normal limits for functional tumors in this series. This further demonstrates the oncologic safety and efficacy of this approach.

In conclusion, robotic assistance has been successfully and reproducibly used for resecting adrenal masses in adults. We report the first series of pediatric adrenalectomy using the latest generation da Vinci Xi robot. Our experience demonstrates that robot-assisted adrenalectomy is a safe, effective and viable option in well-selected pediatric patients. Surgical excision can be accomplished with rapid recovery time, relatively low surgical morbidity, and comparable oncologic outcomes. While adhering to sound oncologic principles, a robotic approach provides added advantages of improved visualization, precision and dexterity. Maturing operative experience and larger series may be able to address if this approach can potentially improve surgical outcomes.

Abbreviations

MRI: Magnetic resonance imaging; MIBG: Metaiodobenzylguanidine; FISH: Fluorescent in situ hybridization; CT: Computed tomography.

Acknowledgements

Not applicable.

Authors' contributions

APM and AYC were responsible for study conception and design. APM, EV, PK and AYC participated in the patients' treatment. APM collected the data and organized the reports. APM, EV, PK and AYC participated in analysis of the data. APM drafted the initial version of the manuscript, and AYC helped with critical revisions. APM, EV, PK and AYC contributed to manuscript revisions. All authors read and approved the final version of the manuscript.

Author details

[1] Institute of Urology, University of Southern California, Los Angeles, CA, USA.
[2] Division of Urology, Children's Hospital Los Angeles, Los Angeles, CA, USA.

References

1. Kelleher CM, Smithson L, Nguyen LL, Casadiego G, Nasr A, Irwin MS, Gerstle JT. Clinical outcomes in children with adrenal neuroblastoma undergoing open versus laparoscopic adrenalectomy. J Pediatr Surg. 2013;48(8):1727–32.
2. Bin X, Qing Y, Linhui W, Li G, Yinghao S. Adrenal incidentalomas: experience from a retrospective study in a Chinese population. Urol Oncol. 2011;29(3):270–4.
3. Brunt LM, Doherty GM, Norton JA, Soper NJ, Quasebarth MA, Moley JF. Laparoscopic adrenalectomy compared to open adrenalectomy for benign adrenal neoplasms. J Am Coll Surg. 1996;183(1):1–10.
4. Dokumcu Z, Divarci E, Ertan Y, Celik A. Laparoscopic adrenalectomy in children: a 25-case series and review of the literature. J Pediatr Surg. 2018;53(9):1800–5.
5. Brandao LF, Autorino R, Laydner H, Haber GP, Ouzaid I, De Sio M, Perdona S, Stein RJ, Porpiglia F, Kaouk JH. Robotic versus laparoscopic adrenalectomy: a systematic review and meta-analysis. Eur Urol. 2014;65(6):1154–61.
6. Uwaydah NI, Jones A, Elkaissi M, Yu Z, Palmer BW. Pediatric robot-assisted laparoscopic radical adrenalectomy and lymph-node dissection for neuroblastoma in a 15-month-old. J Robot Surg. 2014;8(3):289–93.
7. Rogers CG, Blatt AM, Miles GE, Linehan WM, Pinto PA. Concurrent robotic partial adrenalectomy and extra-adrenal pheochromocytoma resection in a pediatric patient with von Hippel-Lindau disease. J Endourol. 2008;22(7):1501–3.
8. Hasson HM. A modified instrument and method for laparoscopy. Am J Obstet Gynecol. 1971;110(6):886–7.
9. Wilson TG. Advancement of technology and its impact on urologists: release of the daVinci Xi, a new surgical robot. Eur Urol. 2014;66(5):793–4.
10. Economopoulos KP, Mylonas KS, Stamou AA, Theocharidis V, Sergentanis TN, Psaltopoulou T, Richards ML. Laparoscopic versus robotic adrenalectomy: a comprehensive meta-analysis. Int J Surg. 2017;38:95–104.

15

Comparison of effect between dartos fascia and tunica vaginalis fascia in TIP urethroplasty

Hao Yang[1,2,3], Xiao-xiao Xuan[2,3], Dong-lai Hu[4], Hang Zhang[1,2,3], Qiang Shu[2,3], Xiao-dong Guo[4*] and Jun-fen Fu[2,3*]

Abstract

Background: Tubularized incised plate (TIP) urethroplasty is the most commonly performed procedure for hypospadias. Several flap procedures have been recommended to decrease the postoperative complication rate in TIP repair, but no single flap procedure is ideal. This study aimed to compare the outcomes of dartos fascia (DF) and tunica vaginalis fascia (TVF) as intermediate layers in TIP urethroplasty.

Methods: We searched PubMed, EMBASE, the Cochrane Library, Web of Science, clinicaltrials.gov, and other sources for comparative studies up to April 16, 2020. Studies were selected by the predesigned inclusion criteria. The primary outcomes were postoperative complications. The secondary outcomes were functional and cosmetic outcomes.

Results: The pooled RR with 95% CI were calculated. We extracted the relevant information from the included studies. Only 6 comparative studies were included. No secondary outcomes were reported. The RR of the total complications rate for DF was 2.41 (95% CI 1.42–4.07, $P=0.0001$) compared with TVF in TIP repair. For each postoperative complication, the RRs were 6.48 (2.20–19.12, $P=0.0007$), 5.95 (1.13–31.30, $P=0.04$), 0.62 (0.25–1.52, $P=0.29$), and 0.75 (0.23–2.46, $P=0.64$) for urethrocutaneous fistula, prepuce-related complications, meatal/urethral stenosis, and wound-related complications, respectively.

Conclusions: This meta-analysis reveals that compared to DF, TVF is a better option in TIP repair in terms of decreasing the incidence of the total postoperative complications, urethrocutaneous fistula, and prepuce-related complications. However there is limited evidence for functional and cosmetic outcomes. Overall, larger prospective studies and long-term follow-up data are required to further demonstrate the superiority of TVF over DF.

Keywords: Hypospadias, Urethrocutaneous fistula, Dartos fascia, Tunica vaginalis fascia, Meta-analysis

*Correspondence: guoxiaodong@zju.edu.cn; fjf68@zju.edu.cn
[2] Children's Hospital, Zhejiang University School of Medicine, Hangzhou, China
[4] Department of Pediatric Surgery, Zhejiang University Jinhua Hospital, Jinhua, China
Full list of author information is available at the end of the article

Background

Hypospadias, resulting from the disruption of the normal urethral formation, is one of the most common congenital malformations in male infants, with an overall predicted prevalence of 20.9 cases per 10,000 male live births around the world [1]. The international total prevalence increased 1.6 times from 1980–2010, by 0.25 cases per 10,000 births per year [1]. The current purpose of hypospadias surgery is to improve the functional and cosmetic outcomes while minimizing the incidence of postoperative complications and avoiding reoperations. The tubularized incised plate (TIP) urethroplasty is the most commonly performed procedure for hypospadias [2]. Additional urethral coverage is now routinely used by most paediatric urologists to reduce the incidence of postoperative complications [3]. Dartos fascia (DF) and tunica vaginalis fascia (TVF) are the two most widely used urethral coverages with good surgical results while results reported by different studies vary [4–6]. At present, there has been no consensus on the better choice between the DF and TVF flap techniques or on the short- and long-term outcomes of both techniques [3]. This meta-analysis aimed to compare the outcomes of TVF and DF as intermediate layers in TIP hypospadias repair.

Methods

Registration

This study is registered with PROSPERO, registration number CRD42019148554. The completed PRISMA checklist for NMA was presented in the Appendices (Additional file 1: Table S1).

Search strategies

Four electronic databases were searched up to April 16, 2020, including PubMed, EMBASE, Cochrane Central and Web of Science. The searching strategy in PubMed was presented as follows: (((((((hypospadias repair[Title/Abstract]) OR hypospadias surgery[Title/Abstract]) OR tubularized incised plate[Title/Abstract]) OR TIP[Title/Abstract]) OR tubularised incised plate[Title/Abstract]) OR Snodgrass repair[Title/Abstract]))) AND (((((((urethral cover*[Title/Abstract]) OR soft tissue cover*[Title/Abstract]) OR additional cover*[Title/Abstract]) OR subcutaneous flap*[Title/Abstract]) OR flap cover*[Title/Abstract]) OR dartos[Title/Abstract]) OR tunica vaginalis[Title/Abstract]). We also screened clinicaltrials.gov, some international professional conference abstract (such as the Society for Pediatric Urology, European Society for Paediatric Urology, Asia–Pacific Association of Pediatric Urologists, American Pediatric Surgical Association and World Federation of Associations of Pediatric Surgery) and the references of included articles and published reviews to identify additional relevant publications.

Inclusion criteria

The studies were selected according to the following criteria: (1) participants were diagnosed with primary hypospadias and received TIP urethroplasty, (2) the study compared TV with DVF, (3) the study reported the incidence of postoperative complications with/without functional or cosmetic outcomes, (4) the article was written in English, and (5) the study was a randomized controlled trial (RCT), quasi-RCT, non-RCT, retrospective, prospective, or concurrent cohort study. Studies with the full text unavailable, ineligibile study types (single-arm trials, reviews, expert opinions, comments, letters to the editor, case report/series, studies on animals and conference reports), or no outcome of interest reported were excluded. Reoperations, non-TIP repair, fistula repair, patients with severe chordee that required UP excision or two-stage repair were also excluded. Complications were defined as urethrocutaneous fistula, meatal/urethral stenosis, wound-related complications (wound dehiscence, wound infection, or meatal retraction), prepuce-related complications (prepuce fistula, prepuce dehiscence, skin necrosis, or phimosis), testis-related complications (testicular ascent, torsion, infection, or atrophy), and urinary tract infection (UTI). Functional outcomes included urinary stream direction, maximum flow rate, voided volume, average flow rate, voiding time, flow curve shape, and residual urine. Cosmetic outcomes included HOSE (hypospadias objective scoring evaluation) score [7], PPPS (Pediatric Penile Perception Score) [8], and HOPE (Hypospadias Objective Penile Evaluation) score [9]. The primary outcomes were postoperative complications. The secondary outcomes were functional and cosmetic outcomes.

Data extraction and quality assessment

Two independent authors (HY, QS) screened all retrieved titles and abstracts according to the pre-described inclusion criteria to identify potentially eligible studies. After screening, we accessed the full text to determine the final included studies independently. The following data from each included study were extracted: study characteristics (first author, published year, study design, hypospadias type, surgery type, and follow-up time) and patient characteristics (patient numbers, patient age, incidence of each complication, evaluation methods and corresponding values of functional and cosmetic outcomes). For the whole process, discrepancies were resolved by discussion between the two reviewers and re-evaluation with a third author (XG). The methodological quality of all included studies were independently assessed using the 27-item Downs and Black scale [10], a validated tool for evaluating randomized and nonrandomized studies, which consists of 4 aspects: study reporting, external validity, internal validity, and the power of the study, and the total scores ranged from 0 to 32. We used the following criteria to assess the risk of bias of study: low-risk study (total score ranged from 24 to 32), moderate-risk study (total score ranged from 16 to 23) and high-risk study (total score ranged from 0 to 15). Interrater consistency for the

Downs and Black score assessment was analyzed using the Kappa statistic, in which the power of the Kappa value was interpreted as poor (Kappa value ≤ 0.40), good (Kappa value ranged from 0.40–0.75), and excellent (Kappa value > 0.75) agreement.

Statistical analysis

We used RevMan 5.3 (Cochrane Library, Oxford, UK) and STATA 13.1 (Corp LP, College Station, TX, USA) software programs to perform this meta-analysis and relevant subgroup analyses. Kappa statistic was performed using IBM SPSS Statistics 23.0 software (IBM Corp., Armonk, NY, USA). The standardized mean difference (SMD) was calculated as the effect size for continuous outcomes and the risk ratio (RR) was calculated for dichotomous outcomes, both with 95% confidence intervals (CI). The Mantel–Haenszel method was used to calculate pooled RR [11]. Heterogeneity was evaluated by the Cochrane's Q-statistic and the I^2 statistic [12]. A random-effects model was used if heterogeneity was significant (the Q statistic was significant or I^2 values > 50%). Otherwise, a fixed-effects model would be used. We used the funnel plot and Egger's test to detect publication bias if at least 10 studies were available [12, 13]. Sensitivity and subgroup analyses were performed to assess the robustness of the results and to find the possible sources of heterogeneity. Several subgroup analyses were conducted, including different hypospadias types, study design, and other available groups. A P value < 0.05 was considered to be statistically significant.

Results

Literature selection and study characteristics

Of 680 database article titles and 57 trial register titles screened, 330 abstracts were reviewed, 13 full texts were reviewed, and 6 articles [14–19] met our inclusion criteria and were included in our meta-analysis (Fig. 1). The 6 comparative studies involved a total of 353 hypospadias patients (145 patients in the TVF group and 208 in the DF group). One study [15] was retrospective, and 5 [14, 16–19] were prospective. Two studies included distal and midshaft hypospadias [14, 18], and 4 [15–17, 19] included all types of hypospadias. All studies performed a one-stage TIP urethroplasty for primary hypospadias (Table 1). Of the included studies, 71/353 (20.11%) reported a postoperative complication: 34/353 (9.63) reported urethrocutaneous fistula, 15/353 (4.25) meatal/urethral stenosis, 12/353 (3.40%) prepuce-related complications, and 9/353 (2.55%) wound-related complications. Only 1 children had a mild testis torsion in DF group, and no instances of damage to testicular vessels, vas deferens, scrotal abscess or haematoma were reported in the included studies (Table 2).

Assessment of methodological quality

Because only 1 RCT, 2 non-RCTs (1 non-randomized trial and 1 controlled before-after trial) and 3 cohort studies were included, we used the Downs and Black scale [10] for assessing methodological quality instead of the Cochrane Collaboration tool for RCT, the NOS (Newcastle–Ottawa Scale) for cohort studies, and MINORS (Methodological Index for Nonrandomized Studies) for non-RCTs.

For the detailed Down and Black scale items and scores of 2 independent raters see Additional file 1: Table S2. The mean Down and Black scores ranged from 16 to 25.5. Strengths included study reporting and external validity. Weaknesses included internal validity and the power of the study. The Kappa value of the interrater consistency for the Downs and Black score assessment was 0.571 ($P = 0.121$), which means we are in good agreement.

Meta-analysis

A total of 6 comparative studies [14–19], comprising 353 hypospadias children with repaired TIP, were included. All studies reported the incidence of postoperative complications. The RR of the total complications rate for DF was 2.41 (95% CI 1.42–4.07, $P = 0.0001$) compared with TVF in TIP repair for hypospadias. The heterogeneity was not statistically significant ($P = 0.13$, $I^2 = 42\%$), and the fixed-effect model was used for analysis (Fig. 2). The RRs were 6.48 (2.20–19.12, $P = 0.0007$), 5.95 (1.13–31.30, $P = 0.04$), 0.62 (0.25–1.52, $P = 0.29$), and 0.75 (0.23–2.46, $P = 0.64$) for urethrocutaneous fistula, prepuce-related complications, meatal/urethral stenosis, and wound-related complications, respectively, when comparing DF to TVF (Fig. 3). The sources of heterogeneity were all statistically not significant (all I^2 values were equal to 0%). No functional or cosmetic outcomes were reported in any of the included studies.

Since only 6 studies were included in this meta-analysis, we did not perform further analysis for publication bias. Sensitivity analyses were conducted by changing the model to a random-effect model and re-performing meta-analyses after omitting each study. The results of sensitivity analyses indicated that changing the model to a random-effect model and omitting any one study did not significantly influence our results, which stabilized the meta-analysis results (Additional file 1: Figs. S1 and S2). Subgroup analyses for postoperative complications of TIP between DF and TVF were conducted and the results are summarized in Table 3.

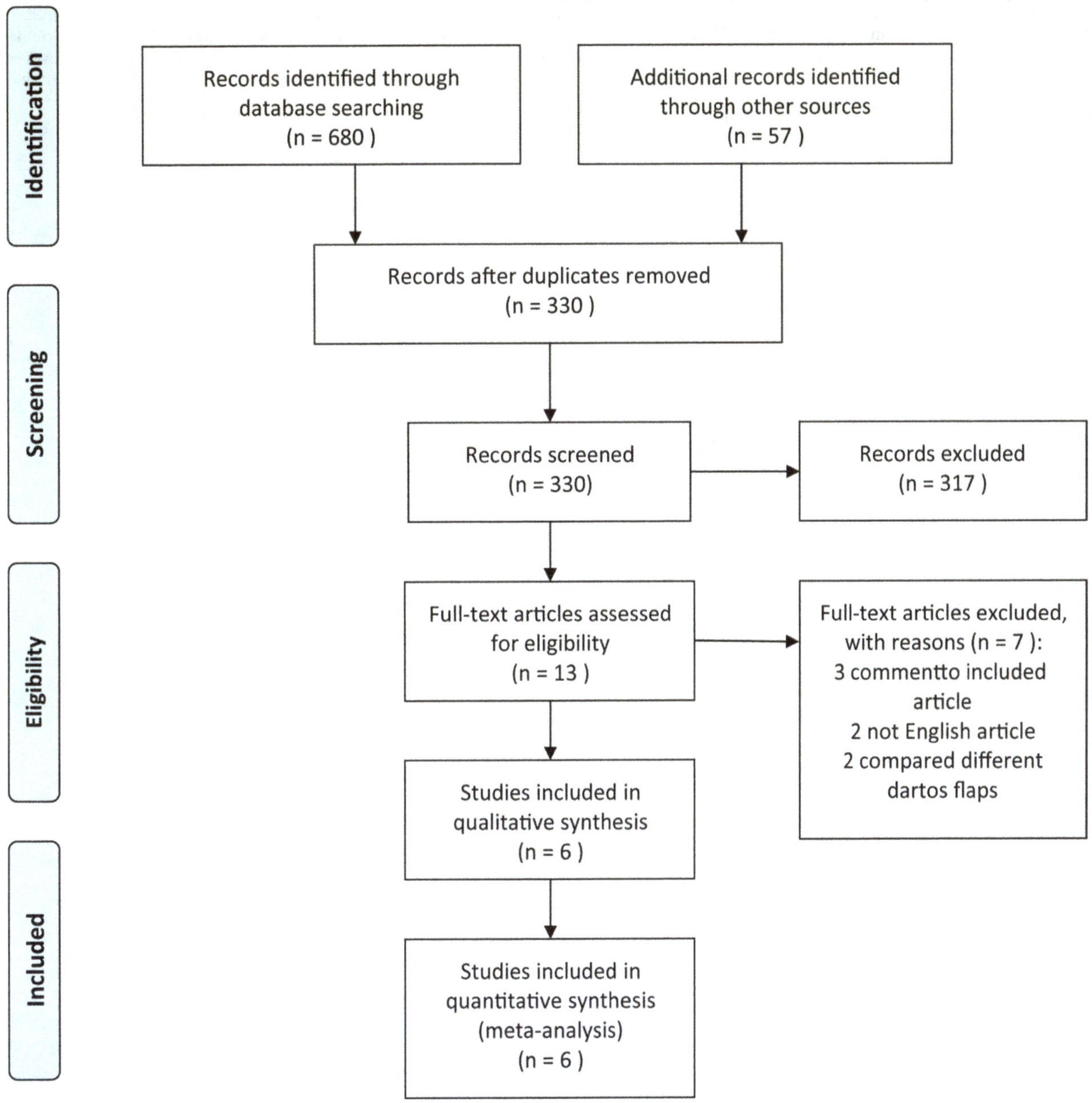

Fig. 1 Flow diagram of study identification and screening for final inclusion

Discussion

This meta-analysis was the first comprehensive synthesis of evidence for currently available comparisons between DF and TVF flap techniques for TIP urethroplasty in primary hypospadias patients in comparative studies. We included 6 comparative studies, comprising 353 hypospadias patients who received TIP repair with the use of DF or TVF flaps. Evidence of our findings came from the pooled estimate size for the primary outcomes, which showed that TVF was better than DF for the repair of hypospadias in terms of total postoperative complications, urethrocutaneous fistula, and wound-related complications. No significant difference was found in meatal/urethral stenosis and prepuce-related complications. No significant difference was found in different hypospadias type, study design, and perioperative use of antibiotics subgroups. Additional, sensitivity analyses verified the robustness of the results in this meta-analysis.

Table 1 Summarizes the primary characteristics of the included trials

Author, year	Study design	Hypospadias type	Total number of patients	Mean age (range) (year)	Follow-up (mo)	Perioperative use of antibiotics	Postoperative complications	Functional and cosmetic outcomes
Babu 2013 [14]	Pro	Distal and midshaft	83	1.06 (0.75–1.6)	12	Intravenous + oral antibiotics	DF: 11 urethrocutaneous fistula, 4 meatal stenosis, 6 skin necrosis, 2 glans dehiscence TVF: 1 urethrocutaneous fistula, 1 glans dehiscence, 4 meatal stenosis	NA
Basavaraju 2017 [15]	Retro	Distal, midshaft and proximal	83	3.44 (1.6–12)	6–36	Intravenous + oral antibiotics	DF: 11 urethrocutaneous fistula, 1 meatal stenosis, 3 glans dehiscence TVF: 0	NA
Chatterjee 2004 [16]	Pro	Distal, midshaft and proximal	49	4.6 (1–22)	12–48(mean 24)	No	DF: 3 urethrocutaneous fistula TVF: 1 wound dehiscence	NA
Dhua 2012 [17]	Pro	Distal, midshaft and proximal	50	3.21 (1–12)	NA	Intravenous + oral antibiotics	DF: 3 urethrocutaneous fistula, 3 skin necrosis TVF: 1 wound dehiscence	NA
Gajbhiye 2018 [18]	Pro	Distal and midshaft	48	1.75 (1.5–4.33)	6–18	Intravenous + oral antibiotics	DF: 3 urethrocutaneous fistula, 3 skin necrosis TVF: 1 wound dehiscence	NA
Kurbet 2018 [19]	Pro	Distal, midshaft and proximal	40	4.85 (0.75–18)	>6	No	DF: 2 urethrocutaneous fistula, 2 meatal stenosis, 1 urethral stricture TVF: 2 meatal stenosis, 1 urethral stricture, 1 mild testis torsion	NA

Pro prospective, *Retro* retrospective, *TIP* tubularized incised plate, *TVF* tunica vaginalis fascia, *DF* dartos fascia, *NA* not available

Reoperation for failed hypospadias or fistula repair has been considered a serious problem because the dense fibrotic tissue causes difficulties in wound healing and increases the rate of complications [20]. Over 300 surgical methods and modifications have been developed for repairing the hypospadias, while various complications have occurred, especially urethrocutaneous fistula, one of the most common complications of these techniques [21]. In our study, the incidence of urethrocutaneous fistula was 9.63%, followed by meatal/urethral stenosis (4.25%), consistent with the 7.50% (fistula) and 4.40% (stenosis) incidence rates in a systematic review [22]. Patient age, glans size, urethral defect length, urethral operation history, surgical procedure, type of surgical

Table 2 Complications of TIP hypospadias repair in all included studies ($N = 353$)

Complication	n (%)	n/N
Urethrocutaneous fistula	34 (47.89)	9.63%
Meatal/urethral stenosis	15 (21.13)	4.25%
Prepuce-related complications	12 (16.90)	3.40%
Wound-related complications	9 (12.68)	2.55%
Testis-related complications	1 (1.41)	0.28%
Urinary tract infection	0 (0)	0
Total complications	71 (100)	20.11%

n number of complication, *N* number of total cases

repair, chordee degree, magnification technique, caudal anesthesia, preoperative hormonal stimulation, and other many factors may relate to the development of complications postoperatively [21–25]. Additional soft coverages on the neourethra are also introduced to avoid these complications, especially to decrease the incidence of postoperative urethrocutaneous fistula. TVF, DF, Buck's fascia, spongious tissue, external spermatic fascia, adipose tissue of the scrotum, adipose tissue of the spermatic cord, and a combination of tissues and platelet-rich plasma are used in different studies [26–32] with various outcomes. Among them, TVF and DF are the most popular flaps used in the repair of hypospadias and fistula.

Objective and comprehensive assessments of the outcome of hypospadias repair may have a major impact on future clinical practice. Evaluations of outcome after hypospadias repair include complication rate, cosmetic outcome, functional outcome, and even the effects on psychology. In this study, we focused on assessing the effect of DF and TVF on the outcomes of complication rate after TIP urethroplasty in primary hypospadias. For functional and cosmetic results in our meta-analysis, the conclusions are uncertain due to the limited evidence. The assessment methods of cosmetic and functional outcomes in most published studies were thought to be prone to bias, subjectivity, or inaccuracy. Several assessment methods have been applied for evaluating cosmetic outcomes after TIP repairs, such as HOSE, PPPS, and HOPE [7–9]. However, all of them are retrospectively assessed, and which method is the most reliable and valid to assess the outcome is uncertain. From the practical point of view, it is highly recommended that standardized assessment tools be used for comparability and reproducibility and to build up a prospective database that does not currently exist. Moreover, there are many measurement indexes applied for the assessment of functional outcome in TIP repair, including urinary stream direction, maximum flow rate, voided volume, average flow rate, voiding time, flow curve shape, and residual urine. However, the significance of these measurement indexes remains uncertain until long-term follow-up studies clarify the significance of abnormal flow parameters [33]. Moreover, the assessment of functional outcomes in non-toilet-trained boys is difficult. Therefore, large prospective studies and uniform assessment criteria for functional and cosmetic evaluation are needed. Other outcomes, such as life quality, sexual function, and sexual psychology, are also not reported in any of the included studies.

DF is a layer of connective tissue found in the penile dorsal or ventral area, foreskin, and scrotum and can be used in hypospadias or fistula repair in different techniques [34, 35]. TVF can be harvested through a penile incision by degloving up to the root of the penis [26] or with an additional scrotal incision that reaches and covers the neourethra through a subcutaneous scrotal tunnel [36]. Excellent vascularity, easy availability and adequate source are advantages of DF, making this flap technique more popular for many paediatric urologists, especially young surgeons. Penile rotation and preputial skin necrosis are commonly reported relevant complications in the use of DF and can be avoided by careful operation and technical improvement. However, harvest of TVF may

Study	DF Events	DF Total	TVF Events	TVF Total	Weight	Risk Ratio M-H, Fixed, 95% CI
Babu 2013	23	62	6	21	51.3%	1.30 [0.61, 2.75]
Basavaraju 2017	15	57	0	26	3.9%	14.43 [0.90, 232.36]
Chatterjee 2004	3	20	1	29	4.7%	4.35 [0.49, 38.88]
Dhua 2012	6	25	1	25	5.7%	6.00 [0.78, 46.29]
Gajbhiye 2018	6	24	1	24	5.7%	6.00 [0.78, 46.14]
Kurbet 2018	5	20	5	20	28.6%	1.00 [0.34, 2.93]
Total (95% CI)		**208**		**145**	**100.0%**	**2.41 [1.42, 4.07]**
Total events	58		14			

Heterogeneity: Chi² = 8.59, df = 5 (P = 0.13); I² = 42%
Test for overall effect: Z = 3.27 (P = 0.001)

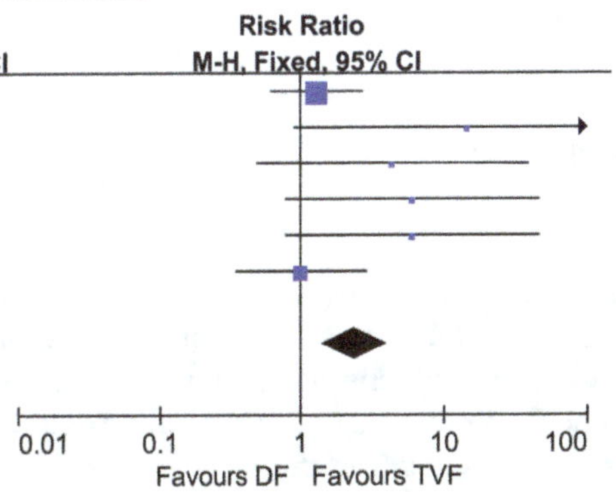

Fig. 2 Forest plot of the comparisons the total complications between DF and TVF flap techniques. *DF* dartos fascia, *TVF* tunica vaginalis fascia

Subgroup	DF Events	DF Total	TVF Events	TVF Total	Weight	Risk Ratio M-H, Fixed, 95% CI
1.1 urethrocutaneous fistula						
Babu 2013	11	62	1	21	6.8%	3.73 [0.51, 27.16]
Basavaraju 2017	11	57	0	26	3.1%	10.71 [0.65, 175.08]
Chatterjee 2004	3	20	0	29	1.9%	10.00 [0.54, 183.61]
Dhua 2012	3	25	0	25	2.3%	7.00 [0.38, 128.87]
Gajbhiye 2018	3	24	0	24	2.3%	7.00 [0.38, 128.61]
Kurbet 2018	2	20	0	20	2.3%	5.00 [0.26, 98.00]
Subtotal (95% CI)		**208**		**145**	**18.7%**	**6.48 [2.20, 19.12]**
Total events	33		1			
Heterogeneity: Chi² = 0.54, df = 5 (P = 0.99); I² = 0%						
Test for overall effect: Z = 3.38 (P = 0.0007)						
1.2 meatal/urethral stenosis						
Babu 2013	4	62	4	21	27.3%	0.34 [0.09, 1.24]
Basavaraju 2017	1	57	0	26	3.1%	1.40 [0.06, 33.18]
Chatterjee 2004	0	20	0	29		Not estimable
Dhua 2012	0	25	0	25		Not estimable
Gajbhiye 2018	0	24	0	24		Not estimable
Kurbet 2018	3	20	3	20	13.7%	1.00 [0.23, 4.37]
Subtotal (95% CI)		**208**		**145**	**44.1%**	**0.62 [0.25, 1.52]**
Total events	8		7			
Heterogeneity: Chi² = 1.49, df = 2 (P = 0.47); I² = 0%						
Test for overall effect: Z = 1.05 (P = 0.29)						
1.3 wound-related complications						
Babu 2013	2	62	1	21	6.8%	0.68 [0.06, 7.10]
Basavaraju 2017	3	57	0	26	3.1%	3.26 [0.17, 60.89]
Chatterjee 2004	0	20	1	29	5.6%	0.48 [0.02, 11.13]
Dhua 2012	0	25	1	25	6.8%	0.33 [0.01, 7.81]
Gajbhiye 2018	0	24	1	24	6.8%	0.33 [0.01, 7.80]
Kurbet 2018	0	20	0	20		Not estimable
Subtotal (95% CI)		**208**		**145**	**29.3%**	**0.75 [0.23, 2.46]**
Total events	5		4			
Heterogeneity: Chi² = 1.56, df = 4 (P = 0.82); I² = 0%						
Test for overall effect: Z = 0.47 (P = 0.64)						
1.4 prepuce-related complications						
Babu 2013	6	62	0	21	3.4%	4.54 [0.27, 77.33]
Basavaraju 2017	0	57	0	26		Not estimable
Chatterjee 2004	0	20	0	29		Not estimable
Dhua 2012	3	25	0	25	2.3%	7.00 [0.38, 128.87]
Gajbhiye 2018	3	24	0	24	2.3%	7.00 [0.38, 128.61]
Kurbet 2018	0	20	0	20		Not estimable
Subtotal (95% CI)		**208**		**145**	**8.0%**	**5.95 [1.13, 31.30]**
Total events	12		0			
Heterogeneity: Chi² = 0.06, df = 2 (P = 0.97); I² = 0%						
Test for overall effect: Z = 2.11 (P = 0.04)						

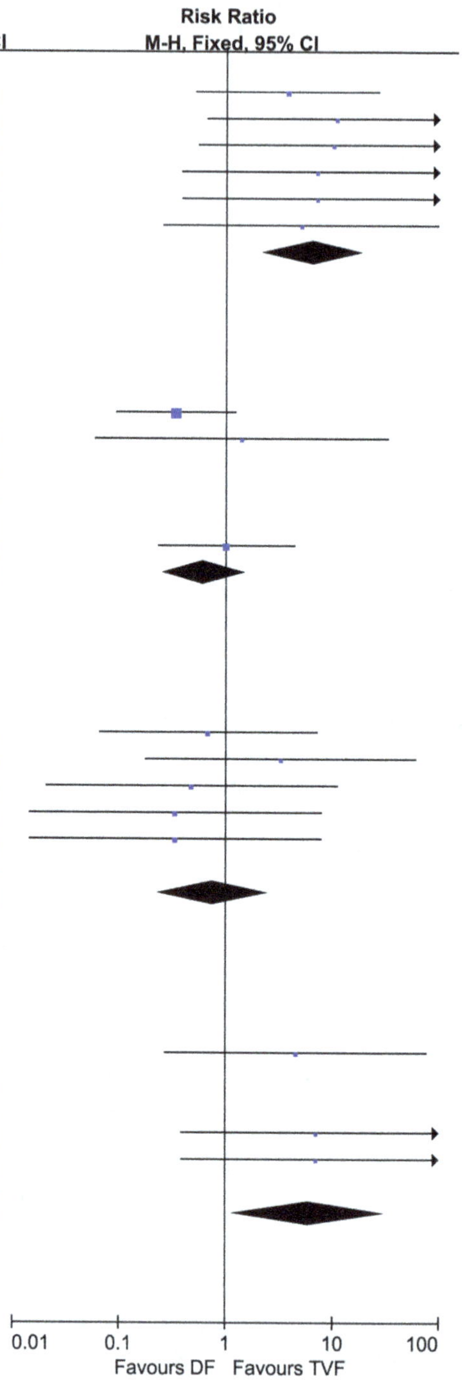

Fig. 3 Forest plot of the comparisons each complication between DF and TVF flap techniques. *DF* dartos fascia, *TVF* tunica vaginalis fascia

damage the vas deferens or vessels of the testicles, resulting in scrotal abscess or scrotal haematoma, but were ultimately not reported in any of the included studies. Snodgrass described additional interposition of vascularized tissues between the tubularized plate and the glans closure dissected from the dorsal preputial and shaft skin [2]. Duckett has described that when dartos is separated from the skin, it compromises the vascularity of the overlying skin [37]. Thus, the dissection of DF may compromise the vascularity of the preputial skin covering and result in subsequent skin necrosis, which is consistent with the conclusion of our outcomes. The blood supply of

Table 3 Subgroup analyses for postoperative complications in meta-analysis

Subgroup	Total complications		Urethrocutaneous fistula		Meatal/urethral stenosisMeatal/urethral stenosis		Prepuce-related complications		Wound-related complications	
	RR (95% CI)	P	RR (95% CI)	P	RR (95% CI)	P	RR (95% CI)	P	RR (95% CI)	P
All patients	*2.41 (1.42–4.07)*		*6.48 (2.20–19.12)*		0.62 (0.25–1.52)		*5.95 (1.13–31.30)*		0.75 (0.23–2.46)	
Hypospadias type										
D & M	1.77 (0.89–3.53)	0.26	4.55 (0.90–23.05)	0.59	0.34 (0.09–1.24)	0.22	5.53 (0.73–41.82)	0.90	0.51 (0.08–3.27)	0.60
D, M & P	*3.25 (1.45–7.30)*		*8.32 (1.91–36.31)*		1.07 (0.28–4.10)		7.00 (0.38–128.87)		0.97 (0.20–4.63)	
Study design										
Retro	14.43 (0.90–232.26)	0.16	10.71 (0.65–175.08)	0.68	1.40 (0.06–33.28)	0.59	–	–	3.26 (0.17–60.89)	0.24
Pro	*1.92 (1.13–3.26)*		*5.63 (1.77–17.97)*		0.56 (0.22–1.43)		*5.95 (1.13–31.30)*		0.45 (0.11–1.90)	
Perioperative use of antibiotics										
Yes	*2.88 (1.51–5.46)*	0.24	*6.26 (1.76–22.22)*	0.90	0.45 (0.14–1.43)	0.40	–	–	0.82 (0.23–2.96)	0.76
No	1.47 (0.58–3.71)		7.26 (0.93–56.54)		1.00 (0.23–4.37)		*5.95 (1.13–31.30)*		0.48 (0.02–11.13)	

Statistically significant results are italicized

Retro retrospective, *Pro* prospective, *P p* value for interaction, *D, M & P* distal, midshaft and proximal

the neourethra tissue may be affected due to the dissection and utilization of DF, which mainly comes from the shortage of dartos or preputial skin necrosis. Although skin necrosis was inconsequential in the long run, it did cause anxiety and distress to the families and resulted in more hospital visits. Moreover, dissection to raise DF may damage the intrinsic blood supply to the outer skin, which is transposed ventrally to provide skin cover and may consequently devitalize, leading to skin necrosis, and fistula formation. However, this is rarely affected in the TVF technique, as its ventral skin covering is almost never compromised. All of these factors can theoretically explain the advantage of TVF over DF. We performed this meta-analysis to prove the advantages of TVF over DF with the data.

The results of our meta-analysis were partially consistent with the results of a systematic review by Fahmy et al. [3]. However, there were several differences between the two studies. The study of Fahmy et al. included not only comparative studies but case series, which weakened the evidence. In addition, the literature retrieval process should be as comprehensive as possible, while there was only one database (PubMed) employed in his study. Our analysis included only comparative studies and searched 4 databases (PubMed, EMBASE, the Cochrane Library and Web of Science), a clinical trial register (clinicaltrials.gov) and several international meeting abstract archives. All of these sources enhanced our evidence.

There are several limitations in our meta-analysis. First, although a comprehensive retrieval was performed, only limited studies were included, and most included studies were nonrandomized clinical trials/studies without reporting prospective power calculations and non-inclusion of consecutive patients, which might bias the results. Given the diversity of types of included studies, the level of evidence for our findings is not high. Second, the duration of follow-up varied, ranging from 6 to 48 months. The relatively short length of follow-up limited the present study, as it is known that long-term follow-up is necessary to determine the true complication rate of hypospadias repair and Spinoit et al. [38] stated in their study that only 47.37% of complications appeared in the first year. Third, the definition of complications was inconsistent among all included studies which indicated that reporting complications also depended on different factors and a publication bias existed. A survey of North American paediatric urologists clearly showed that there is a discrepancy between complication rates reported in the literature and participants' operative outcomes, regardless of practice setting, operative volume, or time in practice [39]. In addition, research aimed at studying the effects of different flaps on urethrocutaneous fistula postoperatively may result in bias in other complications. Last, other than follow-up periods and complications criteria, differences in other clinical characteristics, including study settings, patient age, thickness and width of flap, and hypospadias type existed, although the statistical heterogeneity was not high. The contribution of these differences to the outcomes was unknown. We performed subgroup analyses to identify potential sources of heterogeneity, but no significant results were found due to the limited number of studies.

Although many uncontrollable confounding factors may affect the hypospadias surgery outcomes, especially the wide variability for individual surgical experience and complexity for hypospadias cases, additional large sample size, well-designed, single-urologist prospective studies need to be conducted for optimal comparisons between these two flap techniques.

Conclusions

This meta-analysis revealed that compared to DF, TVF is a better option in TIP repair in terms of decreasing the incidence of the total complications, urethrocutaneous fistula, and prepuce-related complications. There is limited evidence for functional and cosmetic outcomes. However, there was substantial heterogeneity between studies indicating a lack of clarity in this field. There remains a need for high-quality prospective comparative trials for reliable evidence and clinical utility.

Supplementary information

Additional file 1. Supplemental Table 1. PRISMA Checklist. **Supplemental Table 2.** Down and Black scale and scores for included studies. **Supplemental Figure 1.** Sensitivity analysis by changing the model to a random-effect model. (**a**) total complications, (**b**) each complication. **Supplemental Figure 2.** Sensitivity analysis by omitting each study. (**a**) total complications, (**b**) urethrocutaneous fistula, (**c**) meatal/urethral stenosis, (**d**) wound-related complications, (**e**) prepuce-related complications.

Abbreviations

TIP: Tubularized incised plate; DF: Dartos fascia; TVF: Tunica vaginalis fascia; RCT : Randomized controlled trials; RR: Risk ratio; CI: Confidence intervals.

Acknowledgements

Not applicable.

Authors' contributions

Manuscript writing and editing: HY, XX, DH, QS, XG and JF. Manuscript revision: HY, XG and JF. Project development: XG. Rewrote project development: JF. Data collection: HY, DH, XX and QS, data management/analysis: HY and HZ. XG and JF contributed equally to this work. All authors reviewed the manuscript. All authors read and approved the final manuscript.

Author details

[1] Zhejiang University School of Medicine, Hangzhou, China. [2] Children's Hospital, Zhejiang University School of Medicine, Hangzhou, China. [3] National Clinical Research Center for Child Health, Hangzhou, China. [4] Department of Pediatric Surgery, Zhejiang University Jinhua Hospital, Jinhua, China.

References

1. Yu X, Nassar N, Mastroiacovo P, Canfield M, Groisman B, Bermejo-Sánchez E, et al. Hypospadias prevalence and trends in international birth defect surveillance systems, 1980–2010. Eur Urol. 2019;76(4):482–90.
2. Snodgrass W. Tubularized incised plate urethroplasty in distal hypospadias. J Urol. 1994;151(2):464–5.
3. Fahmy O, Khairul-Asri MG, Schwentner C, Schubert T, Stenzl A, Zahran MH, et al. Algorithm for optimal urethral coverage in hypospadias and fistula repair: a systematic review. Eur Urol. 2016;70(2):293–8.
4. Cheng EY, Vemulapalli SN, Kropp BP, Pope JC 4th, Furness PD 3rd, Kaplan WE, et al. Snodgrass hypospadias repair with vascularized dartos flap: the perfect repair for virgin cases of hypospadias? J Urol. 2002;168(4 Pt 2):1723–6 (discussion 1726).
5. Chandrasekharam VV. Comparative study of dartos fascia and tunica vaginalis pedicle wrap for the tubularized incised plate in primary hypospadias repair. BJU Int. 2005;95(6):909–10.
6. Landau EH, Gofrit ON, Meretyk S, Katz G, Golijanin D, Shenfeld OZ, et al. Outcome analysis of tunica vaginalis flap for the correction of recurrent urethrocutaneous fistula in children. J Urol. 2003;170(4 Pt 2):1596–9159 (discussion 1599).
7. Holland AJ, Smith GH, Ross FI, Cass DT. HOSE: an objective scoring system for evaluating the results of hypospadias surgery. BJU Int. 2011;88(3):255–8.
8. Weber DM, Schönbucher VB, Landolt MA, Gobet R. The Pediatric Penile Perception Score: an instrument for patient self-assessment and surgeon evaluation after hypospadias repair. J Urol. 2008;180(3):1080–4.
9. van der Toorn F, de Jong TP, de Gier RP, Callewaert PR, van der Horst EH, Steffens MG, et al. Introducing the HOPE (Hypospadias Objective Penile Evaluation)-score: a validation study of an objective scoring system for evaluating cosmetic appearance in hypospadias patients. J Pediatr Urol. 2013;9(6 Pt B):1006–16.
10. Downs SH, Black N. The feasibility of creating a checklist for the assessment of the methodological quality both of randomised and non-randomised studies of health care interventions. J Epidemiol Commun Health. 1998;52(6):377–84.
11. Mantel N, Haenszel W. Statistical aspects of the analysis of data from retrospective studies of disease. J Natl Cancer Inst. 1959;22(4):719–48.
12. Higgins JPT, Green S. Cochrane handbook for systematic reviews of interventions version 5.1.0. https://handbook-5-1.cochrane.org/; 2011. Accessed 25 Mar 2020.
13. Egger M, Davey Smith G, Schneider M, Minder C. Bias in meta-analysis detected by a simple, graphical test. BMJ. 1997;135(7109):629–34.
14. Babu R, Hariharasudhan S. Tunica vaginalis flap is superior to inner preputial dartos flap as a waterproofing layer for primary TIP repair in midshaft hypospadias. J Pediatr Urol. 2013;9(6 Pt A):804–7.
15. Basavaraju M, Balaji DK. Choosing an ideal vascular cover for Snodgrass repair. Urol Ann. 2017;9(4):348–52.
16. Chatterjee US, Mandal MK, Basu S, Das R, Majhi T. Comparative study of dartos fascia and tunica vaginalis pedicle wrap for the tubularized incised plate in primary hypospadias repair. BJU Int. 2004;94(7):1102–4.
17. Dhua AK, Aggarwal SK, Sinha S, Ratan SK. Soft tissue covers in hypospadias surgery: is tunica vaginalis better than dartos flap? J Indian Assoc Pediatr Surg. 2012;17(1):16–9.
18. Gajbhiye V, Singh N, Singh S, Verma RS. Tunica vaginalis flap (TVF) as an alternative to dartos flap in primary hypospadias repair-our experience. J Evol Med Dent Sci. 2018;7(16):1970–3.
19. Kurbet SB, Koujalagi RS, Geethika V, Nagathan V. A 1-year randomized controlled trial to compare the outcome of primary repair of hypospadias with vascular cover using tunica vaginalis flap with those using preputial dartos fascia. Afr J Paediatr Surg. 2018;15(1):42–7.
20. Snodgrass W, Bush NC. Re-operative urethroplasty after failed hypospadias repair: how prior surgery impacts risk for additional complications. J Pediatr Urol. 2017;13(3):289.e1-6.
21. Dokter EM, Mouës CM, Rooij IALMV, Biezen JJV. Complications after hypospadias correction: prognostic factors and impact on final clinical outcome. Eur J Pediatr Surg. 2018;28(2):200–6.
22. Hardwicke JT, Bechar JA, Hodson J, Osmani O, Park AJ. Fistula after single-stage primary hypospadias repair: a systematic review of the literature. J Plast Reconstr Aesthet Surg. 2015;68(12):1647–55.
23. Yildiz T, Tahtali IN, Ates DC, Keles I, Ilce Z. Age of patient is a risk factor for urethrocutaneous fistula in hypospadias surgery. J Pediatr Urol. 2013;9(6 Pt A):900–3.
24. Bush NC, Villanueva C, Snodgrass W. Glans size is an independent risk factor for urethroplasty complications after hypospadias repair. J Pediatr Urol. 2015;11(6):355.e1-5.
25. Rynja SP, de Jong TPVM, Bosch JLHR, de Kort LMO. Testosterone prior to hypospadias repair: Postoperative complication rates and long-term cosmetic results, penile length and body height. J Pediatr Urol. 2018;14(1):31.e1-8.
26. Snow BW. Use of tunica vaginalis to prevent fistula in hypospadas. J Urol. 1986;136(4):861–3.
27. Churchill BM, van Savage JG, Khoury AE, McLorie GA. The dartos flap as an adjunct in preventing urethrocutaneous fistula in repeat hypospadias surgery. J Urol. 1996;156(6):2047–9.

28. Yerkes EB, Adams MC, Miller DA, Pope JC 4th, Rink RC, Brock JW 3rd. Y-to-I Wrap: Use of the distal spongiosum for hypospadias repair. J Urol. 2000;163(5):1536–8 (discussion 1538-9).
29. Yamataka A, Ando K, Lane GJ, Miyano T. Pedicled external spermatic fascia flap for urethroplasty in hypospadias and closure of urethrocutaneous fistula. J Pediatr Surg. 1998;33(12):1788–9.
30. Seo S, Ochi T, Yazaki Y, Okawada M, Doi T, Miyano G, et al. Soft tissue interposition is effective for protecting the neourethra during hypospadias surgery and preventing postoperative urethrocutaneous fistula: a single surgeon's experience of 243 cases. Pediatr Surg Int. 2015;31(3):297–303.
31. Bilici S, Sekmenli T, Gunes M, Gecit I, Bakan V, Isik D. Comparison of dartos flap and dartos flap plus spongioplasty to prevent the formation of fistulae in the Snodgrass technique. Int Urol Nephrol. 2011;43(4):943–8.
32. Mahmoud AY, Gouda S, Gamaan I, Baky Fahmy MA. Autologous platelet-rich plasma covering urethroplasty versus dartos flap in distal hypospadias repair: a prospective randomized study. Int J Urol. 2019;26(4):475–80.
33. Springer A. Assessment of outcome in hypospadias surgery: a review. Front Pediatr. 2014;2:2.
34. Jia W, Liu GC, Zhang LY, Wen YQ, Fu W, Hu JH, et al. Comparison of tubularized incised plate urethroplasty combined with a meatus-based ventral dartos flap or dorsal dartos flap in hypospadias. Pediatr Surg Int. 2016;32(4):411–5.
35. Erol A, Kayikci A, Memik O, Cam K, Akman Y. Single vs. double dartos inter position flaps in preventing urethrocutaneous fistula after tubularized incised plate urethroplasty in primary distal hypospadias: a prospective randomized study. Urol Int. 2009;83(3):354–8.
36. Pescheloche P, Parmentier B, Hor T, Chamond O, Chabaud M, Irtan S, et al. Tunica vaginalis flap for urethrocutaneous fistula repair after proximal and mid-shaft hypospadias surgery: a 12-year experience. J Pediatr Urol. 2018;14(5):421.e1-6.
37. Duckett JW. Hypospadias. In: Walsh PC, Retik AB, Vaughan ED, Wein AJ, editors. Campbell's urology. Philadelphia: Academic; 1998. p. 2094–116.
38. Spinoit AF, Poelaert F, Groen LA, Van Laecke E, Hoebeke P. Hypospadias repair at a tertiary care center: long-term followup is mandatory to determine the real complication rate. J Urol. 2013;1899(6):2276–81.
39. Prasad MM, Marks A, Vasquez E, Yerkes EB, Cheng EY. Published surgical success rates in pediatric urology–fact or fiction? J Urol. 2012;188(4 Suppl):1643–7.

16

Retrograde ureteric stent insertion from percutaneous suprapubic access to the bladder in renal transplant recipients with ureteric stenosis: A novel minimally invasive technique

Jian-Hui Wu[1], Chun-Bai Mo[2], Li Dong-Zhai[3], Fei Luo[4], Qing-Tong Ma[1] and Shi-Qiang Yang[1*]

Abstract

Background: Ureteric stricture is a common and salvaging complications after renal transplantation. Two treatment methods are usually used, retrograde ureteral stent placement and percutaneous nephrostomy. The former has a higher failure rate, the latter has a great risk. Therefore, a safe and reliable treatment is needed.

Case presentation: A technique of retrograde insertion of ureteral stent was established, which was applicable in three transplant recipients with post-transplant ureteral stenosis, and the data was retrospectively recorded. The patients are 2 men and 1 woman, ages 44, 27 and 32 years. These patients underwent a total of five times of retrograde insertion of ureteral stent between 2018 and 2019. None of these patients had any postoperative complication, but all patients had complete recovery from oliguric status within two weeks.

Conclusions: The retrograde ureteric stent insertion by percutaneous suprapubic access to the bladder (RUS-PSAB) was demonstrated feasibility and safety in a case series with short-term follow-up. However, larger prospective studies are needed.

Keywords: Kidney transplantation, Ureteral obstruction, Stent, Complications, Ureteral calculi, Kidney calculi, Retrospective studies

Background

Urological complications occupy 2–14% of all complications during renal transplantation [1, 2]. The incidence of ureteric stricture after kidney transplantation can reach up to 3% [2]. Among all ureteric stricture cases, 73% occur at the distal end, involving the ureteroneocystostomy [3]. When patients who received a kidney present with hydronephrosis due to obstructing stones or ureteric stricture, they should undergo the insertion of either a nephrostomy or a ureteral stent as soon as possible. Conventionally, ureteral catheterization under a cystoscope has been considered an initial approach before percutaneous renal puncture with drainage [4, 5]. Several reports have suggested that nephrostomy placement is cost-saving and safe. However, in the experience of the investigators, most candidates are reluctant to undergo percutaneous renal drainage due to hidden risks. A randomized study revealed that there was no significant difference between nephrostomy and ureteral stenting [6]. Furthermore, retrograde ureteral stent placement in transplant recipients can be time-consuming

*Correspondence: yangshiqiang009@126.com
[1] Department of Urology, Tianjin First Central Hospital, No. 24 Fukang Road, Nankai District, Tianjin 300192, China
Full list of author information is available at the end of the article

and technically difficult. In the present study, we report our experience in using retrograde ureteral stent insertion through percutaneous suprapubic access to the bladder (RUS-PSAB) to successfully relieve ureteral obstruction in three patients with confirmed allograft hydronephrosis.

Case presentation

Patient 1 was a 44-year-old Chinese male with end-stage renal disease (ESRD) of unknown origin and a blood type of AB (Rh+). Before accepting renal transplantation from his 59-year old father with a blood type of B (Rh+), the patient has been on hemodialysis for more than one year. During surgery, the graft renal vein and artery were anastomosed to the patient's right external iliac vein and artery, respectively, using 5-0 polypropylene in an end-to-side manner. Then, a 6-Fr 13-cm double-J stent was placed, and the transplanted ureter was anastomosed to the recipient bladder using the Lich-Gregoire technique, which incorporated a 5-0 polyglactin interrupted suture. The patient's postoperative immunosuppression regimen consisted of tacrolimus, mycophenolate mofetil and prednisolone. Four weeks after the transplantation, the double-J stent was removed by cystoscope under local anesthesia. The patient's serum creatinine (s-CR) at discharge was 75 μmol/L (normal range: 45–84 μmol/L).

At five years post-transplantation, the ultrasound revealed multiple calculi at renal calices (Fig. 1). Watchful waiting was suggested, since the patient was asymptomatic with normal s-CR. After four months, the patient was admitted for swelling pain that involved the renal allograft and decreased urine output. The allograft ultrasound revealed severe hydronephrosis, and the computed tomography (CT) demonstrated a 10-mm calculus obstructing the ureterocystostomic site. The patient underwent a cystoscopy for ureteral stenting, but failed. Since the transplanted ureteral orifice was located at the dome of the bladder, which formed an oblique angle between the orifice and cystoscopic access site, the intubation from a different plane carried a low probability of success. Prior to the percutaneous nephrostomy (PCN), percutaneous cystostomy was performed at a position relative to the ureteral orifice of the renal allograft using an 18-G needle (cook), in order to correct the oblique intubation angle. Under cystoscope guidance, the channel size was expanded step by step to 10F, followed by the placement of an expanded sheath close to the edge of the transplanted ureteral orifice. One retrograde guidewire was passed into the transplanted ureteral orifice, and a double-J tube (Black Silicone Filiform DP Ureteral Stent Set Wire Guide with Hydrophilic Coating, Cook Incorporated, USA) was successfully inserted into the allograft along the guidewire. After two weeks, a retrograde ureteroscope was inserted and reached the calculus, and Holmium-yttrium aluminum garnet (Ho-YAG) laser lithotripsy was performed (VersaPulse ® PowerSuite

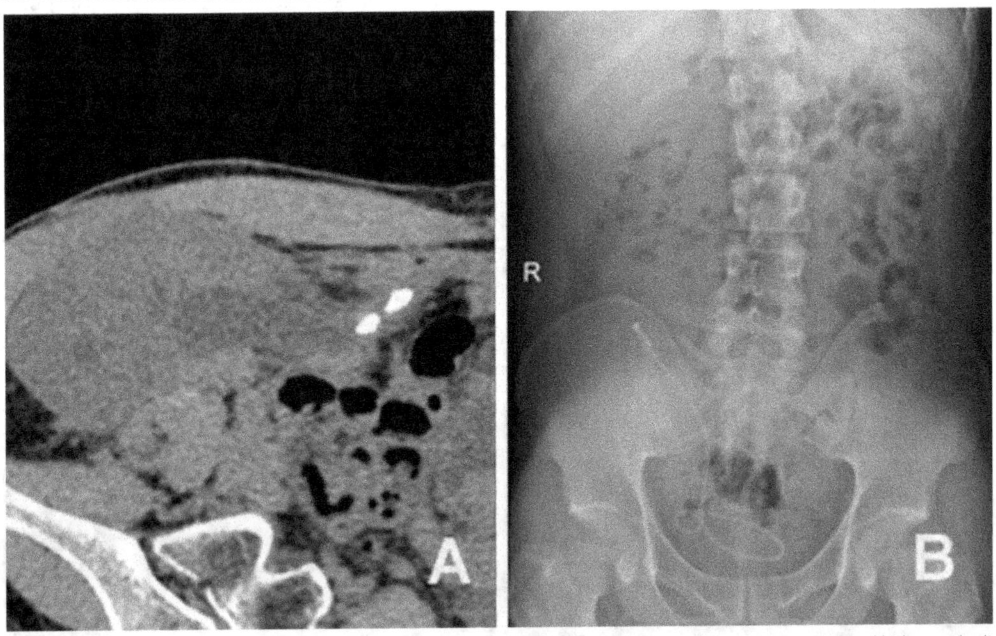

Fig. 1 The placement of a double-J stent in a 39-year-old Chinese male developing ureterovesical junction stenosis and kidney calculi. **a** The computed tomography revealed multiple allograft stones. **b** The KUB film revealed that the double-J stent was inserted into the pelvis of the renal allograft

TM 100+W, Lumenis Surgical, USA). Although the lithotripsy was successfully performed at the first time, the ureter could not be reached through the conventional route of the ureteroscope again for subsequent calculus fragment removal. After several failed attempts, the surgeons repeated the trans-vesical puncture to place the double-J tube similar to the first treatment session. After 1 month, the double-J tube was removed using a cystoscope, and there were few stone residues left in the allograft, with diameters of < 4 mm. The patient's s-CR remained at 85 μmol/L (Fig. 1).

Patient 2 was a 32 years old woman with ESRD secondary to IgA nephropathy, hypertension and renal anemia. This patient was admitted for renal transplantation from a deceased donor on April 2019. The donor was a 38-year-old man who died from traffic accident-related craniocerebral trauma. The donor and recipient were blood-group compatible based on a 5 HLA antigen match, and both flow microcytotoxicity and direct microcytotoxicity cross-match were negative. The panel reactivity for the recipient was 2%. The renal allograft vessels were anastomosed side-to-end to the recipient's external iliac vessels using two 5/0 prolene running sutures. After placing a double-J stent, the transplanted ureter was anastomosed to the bladder according to the Lich-Gregoire technique using 5/0 polydioxanone sutures. The duration of this procedure was 110 min, with 20 mL of blood loss. The postoperative immunosuppression regimen consisted of tacrolimus, mycophenolate mofetil and prednisolone. At the 14th postoperative day, the double-J stent was removed, and the patient's s-CR decreased to within the normal level. However, at 20 days after the transplantation, the patient was readmitted due to high fever, oliguria and allograft area pain. The examination of this recipient revealed elevated s-CR, urea nitrogen and uric acid, with electrolyte disturbance. The urine culture grew *Escherichia coli* with positive extended-spectrum beta-lactamase. Ultrasonography revealed a mildly hydronephrotic allograft and complete ureteral dilatation. The patient's condition improved after intravenous Sulperazone treatment. However, after 1 month, the patient's s-CR remained elevated during the outpatient test, and the magnetic resonance imaging (MRI) identified a pelvic lymphocoele arising from the right pelvic cavity, which compressed the allograft ureter. Cystoscopic intubation was attempted to decompress the patient's collecting system prior to performing the PCN, but failed. Based on the successful experience in patient 1, the trans-vesical puncture was repeated to place the double-J stent, and the procedure succeeded. The patient finally recovered her renal function after ultrasound-guided puncture and pelvic lymphocoele drainage. The double-J stent was retained for 3 months, and removed using a cystoscope (Fig. 2).

Patient 3 was a 27 years old Chinese male diagnosed with ESRD, who received twice a week of hemodialysis for two years. The patient's blood type was B (Rh+), which was the same as that of the donor. The donor was the patient's 52-year-old healthy mother. Ureter and bladder anastomosis were performed using the Lich-Gregoire method. The patient's postoperative immunosuppression regimen consisted of tacrolimus, mycophenolate mofetil and steroid. At the 14th postoperative day, the double-J stent was smoothly removed using a cystoscope.

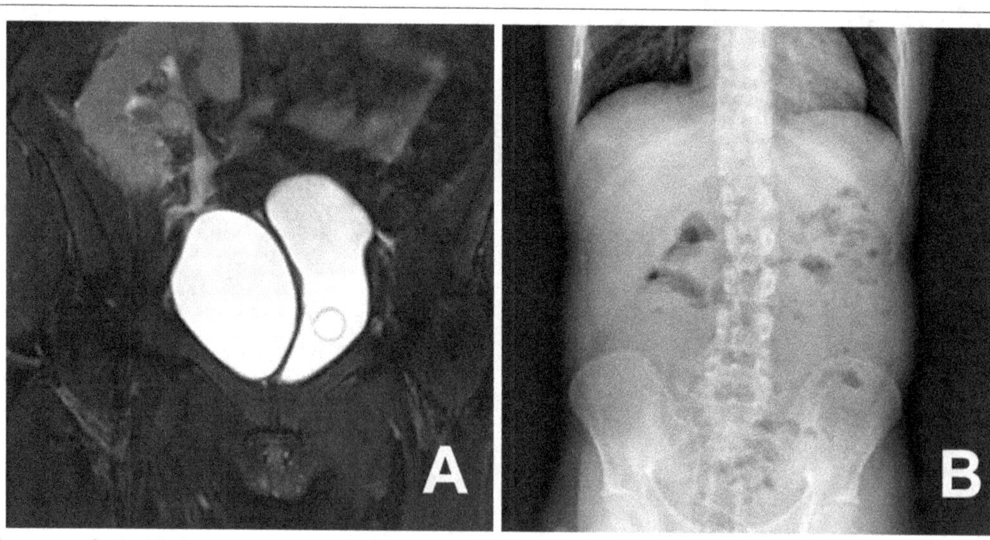

Fig. 2 The placement of a double-J stent in a 32-year-old female with a right pelvic lymphocoele compressing the ureter. **a** The placement of a double-J stent into the pelvis of the renal allograft. **b** The KUB film revealed that the stent was inserted into the pelvis

At discharge, the patient's renal function returned to normal. At the 22nd postoperative day, the patient was hospitalized due to high fever. The ultrasound merely revealed perirenal effusion, and the patient was discharged after antibiotic treatment. However, at 2 months after the operation, the ultrasound examination revealed a hydronephrotic allograft. Despite the patient's asymptomatic status, the patient remained hospitalized, and the admission s-CR was slightly elevated at 114 μmol/L, with normal serum urea, uric acid and calcium. The patient's serum inorganic phosphorus and magnesium levels slightly decreased at 0.67 mmol/L (normal range: 0.85–1.51 mmol/L) and 0.70 mmol/L (normal range: 0.75–1.02 mmol/L), respectively. The patient underwent transurethral cystoscope catheterization under general anesthesia, but failed. The patient was discharged with watchful waiting. At 3.5 months after the transplantation, the patient was admitted for the third time due to fever, oliguria and elevated s-CR. The ultrasonography revealed hydronephrosis with multiple ureteral calculi. The patient underwent cystoscopy with stenting, but failed again due to difficulty of access (the ureteral opening located at the bladder top, near the pubic symphysis) and ureteral opening stenosis. Therefore, trans-vesical puncture was attempted to place the double-J tube again, which was successful. The recovered smoothly after the operation. For the ureteral calculi treatment, ureteroscopy was performed after two weeks. However, the retrograde ureteroscopy through either urethra, or cystostomy access to enter the allograft ureter failed. The investigators resorted to the original approach again for double-J stenting, and was successful. The patient is presently waiting for the lithotripsy (Fig. 3).

Discussion and conclusions

Renal transplantation is the definitive treatment for patients with ESRD. However, ureteroneocystostomy stenosis and allograft lithiasis are potentially devastating complications [7, 8]. According to recent reports, ureteroneocystostomy stenosis is the most common urologic complication during renal transplantation [8, 9], while allograft lithiasis is another uncommon but difficult-to-treat complication [10]. These complications can lead to renal damage resulting from urinary obstruction and mortality due to infection. Several studies have demonstrated that most cases can be endoscopically managed if patients with hydronephrosis after renal transplantation do not prefer active surveillance or surgery [2, 11, 12]. The timely and effective decompression of obstructed ureters is frequently challenging due to the un-physiologic location of the ureteroneocystostomy [13]. For patients with significant hydronephrosis with renal function decline and sepsis, the prompt insertion of PCN can minimize the morbidity through immediate drainage and decompression, allowing for the diagnosis of the site of obstruction based on antegrade pyelography. However,

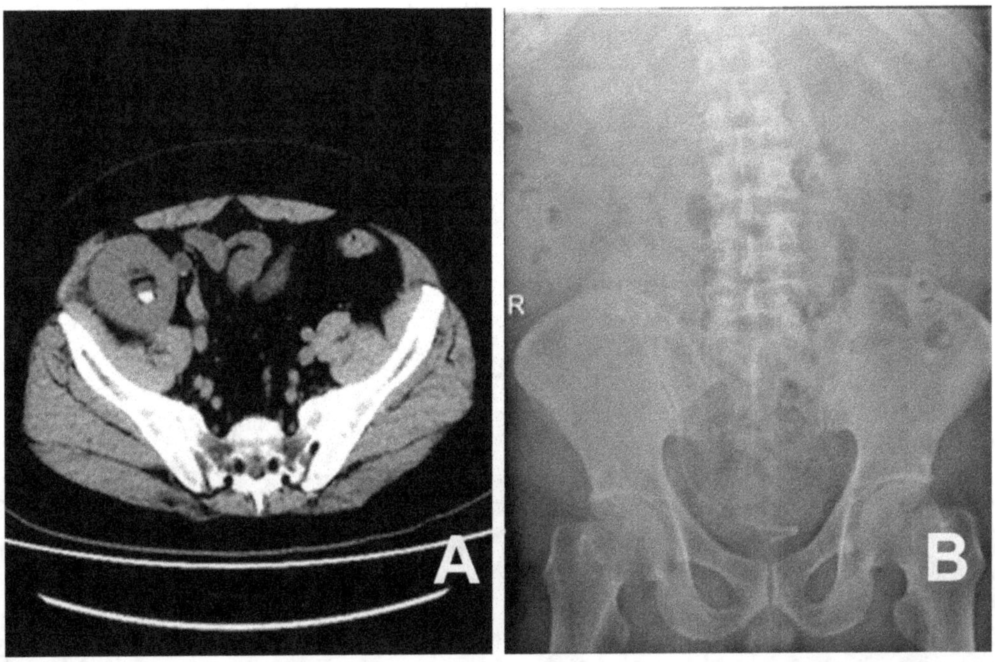

Fig. 3 The placement of a double-J stent in a 27-year-old male developing ureterovesical junction stricture and ureteral calculi. **a** The computed tomography revealed multiple transplant ureteral calculi. **b** The KUB film revealed that the double-J stent was inserted into the pelvis

PCN is associated with a risk of infection, bleeding and graft injuries, causing greater difficulty during the removal and exchange of an indwelling stent. Therefore, it appears more reasonable to use the retrograde ureteral stent placement as a first-line treatment for relieving upper urinary obstruction. Once the retrograde approach fails, the antegrade one can be applied.

The retrograde approach proposed by the investigators has its advantages and disadvantages. This approach is minimally invasive, bloodless and repeatable. On the other hand, the success rate of this approach remains unclear, and the main challenge during stent insertion is the localization of the neo-orifice and the difficulty in advancing the stent through the angulated ureteral route [12]. Furthermore, both the bladder outlet and ureteral orifice are usually located in the triangular region plane of the bladder, and this anatomical alignment facilitates the transurethral ureteral intubation due to the same plane and direction. Halstuch et al. [14] reported that during the placement of a double pigtail stent in the native ureter, the stent would constantly be surrounded by the ureteral wall, and any forward pressure applied to the stent promote forward movement. However, the allograft ureter frequently goes into the dome of the bladder at an oblique angle, which makes the ureteral orifice intubation difficult for the following three reasons. First, directing a wire to a ceiling oriented orifice can be challenging. Second, advancing the stent over a guidewire tends to recoil back. Third, the guidewire can easily slide out of the neo-orifice while attempting to pass a ureteral catheter through the wire. At present, few reports have described the retrograde approach of ureteral intubation for transplant kidneys [15]. Elias Hyams et al. reported a retrograde technique for accessing an angle-tipped angiographic catheter. That is, they used a Kumpe or Berenstein catheter to advance a flexible tipped guidewire retrograde into the collecting system under fluoroscopic guidance [16]. From an anatomical perspective, the neo-orifice of the allograft on the right (or left) side of the pelvic cavity resembles the right (or left) ureteral orifice of the native kidney projecting onto the anterior bladder wall (Fig. 4). For instance, in projecting the bladder outlet to the anterior wall of the native bladder, the intubation would be carried out on a triangular-like plane, which is similar to the trigone of the native bladder. In this scenario, the central or left (or right) anterior wall of the native bladder would be selected as the catheter entry site, which is closer and below the neo-orifice (Fig. 5). Using the approach outlined above, a total of five successful RUS-PSABs were performed in three patients with ureteral obstruction after renal transplantation. The investigators consider that two major factors influence the success of the RUS-PSAB, which include a sensor

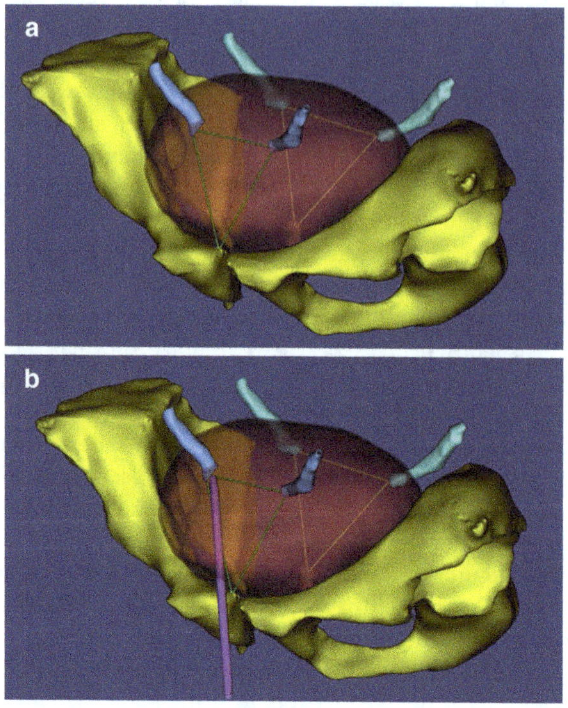

Fig. 4 A 3-dimensional graph illustrates the position of the allograft ureteral and original ureteral orifice. **a** The anatomical relationship between the transplant ureteral orifice and the original ureteral orifice upon projection. **b** Introduction of the access by percutaneous suprapubic cystotomy to the ureter orifice of the allograft and the retrograde placement of a double-J stent into the allograft pelvis

straight tip guidewire (0.035-inch [150 cm]; Boston Scientific, USA) and a double-J tube (Black Silicone Filiform DP Ureteral Stent Set Wire Guide with Hydrophilic Coating, Cook Incorporated, USA).

Zavos et al. [17] reported the ureteropelvic stenosis of renal allografts in 12.5% of transplant recipients, while ureteral obstruction and ureterovesical stricture were found in 28.1% and 30.2% of transplant recipients, respectively. Halstuch et al. [14] reported that the ureterovesical anastomotic stricture had an incidence of 1–4.5% after renal transplantation. Ozkaptan et al. [11] reported that ureterovesical anastomotic obstruction followed by ureteral stenosis was the most common reason for urinary tract stenosis. Etiological factors for ureteral strictures in existing studies include ureteral devascularization, allograft ureterolithiasis, urinary leakage, allograft rejection, ureteral BK virus infection, compression of the ureter by hematoma or lymphoceles, and surgical complications. Ureteral stricture appears to be a common complication in transplant recipients. Indeed, surgeons should provide more attention to the angle between the ureterovesical junction and stricture, and evaluate whether this is too acute. If so, the wire or stent insertion

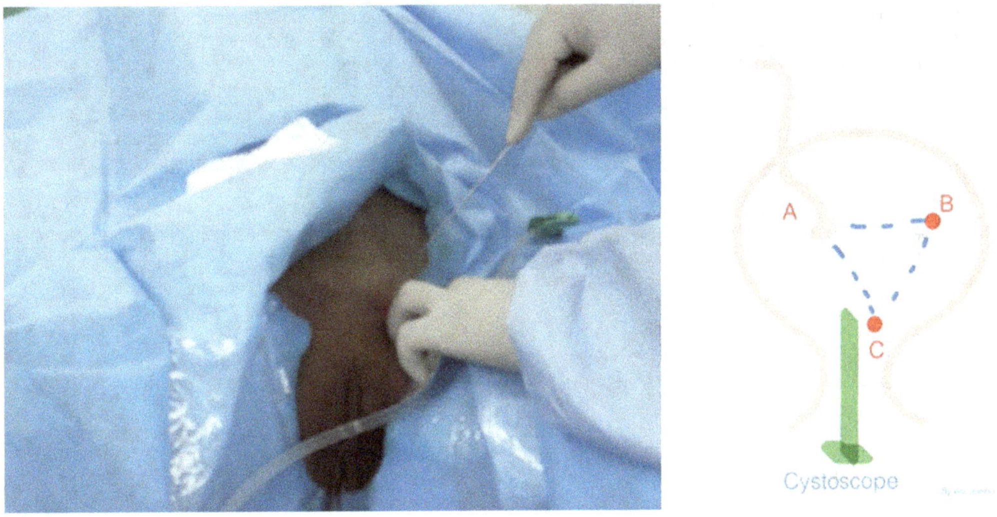

Fig. 5 Selection of the puncture site for the suprapubic cystostomy: under cystoscopic monitoring, the location of the vesicostomy puncture site should be selected between points B and C

may fail with or without ureteral stenosis. Many ureteroneocystostomy approaches have been described, each with its advantages and disadvantages [8, 18, 19]. The investigators suggest adjusting the vesico-ureteric anastomosis farther away from the suprapubic area after distending the bladder.

There are no practice guidelines for treating post-transplant ureteral stenosis and calculi, and the experience of the urological team has become instrumental. The present case series is the first to describe the approach for the successful RUS-PSAB among patients receiving renal transplantation with ureteral stricture. The experience of the investigators supports the feasibility of the RUS-PSAB approach for allograft obstruction relief. The absence of complications in these three patients was reassuring, but complications from the cystectomy should still be considered. Furthermore, this approach is compatible with procedures, such as ureteroscopic laser lithotripsy. In the third patient, a flexible ureterorenoscopy (F-URS) were planned.

Semi-rigid ureteroscopes were used to attempted to pass through the percutaneous cystotomy access into the transplanted ureter, but eventually failed in the third patient. Sometimes, the operator may succeed in the ureteral intubation through the urethra, similar to that described in the first patient. However, the probability of failure remains high. At present, the investigators suggest the use of the RUS-PSAB method or PCN, since there have been many reports of using flexible ureteroscopes(F-URS) to treat urolithiasis in patients receiving renal transplantation [16, 20–22]. Nonetheless, percutaneous cystotomy access may still offers a clear and accurate access for F-URS, and facilitates laser lithotripsy for managing allograft calculi.

These present results indicate that this novel stent placement technique for allograft recipients is frequently successful. Indeed, this treatment entails higher cost due to the use of disposable materials and percutaneous access. However, the investigators consider the additional cost to be justified by its high success rate, safety and absence of severe consequences, resulting from the failed stent insertion. Therefore, this approach is an attractive alternative for ureteral stent replacement among patients receiving renal transplantation. Finally, the present study is limited by the relatively small cohort size and its single-center nature.

Supplementary information

Additional file 1. Retrograde ureteric stent insertion from percutaneous suprapubic access to the bladder in renal transplant recipients with ureteric stenosis.

Abbreviations

RT: Renal transplantation; PCN: Percutaneous nephrostomy; MRI: Magnetic resonance imaging; RUS-PSAB: Retrograde ureteral stent insertion through percutaneous suprapubic access to the bladder; F-URS: Flexible ureteroscopes.

Acknowledgements

Not applicable.

Authors' contributions

JW designed and performed operations and then analyzed and interpreted the patient data regarding the ureteral stricture after the transplant and was a major contributor in writing the manuscript. SY supervised and performed operations of the kidney, and was a major contributor in writing the manuscript. CM analyzed and interpreted the patient data, and provided information on kidney transplant patients. LZ provides anatomical analysis and 3D image construction. FL was a secondary contributor in writing the manuscript. QM was a secondary contributor in writing the manuscript. All authors read and approved the final manuscript.

Author details
[1] Department of Urology, Tianjin First Central Hospital, No. 24 Fukang Road, Nankai District, Tianjin 300192, China. [2] Department of Renal Transplant, Tianjin First Central Hospital, Tianjin 300192, China. [3] Department of Anatomy and Histology, School of Basic Medical Sciences, Tianjin Medical University, Tianjin 300070, China. [4] Department of Urology, Tianjin Union Medical Center, Tianjin 300121, China.

References

1. Streeter EH, Little DM, Cranston DW, Morris PJ. The urological complications of renal transplantation: a series of 1535 patients. BJU Int. 2002;90:627–34.
2. Kwong J, Schiefer D, Aboalsamh G, Archambault J, Luke PP, Sener A. Optimal management of distal ureteric strictures following renal transplantation: a systematic review. Transpl Int. 2016;29:579–88.
3. Jaskowski A, Jones RM, Murie JA, Morris PJ. Urological complications in 600 consecutive renal transplants. Br J Surg. 1987;74:922–5.
4. Bach C, Kabir M, Zaman F, Kachrilas S, Masood J, Junaid I, et al. Endourological management of ureteric strictures after kidney transplantation: stenting the stent. Arab J Urol. 2011;9:165–9.
5. Mostafa SA, Abbaszadeh S, Taheri S, Nourbala MH. Percutaneous nephrostomy for treatment of posttransplant ureteral obstructions. Urol J. 2008;5:79–83.
6. Mano R, Golan S, Holland R, Livne PM, Lifshitz DA. Retrograde endoureterotomy for persistent ureterovesical anastomotic strictures in renal transplant kidneys after failed antegrade balloon dilation. Urology. 2012;80:255–9.
7. Manassero F, Vistoli F, Mogorovich A, Maria DEM, Boggi U, Selli C. Early and late ureteral complications after renal transplant. Minerva Urol Nefrol. 2017;69:613–8.
8. Choi YS, Kim KS, Choi SW, Bae WJ, Hong SH, Lee JY, et al. Ureteral complications in kidney transplantation: analysis and management of 853 consecutive laparoscopic living-donor nephrectomies in a single center. Transplant Proc. 2016;48:2684–8.
9. Krajewski W, Dembowski J, Kołodziej A, Małkiewicz B, Tupikowski K, Matuszewski M, et al. Urological complications after renal transplantation—a single centre experience. Cent European J Urol. 2016;69:306–11.
10. Duty B, Lam M. Management of stone disease in renal transplant kidneys. Smith's textbook of endourology, Fourth Edited. 2019;827–35
11. Özkaptan O, Sevinc C, Balaban M, Karadeniz T. Minimally invasive approach for the management of urological complications after renal transplantation: single center experience. Minerva Urol Nefrol. 2018;70:422–8.
12. Balaban M, Ozkaptan O, Sevinc C, Karadeniz T. Minimally invasive approach to ureteral stricture in transplant kidney by periodic retrograde ureteral stent placement and exchange. Transplant Proc. 2018;50:3405–10.
13. Vashishtha S, Sureka SK, Agarwal S, Srivastava A, Prabhakaran S, Kapoor R, et al. Urethral stricture and stone: their coexistence and management. Urol J. 2014;11:1204–10.
14. Halstuch D, Ehrlich Y, Shenhar C, Mano R, Baniel J, Margel D, et al. Transplant kidney retrograde ureteral stent placement and exchange: overcoming the challenge. Urology. 2018;111:220–4.
15. Gerrard ER Jr, Burns JR, Young CJ, Urban DA, Hammontree LN, El-Galley R, et al. Retrograde stenting for obstruction of the renal transplant ureter. Urology. 2005;66:256–60 (**(discussion 60)**).
16. Hyams E, Marien T, Bruhn A, Quirouet A, Andonian S, Shah O, et al. Ureteroscopy for transplant lithiasis. J Endourol. 2012;26:819–22.
17. Zavos G, Pappas P, Karatzas T, Karidis NP, Bokos J, Stravodimos K, et al. Urological complications: analysis and management of 1525 consecutive renal transplantations. Transplant Proc. 2008;40:1386–90.
18. Dadkhah F, Asgari MA, Tara A, Safarinejad MR. Modified ureteroneocystostomy in kidney transplantation to facilitate endoscopic management of subsequent urological complications. Int Urol Nephrol. 2010;42:285–93.
19. Wasnick RJ, Butt KM, Laungani G, Shirani K, Hong JH, Adamsons RJ, et al. Evaluation of anterior extravesical ureteroneocystostomy in kidney transplantation. J Urol. 1981;126:306–7.
20. Mitsui Y, Wada K, Araki M, Yoshioka T, Ariyoshi Y, Nishimura S, et al. Ureterolithotripsy for a ureteral calculus at the ureteroureterostomy of a renal-transplant recipient. Acta Med Okayama. 2017;71:449–52.
21. Sevinc C, Balaban M, Ozkaptan O, Karadeniz T. Flexible ureterorenoscopy and laser lithotripsy for the treatment of allograft kidney lithiasis. Transplant Proc. 2015;47:1766–71.
22. Basiri A, Simforoosh N, Nikoobakht M, Hosseini Moghaddam MM. The role of ureteroscopy in the treatment of renal transplantation complications. Urol J. 2004;1:27–31.

Circumcision and its alternatives in Germany: An analysis of nationwide hospital routine data

Christina Oetzmann von Sochaczewski[1,2*], Jan Gödeke[1] and Oliver J. Muensterer[1,3]

Abstract

Background/purpose: Circumcisions are among the most frequent operations in children. Health service data on circumcision in the United States has documented an increase in neonatal circumcisions since 2012. We investigated whether a similar effect could be found in Germany, which does not endorse neonatal circumcision.

Methods: We analysed German routine administrative data for operations conducted on the preputium in order to analyse the frequency, age distribution, and time-trends in hospital-based procedures on a nationwide basis.

Results: There were 9418 [95% confidence interval (CI) 8860–10,029] procedures per year, of which 4977 (95% CI 4676–5337) were circumcisions. Age distributions were highly different between both circumcisions (van der Waerden's $\chi^2 = 58.744$, $df=4$, $P<0.0001$) and preputium-preserving operations (van der Waerden's $\chi^2 = 58.481$, $df=4$, $P<0.0001$). Circumcisions were more frequent in the first 5 years of life and above 15 years of age, whereas preputium-preserving procedures were preferred in the age groups between 5 and 14 years of age. The number of circumcisions and preputium-preserving operations decreased in absolute and relative numbers.

Conclusions: The increasing trend towards neonatal circumcision observed in the United States is absent in Germany. The majority of patients were operated after the first year of life and absolute and relative numbers of hospital-based procedures were decreasing. Other factors such as increasing use of steroids for the preferred non-operative treatment of phimosis may play a role. As operations in outpatients and office-based procedures were not covered, additional research is necessary to obtain a detailed picture of circumcision and its surgical alternatives in Germany.

Level of evidence: III.

Keywords: Health services research, Paediatric surgery, Administrative data, Population-based, Penile surgery, Inpatients

Background

Circumcision beyond infancy is among the most frequent paediatric surgical operations in countries that do not encourage neonatal circumcision [1], contrary to those who do [2]. Just recently, the current situation of circumcision in the United States has been described by an increasing proportion of neonates who underwent circumcision. Affirmation of this practice in the guidelines by the American Academy of Paediatrics in 2012 may play a role, as *Many* et al. noted [2]. The guideline of the American Academy of Paediatrics has been criticised, because of a cultural bias that prohibits its applicability in other countries of the developed world [3]. Although this cultural aspect has been recognised before and named the "uniquely American medical enigma" [4]—it is likely that the results of the study by Many et al. [2] will not be transferrable to countries outside the United States. We therefore analysed German routine administrative data for paediatric patients that were treated by circumcision

*Correspondence: c.oetzmann@gmail.com
[2] Sektion Kinderchirurgie, Klinik und Poliklinik für Allgemein-, Viszeral-, Thorax- und Gefäßchirurgie, Universitätsklinikum Bonn, Venusberg-Campus 1, D-53127 Bonn, Germany
Full list of author information is available at the end of the article

or its preputium-preserving alternatives irrespective of the operating department in order to report data for a country that does not endorse neonatal circumcision.

Methods

Routine data from German hospital reimbursement

We bought data files—in the form of separate Microsoft Excel sheets for every included year—from the *Statistisches Bundesamt* (Federal Statistics Office) including principal diagnoses and procedures of the German Modification of the International Classification of Diseases—Version 10 for the years 2005–2017. Data were analysed all operations conducted on the preputium (5–640) with its respective sub-classifications: frenulotomies (5–640.0), dorsal slit (5–640.1), circumcision (5–640.2), frenulum- and preputioplasty (5–640.3), and freeing of preputial adhesions (5–640.5), whereas repositions of a paraphimosis under anaesthesia (5–640.4) were excluded. These data files are stratified in the mandatory age-groups of all administrative statistics: The first year of life, the ages 1–4, 5–9, 10–14, and 15–19 years. The properties and pitfalls of these data have been described in detail elsewhere [5]. In brief, the national hospital statistic became mandatory in 2002 for every hospital that is reimbursed via the German system of diagnosis related groups, any licenced hospital with all its somatic departments, excluding only psychiatric departments, and can be obtained from 2005 onward [6]. Due to the mandatory nature, missing data for discharge information—principal diagnoses, procedures, age, sex, and length of stay—of hospitalised patients are almost non-existent [6]. Coding of these data follows standardised formats. Non-coded or incorrectly coded procedures lead to lack of reimbursement [6].

Statistical analysis

Statistical analysis was conducted in R (version 3.5.3) [7] with its generic stats4-package (version 3.5.3) unless indicated otherwise. Procedures per year were evaluated using ordinary least square linear regression as described before for these types of data [8–10]. Linear regression's prerequisites of normality of residuals was checked using the Shapiro–Wilk test and homogeneity of variances was tested via the *F*-test using R's olsrr-package (version 0.5.3) [11]. Differences between age groups were assessed using van der Waerden's test [12] followed by posthoc comparison via Conover–Iman test with the PMCMRplus-package (version 1.4.4) [13] as recommended elsewhere [14]. Confidence intervals for point estimates were calculated via bias-corrected, accelerated bootstrap with 10,000 repetitions using the *groupwise Mean*-function from the car-package (version 2.0.0) [15] as described before [16, 17]. Testing for differences between the relative share of circumcisions and its alternatives was done with Student's *t*-test. Corrections for multiple testing were conducted according to Benjamini–Hochberg [18, 19]. The colour palettes from the viridis-package (version 0.5.3) have been used to generate figures as inclusive as possible for colour-blind readers [20].

Results

There were 122,431 operations on the male prepuce included between 2005 and 2017, which equals 9418 (95% confidence interval: 8860–10,029) procedures per year. The majority of these operations were circumcisions, of which 4977 (95% confidence interval: 4676–5337) were performed annually (Fig. 1). The most frequent preputium-preserving operation was freeing of preputial adhesions with 1840 (95% confidence interval: 1717–1966), followed by 1777 (95% confidence interval: 1713–1844) cases of preputioplasty, 670 (95% confidence interval: 607–734) frenulotomies, and 154 (95% confidence interval: 132–178) dorsal slits (Fig. 2) annually.

We found relevant differences in the distribution of cases among the age groups for both circumcisions (van der Waerden's $\chi^2 = 58.744$, $df = 4$, $P < 0.0001$ with all posthoc comparisons $P < 0.0001$; Table 1) and for the preputium-preserving operations (van der Waerden's $\chi^2 = 58.481$, $df = 4$, $P < 0.0001$ with all posthoc comparisons $P < 0.0001$; Table 2).

The comparison of relative shares of circumcisions and preputium-preserving operations between the age groups revealed that circumcision was more frequent in

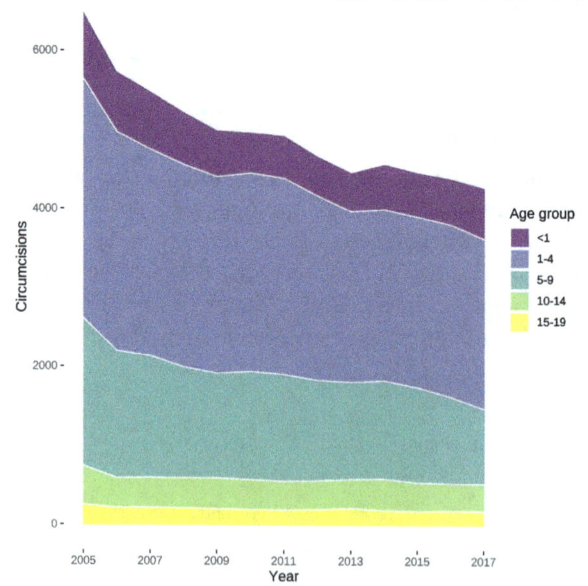

Fig. 1 Cumulative number of circumcisions performed per year in Germany in paediatric age groups between 2005 and 2017

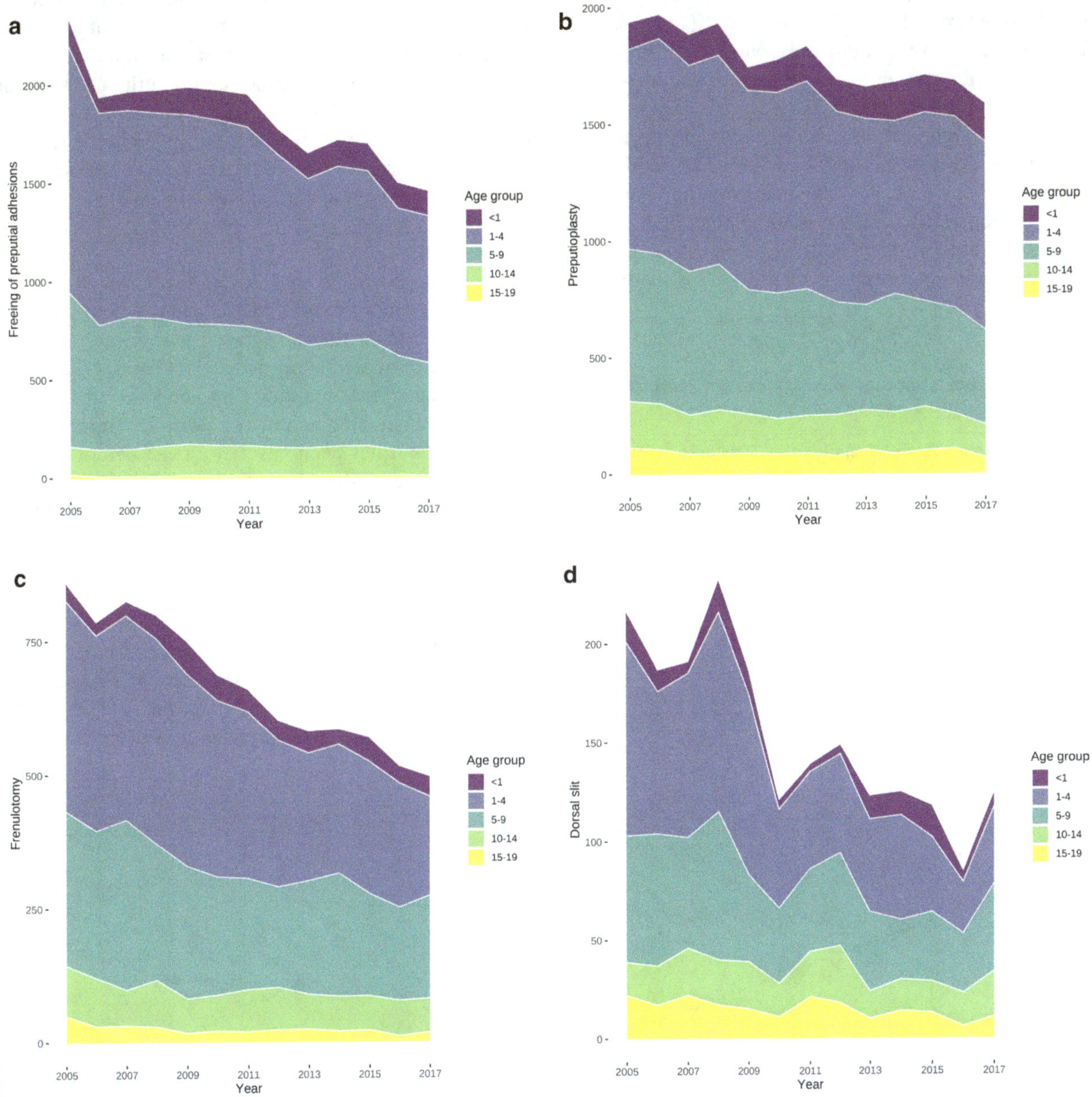

Fig. 2 Cumulative number of preputium-preserving alternative procedures per year in paediatric age groups between 2005 and 2017. **a** Freeing of preputial adhesions. **b** Preputioplasty. **c** Frenulotomy. **d** Dorsal slit

Table 1 Distribution of yearly circumcisions between the age groups

Age group	Mean	95% CI
< 1	621	572–688
1–4	2430	2310–2590
5–9	1330	1230–1480
10–14	383	370–415
15–19	207	197–221

CI confidence interval

Table 2 Distribution of yearly preputium-preserving operations between the age groups

Age group	Mean	95% CI
< 1	319	291–335
1–4	2170	2030–2320
5–9	1400	1290–1520
10–14	408	392–424
15–19	143	134–159

CI confidence interval

the first year of life, in the age-groups between 1 and 4 years, and between 15 and 19 years of age (all $P<0.0001$; Table 3), whereas preputium-preserving operations were more frequent between the older age groups of 5–9 and 10–14 years (both $P<0.0001$; Table 3).

There was a relevant decrease of circumcisions among patients in all age groups between 2005 and 2017 (Fig. 3a), which was also true for preputium-preserving operations with the exception of the first year of life whose numbers increased over time (Fig. 3b). This increase in absolute numbers of procedures in the first year of life could be related to an increasing number of live births since 2011, because the numbers of circumcisions per 100,000 boys in their first year of life decreased (Fig. 4a) and remained stable for preputium-preserving operations (Fig. 4b). Similar to absolute numbers, the relative numbers of procedures also dropped in the remaining age-groups for both circumcision (Fig. 4a) and its preputium-preserving alternatives (Fig. 4b).

Table 3 Relative share of operations between the age groups

Age group	Circumcision (%)	Preputium-preserving (%)	Difference (%)	95% CI
<1	65.7	34.3	31.4	26.7–36.2
1–4	52.9	47.1	5.7	4.9–6.7
5–9	48.8	51.2	- 2.4	- 3.5 to - 1.4
10–14	48.4	51.6	- 3.2	- 4.7 to - 1.8
15–19	59.3	40.7	18.5	16.7–20.3

CI confidence interval

Discussion

A recent study demonstrated an increasing frequency of neonatal circumcisions in the United States following publication of the most recent American Academy of Paediatrics guideline on the subject from 2012, which expresses an affirmative stance on neonatal circumcision after more than a decade of equipoise [2]. Interestingly, a similar trend has been described even before the millennium using routine hospital data [21]. In preceding studies, two moderator variables have been identified: Medicaid coverage of circumcision was linked to a 24% higher rate of neonatal circumcision compared to non-Medicaid-coverage, and Hispanic descent was associated to lower circumcision rates [22]. Consequently, the number of neonatal circumcisions dropped in states that withdrew Medicaid coverage for neonatal circumcisions, but remained stable in states that did not [23]. Likewise, this study also demonstrated a reduced frequency

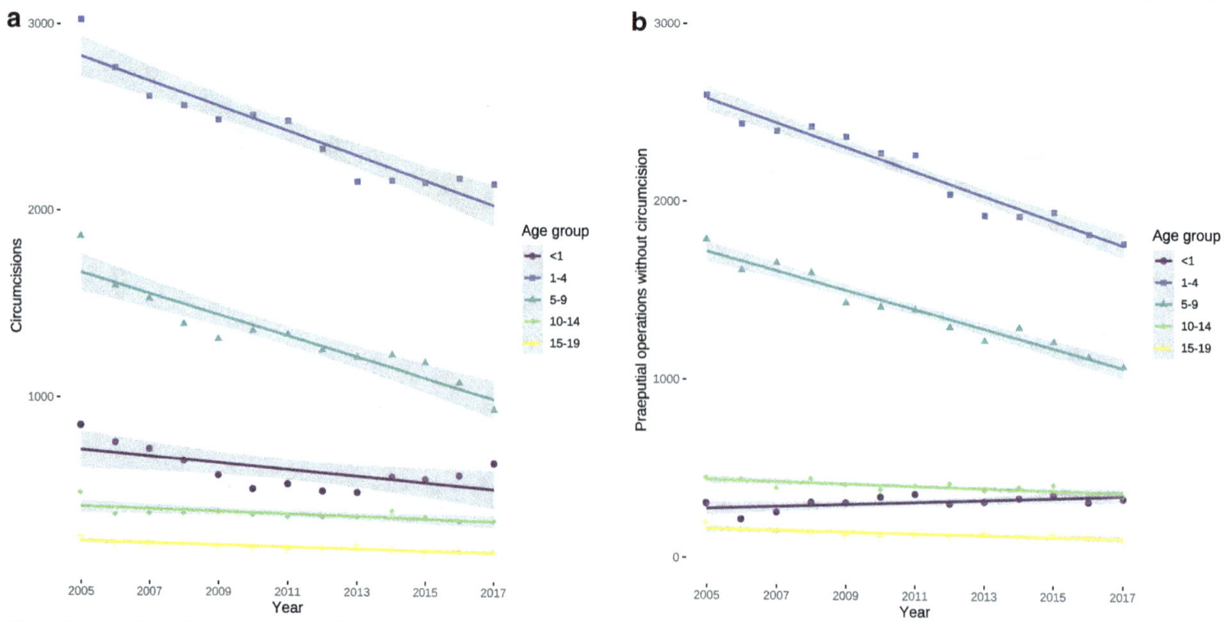

Fig. 3 Hospital-based circumcisions and preputium-preserving operations between 2005 and 2017. **a** Circumcisions. **b** Preputium-preserving operations. Their numbers decreased between 1 and 4 years of age by 68 per year (95% CI 58–78, $P<0.0001$), between 5 and 9 years by 54 yearly procedures (95% CI 46–63, $P<0.0001$), from 10 to 14 years of age by 6 operations per year (95% CI 2–9, $P=0.0035$), and between 15 and 19 years by 4 procedures (95% CI 1–7, $P=0.0075$), but increased in the first year of life by 6 yearly procedures (95% CI 1–12, $P=0.0225$)

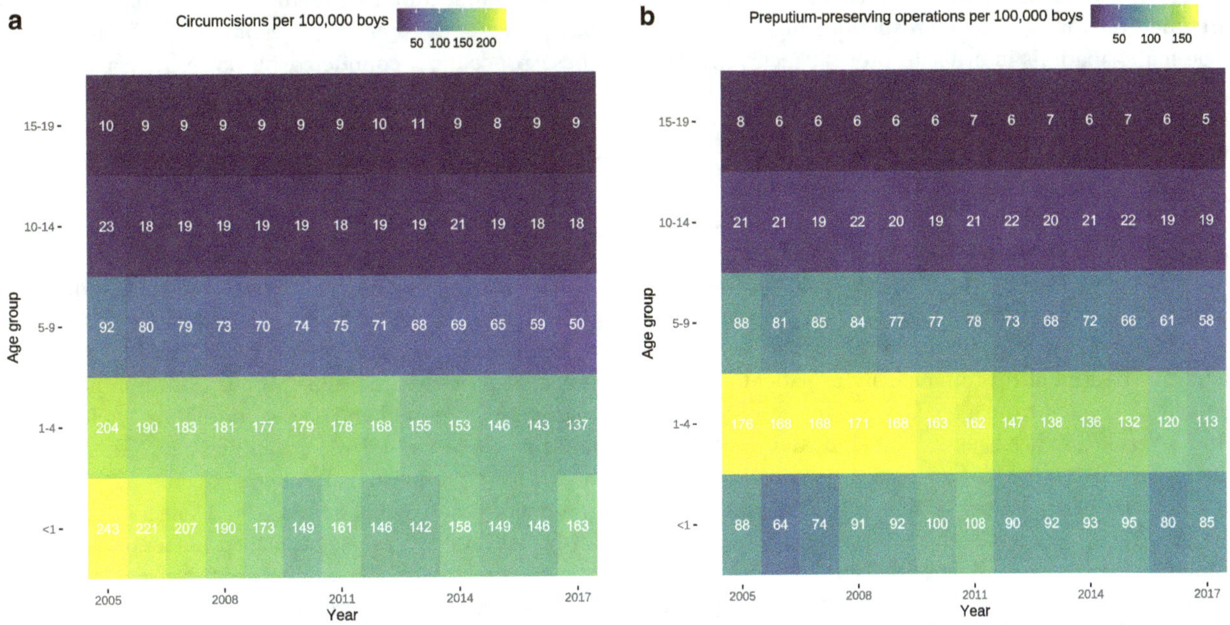

Fig. 4 Hospital-based circumcisions and preputium-preserving operations per 100,000 boys between 2005 and 2017. **a** Circumcisions. **b** Preputium-preserving operations

of neonatal circumcision among children of Hispanic descent and a slightly reduced frequency of neonatal circumcisions among non-Hispanic black children [23]. For Germany, circumcision has been associated to being born into a migrant family, particularly being descended from Turkish families with a more than tripled rate of circumcisions compared to the rest of Germany's paediatric population [24]. Many et al. [2] used the Paediatric Health Information System database that covers free-standing children's hospitals from many states from the United States of America, although particularly those in metropolitan areas, and has been described to be somewhat representative for the whole paediatric population in the United States of America [25]. Of note, the moderator variables were associated with a reduced frequency of neonatal circumcisions, but not an increase, which has not been described for any other potential factor [22, 23].

This is in contrast to other countries such as Australia for which a decreasing rate of circumcision has been described in the same time period [26] and beyond [27]. Similar trends were observed in England [28] and Northern Ireland [29], but large-scale population-based data is scarce and reasons remain unclear. Using nationwide administrative data for hospital reimbursement, we were also able to show a decreasing trend in circumcisions in German hospital-based procedures among all age groups. However, the preputium-preserving operations also showed a declining trend in all age groups, except those in their first year of life. This could be linked to the general reduction in surgical diseases described before, for example in infantile hypertrophic pyloric stenosis [30] or inguinal hernia [31]. An alternative explanation might be a shift of these operations towards outpatient surgery: The vast majority of paediatric surgical departments offer circumcision as an outpatient procedure [32], but this is unlikely as these procedures have been conducted primarily on outpatients even back in the 1980s [33] as it was the case in the United States, too [34]. Although there is no universally accepted age threshold that would preclude outpatient surgery, in Germany, it is uncommon below the age of six months. An individual decision between caretakers, surgeons, and anaesthetists should be reached on whether the procedure can be performed as an outpatient surgery [35]. Consequently, we are confident that the present data covers all operations in neonates, except ritual circumcisions performed by non-physicians, but there is considerable uncertainness in older age groups. This is supported by a cohort of boys that received a preputial operation from an office-based paediatric surgeon, in which none of the patients were operated on in their first year of life [36].

The obvious difference of our data to those by Many et al. is the age distribution between the two cohorts: They reported 67% of all circumcisions in the first year of life, whereas only 12.5% of circumcisions in our cohort were performed in this age group. For the preputium-preserving operations, this number was even smaller with 7.2% of all procedures. This difference is not surprising as the German guideline only recommends circumcision for Lichen sclerosus and high-grade urologic malformations in order to prevent recurrent infections, which leaves only phimosis as a possible indication for surgery and only after a local therapy with steroids has been applied for a sufficient amount of time [37]. Similarly to the observation by Many et al. [2] for circumcisions, the effects of guideline changes could also be observed in Germany, but the other way round: The first step of a local treatment with steroids [37] resulted in a directly observable change in therapy preferences. In 2005, local steroids were never used, but became the definitive treatment for the majority of patients in a single-centre analysis from a tertiary paediatric surgery unit [38]. A result that has been validated in later cohorts [39] and thus reflects the different recommendations made by the German guidelines compared to the guideline by the American Academy of Paediatrics: An affirmative stance towards neonatal circumcision [40] versus primary non-operative treatment that considers a primary circumcision without preceding local steroid therapy in the absence of a balanitis xerotica obliterans or high-grade urinary tract anomalies as not *lege artis* [41]. For the United States of America, there is no recommendation by the American Urological Association towards the use of topical steroids for phimosis [42]. However, results from a cohort treated by an office-based paediatric surgeon before 2015 showed that only 11% of operated boys received preceding treatment with local steroids [36], so guideline compliance may vary between hospital- and office-based surgeons. On the contrary, in a cohort from the Capital region of Denmark, the majority of patients received topical steroids as first-choice treatment of phimosis and had a similar age-distribution as in the our report using administrative data, too [43].

Although ritual circumcisions should in theory not be conducted within the health-care system, it is likely that they are present [44]. Their relevance has been quantified in data from England based on the comparison with the expected incidence of phimosis [28]. Based on the report that in a German cohort of 176 boys treated for phimosis by an office-based paediatric surgeon, the decision for treatment was based on a non-retractable preputium [36], and taking into account that a non-retractable foreskin is present in 50% of first-graders [45], it is unclear how many circumcisions were performed for therapeutic reasons. Non-medically indicated circumcision in boys in Germany can be performed explicitly by discretion of parental custody since 2013. In the first six months of life, circumcision may be performed by non-physicians if this person is designated to do so by a religious community [46]. Consequently, the latter cases will not be represented within our data if there is no immediate major complication that required therapy on an inpatient basis. Currently, there is no estimate on the number of these procedures conducted by non-physicians without adequate anaesthesia [47]. This might be a general issue due to, perceived, profanity of topics like circumcisions, exemplified by unpublished theses with relatively large cohorts examining the efficacy of local steroids [38, 39], whereas small cases series with single digit numbers of patients still easily appear in the international literature if they present something novel or deal with more prestigious diseases [48]. This is important in so far, as truly representative cohort studies found a more than doubled prevalence of circumcision in boys from families with a migrant background and even a more than tripled prevalence in those from Turkish families [24]. This suggests that ritual circumcisions frequently occur.

A major limitation of our data is its sole focus on hospital-based procedures. As described before, circumcision and its alternatives are often conducted on outpatients [33, 34] and office procedures are recompensed to the surgeon via a different way than it is the case for hospitals. Consequently, our data does not offer the full picture of circumcision and its preputium-preserving alternatives as the distribution of procedures may be different in outpatients. The generalisability to other countries that do not endorse neonatal circumcision is therefore unclear due to the different structure of the German health system that favours inpatient-based approaches due to highly different reimbursements compared to office-based procedures [49]. Another limitation is the focus of administrative data used by us on cases instead of patients: The same patient treated with a preputium-preserving procedure might later on reappear in the data with a circumcision, but this cannot be tracked due to the case-based approach of the data. It may thus also be possible that there is no reduction in foreskin surgery, but just a shift towards outpatient-clinics or office-based surgeons, because these procedures cannot be tracked by the administrative data used by us. This limitation would not apply to databases of the statutory health insurances, because they are patient-based instead of case-based. Other limitations are those that are inherent in the use of secondary administrative datasets: Lack of clinical and demographic details due to the focus on reimbursement of hospitals, misclassifications due to coding errors, and systematic errors introduced by variations in coding practice, because the coding is done at the local hospital level.

Other factors such as information of parents on the altered risk of sexually transmitted diseases following circumcision are unlikely to have effects on parental decisions for or against circumcision [50]. Likewise, we also consider potential effects of a vaccination against human papilloma virus diminishable, because this vaccination is only among the lists of services covered from 2019 onwards by the statutory health insurances in Germany that serve around 90% of Germany's population [51].

However, our study offers a first comparator to the study by Many et al. [2] from a country that does not endorse neonatal circumcision despite its limitations. Moreover, it might serve as a vanguard to prompt others to contribute population-based data on circumcision and its preputium-preserving alternatives as it has been done for infantile hypertrophic pyloric stenosis [30] or inguinal hernia [52].

Conclusions

An increasing trend towards neonatal circumcision observed in the United States is absent in Germany. The vast majority of patients were operated after the first year of life for both circumcision and preputium-preserving procedures. The number of both types of procedures was declining over time with the exception of preputium-preserving procedures in the first year of life. Topical steroid therapy as recommended in the local guidelines may play a role in this development. Additional population-based data from countries able to cover both in- and outpatients in their respective registries or administrative data are needed to gain further insight into the epidemiology of these operations. For data from Germany, a combination of hospital-based and office-based procedures is necessary to gain a full insight of the spectrum of preputial surgery. These data might be available at the databases of the statutory health insurances, at least for outpatients operated in hospitals, which would also offer the opportunity to explore the diagnoses that represent the reasons for the surgical procedures.

Acknowledgements
Not applicable.

Authors' contributions
Conceptualisation of the study, data acquisition, analysis and interpretation, and writing: CO. Conceptualisation of the study, interpretation, and writing: OM. Interpretation and critical revision: JG. All authors agree with the submission. All authors read and approved the finalmanuscript.

Author details
[1] Klinik und Poliklinik für Kinderchirurgie, Universitätsmedizin Mainz der Johannes Gutenberg-Universität, Mainz, Germany. [2] Sektion Kinderchirurgie, Klinik und Poliklinik für Allgemein-, Viszeral-, Thorax- und Gefäßchirurgie, Universitätsklinikum Bonn, Venusberg-Campus 1, D-53127 Bonn, Germany. [3] Kinderchirurgische Klinik und Poliklinik, Dr. von Haunersches Kinderspital der Ludwig- Maximilians-Universität München, Munich, Germany.

References

1. Stark E, Steffens J. Stand der ambulant-operativen Kinderurologie. Aktuelle Urol. 2006;37:127–31.
2. Many BT, Rizeq YK, Vacek J, Cheon EC, Johnson E, Hu Y-Y, et al. A contemporary snapshot of circumcision in US children's hospitals. J Pediatr Surg. 2020;55:1134–8.
3. Frisch M, Aigrain Y, Barauskas V, Bjarnason R, Boddy S-A, Czauderna P, et al. Cultural bias in the AAP's 2012 technical report and policy statement on male circumcision. Pediatrics. 2013;131:796–800.
4. Wallerstein E. Circumcision. The uniquely American medical enigma. Urol Clin North Am. 1985;12:123–32.
5. Nimptsch U, Spoden M, Mansky T. Variablendefinition in fallbezogenen Krankenhausabrechnungsdaten—Fallstricke und Lösungsmöglichkeiten. Gesundheitswesen. 2020;82:29–40.
6. Nimptsch U. Disease-specifictrends of comorbidity coding and implications for risk adjustment in hospitaladministrative data. Health Serv Res. 2016;51:981–1001.
7. R Core Team. R: a language and environment for statistical computing. Vienna: R Foundation for Statistical Computing; 2019. Accessed 25 Feb 2019.
8. Schröder A, Muensterer OJ, Oetzmann von Sochaczewski C. Jungen sterben häufiger an nekrotisierender Enterokolitis: Ergebnisse der deutschlandweiten Krankenhausstatistik von 2000 bis 2017. Monatsschr Kinderheilkd. 2020. https://doi.org/10.1007/s00112-020-00877-0.
9. Oetzmann von Sochaczewski C, Muensterer OJ. Laparoscopy for abdominal testes: nationwide analysis of German routine data. J Laparoendosc Adv Surg Tech. 2021;31:236–41.
10. Oetzmann von Sochaczewski C, Muensterer OJ. The incidence of infantile hypertrophic pyloric stenosis nearly halved from 2005 to 2017: analysis of German administrative data. Pediatr Surg Int. 2021. https://doi.org/10.1007/s00383-020-04810-0.
11. Hebbali A. Olsrr: tools for building OLS regression models. 2020. Accessed 14 Apr 2020.
12. van der Waerden BL. Order tests for the two-sample problem and their power. Indag Math Proc. 1952;55:453–8.
13. Pohlert T. PMCMRplus: calculate pairwise multiple comparisons of mean rank sums extended. 2020. Accessed 23 Apr 2020.
14. Luepsen H. Comparison of nonparametric analysis of variance methods: a vote for van der Waerden. Commun Stat Simul Comput. 2018;47:2547–76.
15. Fox J, Weisberg S, Price B, Adler D, Bates D, Baud-Bovy G, et al. Car: companion to applied regression. 2018. Accessed 11 Mar 2020.
16. Oetzmann von Sochaczewski C, Tagkalos E, Lindner A, Lang H, Heimann A, Muensterer O. Technical aspects in esophageal lengthening: an investigation of traction procedures and suturing techniques in swine. Eur J Pediatr Surg. 2019;29:481–4.
17. Baumgart J, Deigendesch N, Lindner A, Muensterer OJ, Schröder A, Heimann A, et al. Using multidimensional scaling in model choice for congenital oesophageal atresia: similarity analysis of human autopsy organ weights with those from a comparative assessment of Aachen Minipig and Pietrain piglets. Lab Anim. 2020;54:576–87.
18. Benjamini Y, Hochberg Y. Controllingthe false discovery rate: a practical and powerful approach to multiple testing. J R Stat Soc Ser B Methodol. 1995;57:289–300.
19. Oetzmann von Sochaczewski C, Deigendesch N, Lindner A, Baumgart J, Schröder A, Heimann A, et al. Comparing Aachen Minipigs and Pietrain piglets as models of experimental pediatric urology to human reference data. Eur Surg Res. 2020;61:95–100.
20. Garnier S, Ross N, Rudis B, Sciaini M, Scherer C. viridis: default color maps from "matplotlib." 2018. Accessed 26 Jan 2021.
21. Centers for Disease Control and Prevention (CDC). Trends in in-hospital newborn male circumcision–United States, 1999–2010. MMWR Morb Mortal Wkly Rep. 2011;60:1167–8.
22. Leibowitz AA, Desmond K, Belin T. Determinants and policy implications of male circumcision in the United States. Am J Public Health. 2009;99:138–45.
23. Torosian T, Quint JJ, Klausner JD. Declinein frequency of Newborn male circumcision after change in medicaid coveragestatus in selected states in the United States. Public Health Rep. 2021. https://doi.org/10.1177/0033354920971719.
24. Kamtsiuris P, Bergmann E, Rattay P, Schlaud M. Inanspruchnahme medizinischer Leistungen: ergebnisse des Kinder- und Jugendgesundheitssurveys (KiGGS). Bundesgesundheitsbl. 2007;50:836–50.
25. Corkum KS, Baumann LM, Lautz TB. Complicationrates for pediatric hepatectomy and nephrectomy: a comparison of NSQIP-P, PHIS,and KID. J Surg Res. 2019;240:182–90.
26. Spilsbury K, Semmens JB, Wisniewski ZS, Holman CDJ. Routine circumcision practice in Western Australia 1981–1999. ANZ J Surg. 2003;73:610–4.

27. Sorokan ST, Finlay JC, Jefferies AL. Canadian Paediatric Society, Fetus and Newborn Committee, Infectious Diseases and Immunization Committee. Newborn male circumcision. Paediatr Child Health. 2015;20:311–5.
28. Cathcart P, Nuttall M, van der Meulen J, Emberton M, Kenny SE. Trends in paediatric circumcision and its complications in England between 1997 and 2003. Br J Surg. 2006;93:885–90.
29. Groves H, Bailie A, McCallion W. Childhood circumcision in Northern Ireland: a barometer of the current practice of general paediatric surgery. Ulster Med J. 2010;79:80–1.
30. Yau A, Cha R, Jayaratnam S, Wilson T, Kukkady A, Evans SM, et al. Declining incidence of pyloric stenosis in New Zealand. ANZ J Surg. 2019;89:1242–5.
31. Han S-R, Kim H-J, Kim N-H, Shin S, Yoo RN, Kim G, et al. Inguinal hernia surgery in Korea: nationwide data from 2007–2015. Ann Surg Treat Res. 2019;97:41–7.
32. Andler W, Lübbers W, Paetzmann-Sietas B, Meyer M, von Seiche J, Schmidt R, et al. Aktuelle Situation der stationären Kinder- und Jugendmedizin in Deutschland: Ergebnisse der 4. Befragung von stationären Einrichtungen der Kinder- und Jugendmedizin. Monatsschr Kinderheilkd. 2007;155:157–66.
33. Steinau G, Tittel A, Schumpelick V. Tageschirurgische (TCH) Eingriffe im Kindesalter an einer chirurgischen Klinik. Zentralbl Chir. 1993;118:25–9.
34. Clair DL, Caldamone AA. Pediatric office procedures. Urol Clin North Am. 1988;15:715–23.
35. Scheuber K, Becke K. Ambulante Anästhesie-Kinder in der ambulanten Anästhesie. Anasth Intensiv Notf. 2013;48:192–9.
36. Eckert K, Janssen N, Franz M, Liedgens P. Die nicht-retrahierbare Vorhaut bei beschwerdefreien Jungen: Eine Indikation zur Zirkumzision? Urologe. 2017;56:351–7.
37. Schmidt A-M, Stehr M. Handlungsempfehlung nach der S2k-Leitlinie Phimose und Paraphimose. Monatsschr Kinderheilkd. 2019;167:1154–6.
38. Reinhard A. Die Therapie der Phimose im Wandel der Zeit. Julius-Maximilians-Universität; 2014. urn:nbn:de:bvb:20-opus-99817.
39. Brönner D. Konservative versus operative Therapie der kindlichen Phimose – Ergebnisse einer monozentrischen retrospektiven Kohortenstudie. Julius-Maximilians-Universität; 2019. urn:nbn:de:bvb:20-opus-182102.
40. Task Force on Circumcision. Male Circumcision. Pediatrics. 2012;130:e756-85.
41. Deutsche Gesellschaft für Kinderchirurgie. Phimose und Paraphimose. S2k-Leitlinie. Nürnberg: Arbeitsgemeinschaft der wissenschaftlichen Fachgesellschaften; 2017. Accessed 25 Jan 2021.
42. Phimosis and Paraphimosis - American Urological Association. Accessed 25 Jan 2021.
43. Sneppen I, Thorup J. Foreskinmorbidity in uncircumcised males. Pediatrics. 2016;137:e20154340-0.
44. Stehr M, Schuster T, Dietz H-G, Joppich I. Die Zirkumzision-Kritik an der Routine. Klin Padiatr. 2001;213:50–5.
45. Hsieh T-F, Chang C-H, Chang S-S. Foreskin development before adolescence in 2149 schoolboys: foreskin development. Int J Urol. 2006;13:968–70.
46. Merkel R, Putzke H. After Cologne: male circumcision and the law. Parental right, religious liberty or criminal assault? J Med Ethics. 2013;39:444–9.
47. Stehr M, Putzke H. Die Entwicklung der Debatte um das Beschneidungsgesetz. Uro-News. 2020;24:32–5.
48. Tijdink JK, Schipper K, Bouter LM, Maclaine Pont P, de Jonge J, Smulders YM. How do scientists perceive the current publication culture? A qualitative focus group interview study among Dutch biomedical researchers. BMJ Open. 2016;6:e008681.
49. Bröckelmann J. Comparison of Hospital- and Office-Based Ambulatory Surgery in Germany: Surgery in small free standing units offers many advantages. Ambul Surg. 2012;17:83–5.
50. Wang ML, Macklin EA, Tracy E, Nadel H, Catlin EA. Updated parental viewpoints on male neonatal circumcision in the United States. Clin Pediatr (Phila). 2010;49:130–6.
51. Takla A, Wiese-Posselt M, Harder T, Meerpohl JJ, Röbl-Mathieu M, Terhardt M, et al. Background paper for the recommendation of HPV vaccination for boys in Germany. Bundesgesundheitsbl. 2018;61:1170–86.
52. Fujiogi M, Michihata N, Matsui H, Fushimi K, Yasunaga H, Fujishiro J. Outcomes following laparoscopic versus open surgery for pediatric inguinal hernia repair: analysis using a national inpatient database in Japan. J Pediatr Surg. 2019;54:577–81.
53. Statistisches Bundesamt. Krankenhäuser-Fallpauschalenbezogene Krankenhausstatistik. Statistisches Bundesamt. Accessed 24 Feb 2021.

18

Hybrid ileal pouch with concomitant anti-refluxing and refluxing ureteroileal anastomosis

Se Young Choi[1,2], Bumjin Lim[3], Byung Hoon Chi[1], Jung Hoon Kim[4], Wonchul Lee[3], Dalsan You[3] and Choung-Soo Kim[3*]

Abstract

Purpose: We report our preliminary experience of using a hybrid ileal pouch, assessing oncologic outcomes, complications, voiding, and renal function.

Methods: The study included 25 patients with bladder cancer treated with radical cystectomy with a hybrid ileal pouch with concomitant anti-refluxing and refluxing anastomosis, performed by a single surgeon. The patients were divided into two groups (first and last cases) according to the surgery date. Postoperative complications, separate renal function by renal scan, voiding function by uroflowmetry with residual urine, and oncologic outcomes were assessed.

Results: The surgery duration was shorter in the last cases than the first cases. The voiding volume increased with time. There were 23 cases of grade 3 complication in 12 patients and one case of grade 4 complication (sepsis). In the first cases, ureterovesical stenosis occurred in five cases, whereas in the last cases, there were no cases of stenosis. In separate renal function, there was no difference between the left and right side or between the first and last cases.

Conclusions: The hybrid ileal pouch showed acceptable oncologic and functional outcomes and complications; therefore, it can be used according to the appropriate surgical situation with a relatively short bowel segment during neobladder construction.

Keywords: Ileal pouch, Urinary diversion, Reflux, Neobladder, Renal function

Introduction

An orthotopic neobladder constructed following radical cystectomy is preferred by patients for physiologic and anatomical reasons. However, there are many complications with this reconstruction, including declining renal function or voiding difficulty, even with experienced surgeons [1, 2]. The ideal orthotopic neobladder preserves renal function and enables the anatomical storage and emptying of urine without an external appliance. The deterioration of renal function is one of the most important adverse events related to urinary diversion, as chronic kidney disease is associated with substantial cardiovascular morbidity and mortality [3]. There is little evidence regarding the impact on renal function of specific types of urinary diversion, that is, anti-refluxing or refluxing techniques. Some authors have suggested that the anti-refluxing type can reduce upper tract scarring by reducing vesicoureteral reflux [4]. Others have maintained that a low-pressure reservoir with a chimney helps to preserve renal function [5]. A recent randomized clinical trial comparing a T-pouch with an anti-refluxing

*Correspondence: cskim@amc.seoul.kr
[3] Department of Urology, Asan Medical Center, University of Ulsan College of Medicine, 88 Olympic-ro 43-gil, Songpa-gu, Seoul 05505, Korea
Full list of author information is available at the end of the article

mechanism versus a Studer pouch did not show significant differences in preservation of renal function at 3 years [6].

Upper tract recurrence following cystectomy has been reported in ~ 5% of cases [7]. Positive ureteral margin at cystectomy has been associated with upper tract recurrence, and the negative conversion may help to decrease the risk of recurrence [8]. The situation of a short remnant ureter occurs because of serial additional resection. The use of a hybrid ileal pouch was introduced to resolve the deficiency of the short ureter. We concerned the effect of anti-refluxing and refluxing ureteroileal anastomosis on separate renal function in the same condition of the neobladder. Here, we report our preliminary experience of radical cystectomy with a hybrid ileal pouch, assessing the oncologic outcomes, complications, voiding, and renal function following surgery.

Materials and methods

The need for informed consent was waived by the Institutional Review Board of the Asan Medical Center owing to the minimal risk of harm. After receiving approval (2018–1041) from the institutional review board at the Asan Medical Center, all methods were carried out in accordance with relevant guidelines and regulations. We retrospectively reviewed the medical records of 25 patients who underwent radical cystectomy and hybrid ileal neobladder construction for bladder cancer between June 2009 and September 2018. In general, patients with favorable performance status and renal function were selected. Before surgery, clinical examination, a laboratory profile, computerized tomography, and a renal scan (^{99m}Tc-diethylene triamine penta-acetic acid or ^{99m}Tc-mercaptoacetyltriglycine), which show separate renal function, were evaluated. The baseline characteristics of patients and tumors and perioperative data including pathology and surgical technique were collected. The first cases (group A; n = 17) were performed between June 2009 and March 2010, and the last cases (group B; n = 8) were performed after May 2016.

All patients had undergone radical cystectomy, urinary diversion, and lymph node dissection. The surgical procedures were performed by one experienced surgeon (C.-S. K.) who had 21.4 cases of the average annual surgeon volume for radical cystectomy over 10 years and had performed > 250 radical cystectomies as the operator before 2009. Between April 2010 and April 2016, the surgeon performed 117 cases of additional radical cystectomy. In general, for the neobladder, an ileal reservoir was constructed with ureteroileal reimplantation in extramural tunnels to prevent reflux (Ghoneim pouch, Fig. 1a) which can be made with a short length of bowel segment ~ 40–50 cm [2]. The most common reason to make a hybrid pouch was due to shortening of the remnant ureter due to additional resection following positive intraoperative frozen section. The surgeon modified the Ghoneim pouch with a Hautmann pouch (Fig. 1b) [9] and constructed the hybrid pouch (Fig. 1c). A 45–60 cm length of ileum was used for the neobladder, which included 6–10 cm of one chimney. A 1-cm-sized

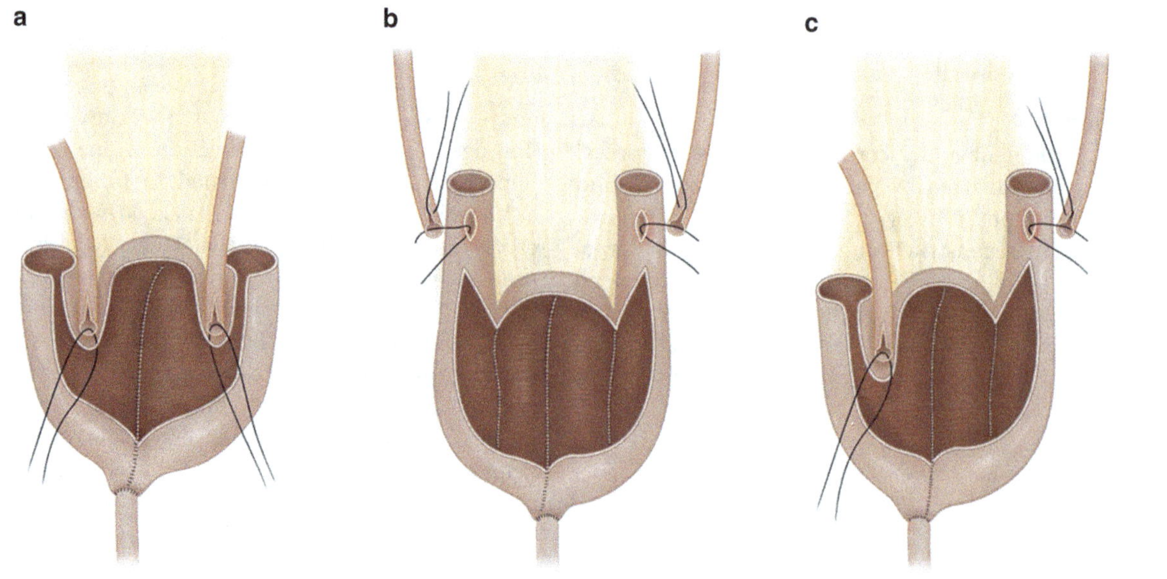

Fig. 1 Concept of the hybrid ileal pouch that was composed of a Ghoneim pouch (anti-refluxing type, (**a**) and Hautmann pouch (refluxing type, **b**) on each side (**c**)

hole was made in the dependent lesion of the neobladder for urethra anastomosis. One ureter was connected to the chimney directly by the refluxing technique, and the other ureter was implanted into the reentrant lesion of the neobladder using the anti-refluxing extramural tunneling technique. In cases of a left-side chimney, the chimney was overlaid on the colon. Ureteral stents were inserted on both sides, and suprapubic cystostomy was maintained until self-voiding following cystography.

Renal function was assessed using the estimated glomerular filtration rate (GFR) calculated with the Chronic Kidney Disease Epidemiology Collaboration equation [10]. We evaluated the separate GFR for each kidney using a renal nucleotide scan. Following radical cystectomy, the patients were generally followed up every 3 months during the first year, every 6 months during years 2–6, and annually thereafter. History taking, physical examination, blood laboratory investigations, urine sedimentation, culture, cytology, renal scan, uroflowmetry with residual urine, and computerized tomography were evaluated. The median duration from the date of surgery to the final follow-up date was 29.8 months (interquartile range [IQR] 18.5–109.3). The follow-up duration of group A and B were 58.1 (IQR 20.8–123.9) months and 25.2 (IQR 14.9–38.1) months ($P=0.086$).

The clinicopathologic characteristics were compared among the three groups using Fisher's exact test for categorical variables and a t-test or Mann Whitney *U* test for continuous variables according to normality by the Kolmogorov–Smirnov test. The characteristics were described as the mean ± standard deviation with IQR or numbers with percentages. Cox proportional-hazard regression was used to compare recurrence and overall survival between groups. All statistical analyses were performed using IBM SPSS Statistics Version 21 (IBM Corporation, Somers, NY, USA) and R version 3.4.3 (R Project for Statistical Computing; http://www.r-project.org/). All *P* values were two-tailed, and $P<0.05$ was considered significant.

Results

The clinical and pathological characteristics of the group A and B are presented in Table 1. There were no differences in baseline characteristics between the group A and B. In the entire cohort, the mean age was 62.3 ± 9.3 years (IQR 57.5–67.0). The majority of patients (88.0%) were male, and 48.0% had a clinical T2 or stage of lower. Among the cohort, 4 patients (16.0%) had clinical lymph nodes and 19 patients (76.0%) had a grade 3 tumor that was obtained at transurethral resection of the bladder tumor. Neoadjuvant chemotherapy was administered to three patients (12.0%).

The duration of surgery was shorter in the group B (389.9 ± 52.8 min) than the group A (499.4 ± 61.7 min, $P<0.001$) (Table 2). There was no difference in hospitalization time ($P=0.092$), T ($P=0.154$), and N stage ($P=0.439$). The majority (88.2%) of group A underwent super-extended lymphadenectomy up to the

Table 1 Clinical and pathological characteristics

	Group A (N = 17)	Group B (N = 8)	Total (N = 25)	p
Age (years)	63.4 ± 7.8 [59.0; 67.0]	60.0 ± 12.0 [50.5; 69.0]	62.3 ± 9.3 [57.5; 67.0]	0.410
Male gender	15 (88.2%)	7 (87.5%)	22 (88.0%)	1.000
Height	165.0 ± 7.9 [161.0; 170.8]	165.5 ± 4.9 [162.7; 169.6]	165.2 ± 7.0 [160.1; 169.7]	0.887
Weight	66.6 ± 8.7 [60.2; 75.3]	64.7 ± 12.8 [56.8; 76.8]	66.0 ± 9.9 [60.2; 76.0]	0.665
Body mass index (kg/m^2)	24.5 ± 3.5 [21.6; 26.4]	22.8 ± 3.5 [20.5; 26.4]	24.0 ± 3.5 [21.3; 26.4]	0.293
Diabetes mellitus	3 (17.6%)	2 (25.0%)	5 (20.0%)	1.000
Hypertension	6 (35.3%)	2 (25.0%)	8 (32.0%)	0.956
Clinical T stage				0.571
≤T2	7 (41.2%)	5 (62.5%)	12 (48.0%)	
≥T3	10 (58.8%)	3 (37.5%)	13 (52.0%)	
Clinical lymph node positive	3 (17.6%)	1 (12.5%)	4 (16.0%)	1.000
Preoperative grade				0.544
G2	3 (20.0%)	0 (0.0%)	3 (12.0%)	
G3	12 (80.0%)	7 (100.0%)	19 (76.0%)	
Neoadjuvant chemotherapy	1 (5.9%)	2 (25.0%)	3 (12.0%)	0.476

Mean ± standard deviation; []: Interquartile range

Table 2 Perioperative characteristics, pathology, and oncologic outcome

	Group A (N=17)	Group B (N=8)	Total (N=25)	*p*
Operation time (min)	499.4±61.7 [464.0; 531.0]	389.9±52.8 [364.5; 424.0]	464.4±77.9 [420.5; 510.0]	**<0.001**
Hospitalization time (days)	54.8±52.6 [32.0; 49.0]	32.1±14.5 [23.5; 33.0]	48.2±45.7 [26.0; 49.0]	0.092
Chimney side				0.694
Left	17 (100.0%)	7 (87.5%)	24 (96.0%)	
Right	0 (0.0%)	1 (12.5%)	1 (4.0%)	
Pelvic lymph node dissection				**<0.001**
Standard	1 (5.9%)	0 (0.0%)	1 (4.0%)	
Extended	1 (5.9%)	8 (100.0%)	9 (36.0%)	
Super-extended	15 (88.2%)	0 (0.0%)	15 (60.0%)	
Pathologic T stage				0.154
≤T2	11 (64.7%)	2 (25.0%)	13 (52.0%)	
≥T3	6 (35.3%)	6 (75.0%)	12 (48.0%)	
Pathologic N stage				0.439
0	14 (82.4%)	5 (62.5%)	19 (76.0%)	
1	1 (5.9%)	0 (0.0%)	1 (4.0%)	
2	1 (5.9%)	1 (12.5%)	2 (8.0%)	
3	1 (5.9%)	2 (25.0%)	3 (12.0%)	
Removed lymph node count	32.6±14.0 [23.0; 39.0]	28.5±10.8 [21.5; 39.0]	31.3±13.0 [22.0; 39.0]	0.475
Number of positive lymph node	0.3±0.7 [0.0; 0.0]	1.4±2.7 [0.0;2.0]	0.6±1.6 [0.0;0.0]	0.532
Postoperative grade				0.513
G2	3 (18.8%)	0 (0.0%)	3 (12.5%)	
G3	13 (81.2%)	8 (100.0%)	21 (87.5%)	
Positive soft margin	0 (0.0%)	1 (12.5%)	1 (4.0%)	0.694
Lymphovascular invasion	3 (17.6%)	4 (50.0%)	7 (28.0%)	0.229
Adjuvant chemotherapy	1 (5.9%)	1 (12.5%)	2 (8.0%)	1.000
Recurrence	5 (29.4%)	4 (50.0%)	9 (36.0%)	0.580
Death	10 (58.8%)	4 (50.0%)	14 (56.0%)	1.000

Bold values indicate statistical significance at $P < 0.05$

Mean ± standard deviation; []: Interquartile range

inferior mesenteric artery, whereas all of the group B had extended lymphadenectomy up to the great vessel bifurcation. In almost all cases, the chimney was on the left side (96.0%). In terms of pathologic T stage, 52.0% of cases were T2 or lower, and 24.0% were N1 or higher. We removed an average of 31.3±13.0 lymph nodes. There was one positive soft tissue margin. During follow-up periods, 9 patients (36.0%) had recurrences and 14 patients (56.0%) succumbed to mortality. There was no upper track recurrence. In Cox analysis, group was not a significant factor in recurrence (hazard ratio [HR] 2.049, 95% confidence interval [CI] 0.548–7.664, p=0.286) and overall survival (HR 4.023, 95% CI 0.934–17.329, P=0.062).

There were no cases in which to keep Foley catheter or clean intermittent catheter. The trends of voiding values of uroflowmetry and residual urine are shown in Fig. 2. There was no statistical difference among the values of peak flow rate and residual urine; however, voiding volume increased from 149.4±19.5 (3 months) to 235.9±29.9 (12 months, P=0.016). The forms of the hybrid ileal pouch at 2 weeks and 1 year post-surgery are shown in Fig. 3. At 2 weeks, ureteral stents were in place on both sides. At 1 year, the pouch appeared larger than that at 2 weeks. Vesicoureteral reflux was observed on the chimney side, but there was no reflux in the anti-refluxing side.

Table 3 shows the complications recorded. A total of 50 complications were reported in 17 patients (68.0%). There were 30 complications during the admission period and 20 complications following discharge. Almost all complications were Clavien grade 2 or 3.

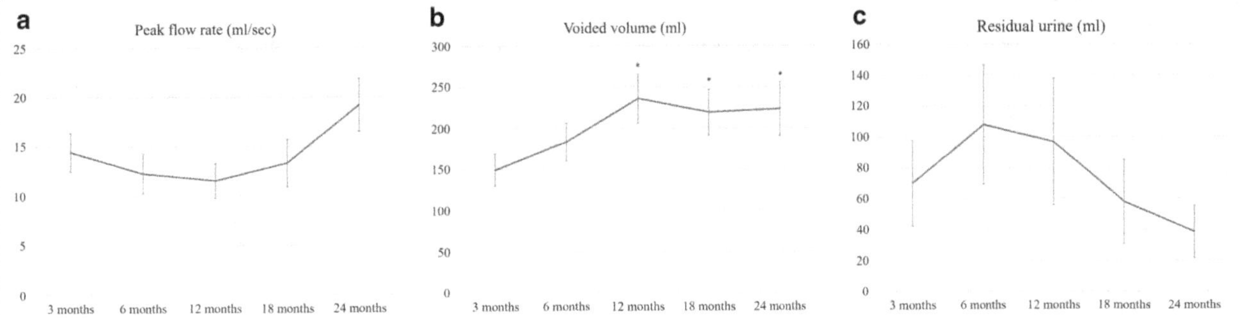

Fig. 2 Peak flow rate (**a**) and voided volume (**b**) of uroflowmetry and residual urine (**c**) following radical cystectomy with a hybrid ileal pouch

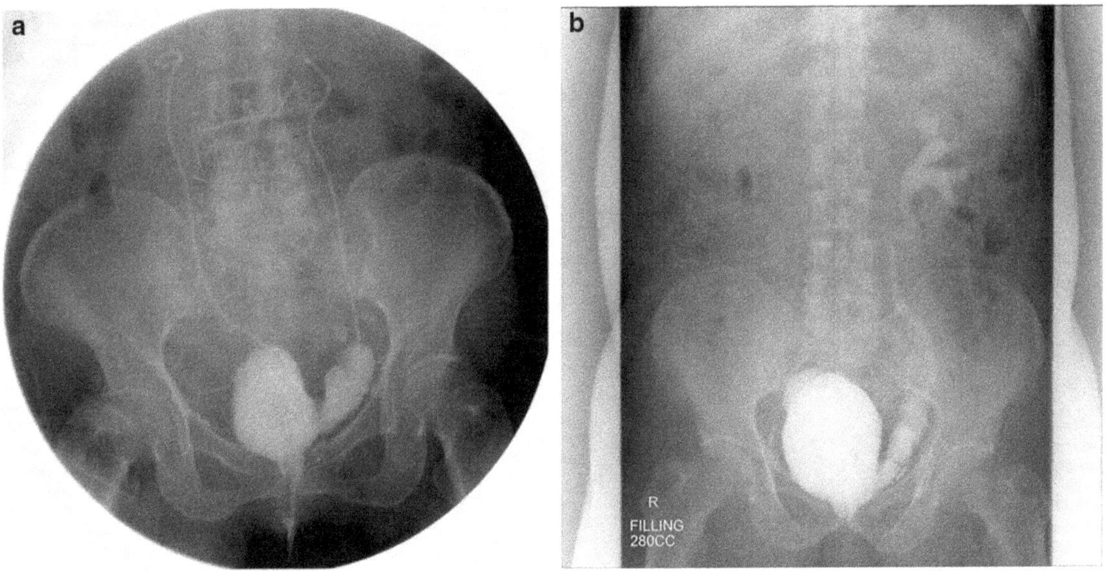

Fig. 3 Representative images of hybrid ileal pouch. Cystography at 2 weeks post-surgery (**a**) and voiding cystourethrography 1 year post-surgery (**b**). *$P < 0.05$ compared with value at 3 months

There were 23 cases of grade 3 in 12 patients (48.0%) and 1 case of grade 4, which was sepsis requiring management in an intensive care unit. Urethrovesical anastomosis leakage was the most common complication. In the group A, there were three cases of left ureterovesical stenosis and two cases of right ureterovesical stenosis. No ureterovesical stenosis was reported in the group B. In the patients with the stenosis, the ipsilateral GFR of the stenosis was significantly decreased (pre-surgery: 40.2 ± 6.9, 1 year: 18.6 ± 10.4, 2 year: 17.0 ± 12.3).

The trends in GFR from pre-surgery to 2 years post-surgery are shown in Fig. 4. The total GFR decreased significantly from pre-surgery (78.0 ± 19.5) to 2 years post-surgery (63.6 ± 15.5, $P = 0.013$). There was no difference between the left and right sides or between the group A and B ($P > 0.05$).

Discussion

Our preliminary results of radical cystectomy with a hybrid ileal pouch showed acceptable oncologic, complication and functional outcomes. There was no upper track recurrence among 24.0% of total recurrences. The recurrence rate can be confounded by the tumor stage. The 5 year recurrence-free survival rate has been reported as 62–68% and upper tract recurrence rates as 2.4–17% [11]. Upper track recurrence can be caused by both metachronous occurrence and intraluminal seeding [12]. Palou et al. reported that vesicoureteral reflux can increase the risk of upper track recurrence following

Table 3 Postoperative complication during follow-up period

	Group A (N = 17)	Group B (N = 8)	Total (N = 25)	Grade 3/4
Short-term complications (during admission)				
Urethrovesical anastomosis leakage	7 (41.2%)	2 (28.6%)	8 (32.0%)	1 (4.0%)
Wound dehiscence	3 (17.6%)	1 (14.3%)	4 (16.0%)	4 (16.0%)
Febrile infection	3 (17.6%)	0 (0.0%)	3 (12.0%)	0 (0.0%)
Ileus	2 (11.8%)	1 (14.3%)	3 (12.0%)	0 (0.0%)
Ureterovesical anastomosis leakage	2 (11.8%)	0 (0.0%)	2 (8.0%)	2 (8.0%)
Neobladder perforation	2 (11.8%)	0 (0.0%)	2 (8.0%)	2 (8.0%)
Abscess	2 (11.8%)	0 (0.0%)	2 (8.0%)	2 (8.0%)
Lymphocele	1 (5.9%)	1 (12.5%)	2 (8.0%)	2 (8.0%)
Ureterovesical stenosis (both)	1 (5.9%)	0 (0.0%)	1 (4.0%)	1 (4.0%)
Urethra stricture	0 (0.0%)	1 (14.3%)	1 (4.0%)	1 (4.0%)
Ileoileal anastomosis perforation	1 (5.9%)	0 (0.0%)	1 (4.0%)	1 (4.0%)
Sepsis	1 (5.9%)	0 (0.0%)	1 (4.0%)	1 (4.0%)
Long-term complications (after discharge)				
Ureterovesical stenosis	5 (29.4%)	0 (0.0%)	5 (20.0%)	5 (20.0%)
Left	3 (17.6%)	0 (0.0%)	3 (12.0%)	
Right	2 (11.8%)	0 (0.0%)	2 (8.0%)	
Fistula	4 (23.5%)	0 (0.0%)	4 (16.0%)	4 (16.0%)
Febrile infection	2 (11.8%)	2 (28.6%)	4 (16.0%)	0 (0.0%)
Small bowel obstruction	0 (0.0%)	1 (14.3%)	1 (4.0%)	1 (4.0%)
Abscess	1 (5.9%)	0 (0.0%)	1 (4.0%)	1 (4.0%)

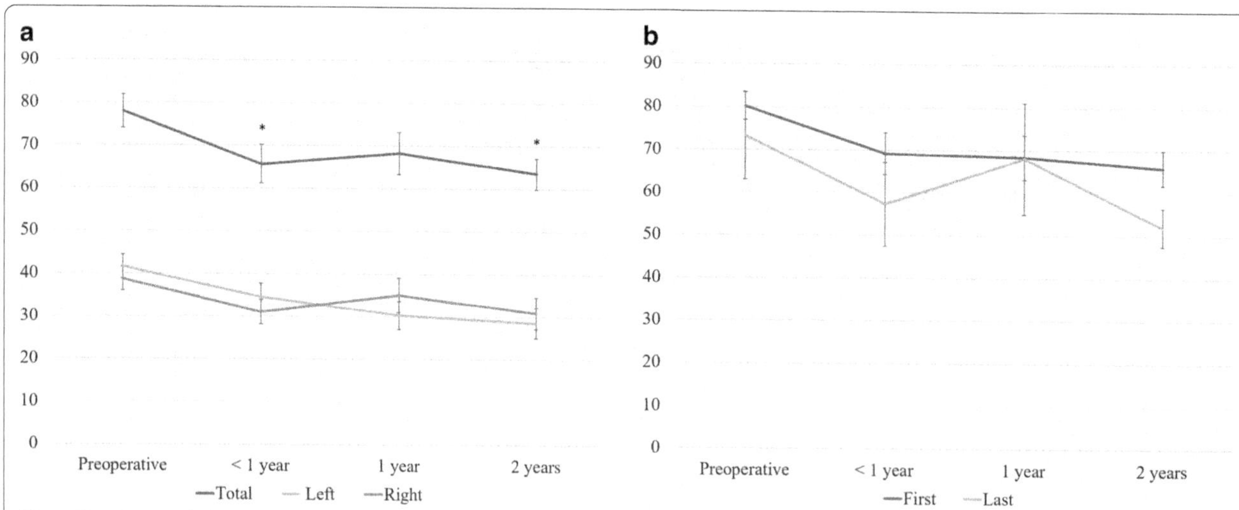

Fig. 4 Trends in total glomerular filtration rate of each renal unit (**a**) and first and last cases (**b**). There was no difference between the left and right sides, or between the first (group A) and last cases (group B). *$P < 0.05$ compared with the mean preoperative value

transurethral resection [13]. In cases of cystectomy, the association between the type of ureteral anastomosis and upper track recurrence is unclear. As recurrence is rare and theoretically no tumor cell is present in the neobladder, urethral recurrence may be associated with the type of diversion between continence and incontinence (5% vs 9%) [14]. However, retrospective cases of urethral or prostate involvement would be avoided in designing a continent-type neobladder; thus, selection bias may be present [14]. Until now, there is no evidence that the neobladder type can increase the urethral recurrence risk. In our study, there was only one case (4%) of urethral recurrence.

In our study, the mortality rate was 56.0%. There were no cases of mortality related to the surgery itself. There was one case of sepsis (grade 4) that was caused by peritonitis following surgery; however, the patient was discharged (hospitalization 103 days) following recovery and survived during the 58 month period without recurrence. In a previous study of 11,933 patients who underwent radical cystectomy, short-term mortality rates were similar between neobladder and ileal conduit after propensity when matching by age, race, gender, stage, facility type, histology, and comorbidity [15].

The complication rate following neobladder reconstruction may be associated with the experience of the surgeon, method of surgery, or condition of the patients. The method of data collection may also influence the assessment of complications. In our study, grade 3 or higher complications were present in 12 patients (48.0%). This rate was higher than reported by others. Hautmann et al. reported an incidence of 21.8% grade 3 or higher complications [9], and Ali-El-Dein et al. reported a 35% incidence of late complications [16]. However, the initial technique may lead to more complications. Gakis et al. reported a 39.2% 90 day complication rate as initial results [17]. Our results were from not only the initial 90 days but also all follow-up periods. In addition, the group B had much fewer complications than the group A. In particular, ureterovesical stenosis decreased from five cases to zero. In the group B, the hospitalization stay was similar to other studies [18]. This may be associated with the modified ureter-fixation technique, with one point of the distal region of the spatulated ureter sutured with full depth from mucosa to serosa, but the other regions of the remnant ureter were sutured on only the mucosa between the ureter and ileum. The anti-refluxing extramural tunnel region should also be sutured on the mucosa only. Although only mucosa was sutured on the regions, there was no ureterovesical anastomosis leakage or neobladder perforation in the group B. In addition, the connection of the mid region of the hybrid pouch to the opened chimney lumen should be positioned in the upper level to the opened chimney prior to closure of the neobladder for sparing chimney lumen with less tension. The upfront chimney beyond the rectum can assist in ensuring the ureter is not angulated or under tension. Although the patients with the ureterovesical stenosis underwent percutaneous nephrostomy or ureteral stent, their ipsilateral GFR was significantly decreased. Therefore, the above techniques about mucosa-to-mucosa and tension-free are important to prevent the stenosis. At last, group B showed relatively acceptable data about complications maintaining renal functions.

The voiding function was maintained reasonably well. At 1 year post-surgery, the void volume reached at least 200 mL. The hybrid pouch was formed into a spherical shape; this spherical shape resembling the original bladder shape may have advantages including constant pressure stresses on the entire wall and prevention of internal folding of the walls. Therefore, the spherical shape may be helpful to voiding function.

We compared the separate renal function of each side. The anti-refluxing types were mainly on the right side, and refluxing types were mainly on the left side. The separate renal function did not differ significantly between the right and left sides. At 2 years, ~ 81.5% of total GFR was preserved. The decreases of GFR are commonly observed following radical cystectomy, and the risk factors include hydronephrosis, pyelonephritis, and ureterovesical stricture [19]. Harraz et al. also reported GFR decreases of ~ 10% after 2 years, with no difference between the refluxing and anti-refluxing type [20]. To establish an ideal pouch to protect renal function, further investigations are required.

This study had some limitations. As a retrospective study, there may have selection bias, including a short remnant ureter. The extent of node dissection was different between 2 groups, because we found the survival gain from super-extended lymphadenectomy was limited [21]. The technique of lymphadenectomy might not be associated with the rates of ureteroileal stricture, because of far region from the lymph node fields. There is also the possibility of the under-reporting of complications; in particular, the presence or degree of incontinence was not surveyed. However, we periodically checked uroflowmetry with residual urine. The small sample size and short follow-up requires additional investigation. In addition, this preliminary technique needs to be established consistently. The comparison of various pouches is difficult because of various patient or tumor characteristics and various surgical techniques. This study can provide clues in distinguishing between anti-refluxing and refluxing types. Use of a hybrid ileal pouch may have advantages for a short remnant ureter, owing to the relatively short length of bowel segment required and anti-refluxing mechanism to prevent direct refluxing infection.

Conclusions

The hybrid ileal pouch had concomitant characteristics of anti-refluxing and refluxing ureteroileal anastomosis. There were no differences in the GFR of each side or in ureterovesical stenosis between the anti-refluxing and refluxing anastomosis side. Skilled techniques may reduce significant complications according to the accumulation of experiences. Our preliminary data of use of a hybrid ileal pouch showed acceptable complication, oncologic, and functional outcomes in patients with bladder cancer. Therefore, the hybrid ileal pouch can be applied according to the appropriate surgical situation with a relatively short bowel segment during neobladder surgery.

Abbreviations
GFR: Glomerular filtration rate; IQR: interquartile range.

Acknowledgements
This manuscript was prepared with the assistance of Enago, an English-language editing company.

Authors' contributions
SYC and C-SK: conception and design. DY and BL: acquisition oof data. WL, JHK and BHC: analysis and interpretation of data. SYC: drafting of manuscript. C-SK: critical revision of the manuscript. SYC and C-SK: obtaining funding. C-SK: supervision. All authors read and approved the final manuscript.

Author details
[1]Department of Urology, Chung-Ang University Hospital, Chung-Ang University College of Medicine, 102, Heukseok-ro, Dongjak-gu, Seoul 06973, Korea. [2]Biomedical Research Institute, Chung-Ang University Hospital, 102, Heukseok-ro, Dongjak-gu, Seoul 06973, Korea. [3]Department of Urology, Asan Medical Center, University of Ulsan College of Medicine, 88 Olympic-ro 43-gil, Songpa-gu, Seoul 05505, Korea. [4]Department of Urology, Hanil General Hospital, Seoul, Korea.

References
1. Hautmann RE, de Petriconi RC, Volkmer BG. 25 years of experience with 1,000 neobladders: long-term complications. J Urol. 2011;185:2207–12.
2. Abol-Enein H, Ghoneim MA. Further clinical experience with the ileal W-neobladder and a serous-lined extramural tunnel for orthotopic substitution. Br J Urol. 1995;76:558–64.
3. Go AS, Chertow GM, Fan D, McCulloch CE, Hsu CY. Chronic kidney disease and the risks of death, cardiovascular events, and hospitalization. N Engl J Med. 2004;351:1296–305.
4. Kristjansson A, Bajc M, Wallin L, Willner J, Mansson W. Renal function up to 16 years after conduit (refluxing or anti-reflux anastomosis) or continent urinary diversion: 2. renal scarring and location of bacteriuria. Br J Urol. 1995;76:546–50.
5. Song C, Kim SC, Park J, Moon DH, Ahn H. Renal function change after refluxing type orthotopic ileal substitution. J Urol. 2011;186:1948–52.
6. Skinner EC, Fairey AS, Groshen S, Daneshmand S, Cai J, Miranda G, et al. Randomized trial of studer pouch versus T-pouch orthotopic ileal neobladder in patients with bladder cancer. J Urol. 2015;194:433–9.
7. Huguet-Perez J, Palou J, Millan-Rodriguez F, Salvador-Bayarri J, Villavicencio-Mavrich H, Vicente-Rodriguez J. Upper tract transitional cell carcinoma following cystectomy for bladder cancer. Eur Urol. 2001;40:318–23.
8. Tollefson MK, Blute ML, Farmer SA, Frank I. Significance of distal ureteral margin at radical cystectomy for urothelial carcinoma. J Urol. 2010;183:81–6.
9. Hautmann RE, de Petriconi RC, Volkmer BG. Lessons learned from 1,000 neobladders: the 90-day complication rate. J Urol. 2010;184:990–4.
10. Matsushita K, Mahmoodi BK, Woodward M, Emberson JR, Jafar TH, Jee SH, et al. Comparison of risk prediction using the CKD-EPI equation and the MDRD study equation for estimated glomerular filtration rate. JAMA. 2012;307:1941–51.
11. Nagele U, Anastasiadis AG, Stenzl A, Kuczyk M. Radical cystectomy with orthotopic neobladder for invasive bladder cancer: a critical analysis of long-term oncological, functional, and quality of life results. World J Urol. 2012;30:725–32.
12. Kakizoe T. Development and progression of urothelial carcinoma. Cancer Sci. 2006;97:821–8.
13. Palou J, Farina LA, Villavicencio H, Vicente J. Upper tract urothelial tumor after transurethral resection for bladder tumor. Eur Urol. 1992;21:110–4.
14. Stein JP, Clark P, Miranda G, Cai J, Groshen S, Skinner DG. Urethral tumor recurrence following cystectomy and urinary diversion: clinical and pathological characteristics in 768 male patients. J Urol. 2005;173:1163–8.
15. Nahar B, Koru-Sengul T, Miao F, Prakash NS, Venkatramani V, Gauri A, et al. Comparison of readmission and short-term mortality rates between different types of urinary diversion in patients undergoing radical cystectomy. World J Urol. 2018;36:393–9.
16. Ali-el-Dein B, Shaaban AA, Abu-Eideh RH, el-Azab M, Ashamallah A, Ghoneim MA. Surgical complications following radical cystectomy and orthotopic neobladders in women. J Urol. 2008;180:206–10.
17. Gakis G, Abdelhafez MF, Stenzl A. The, "I-Pouch": Results of a new ileal neobladder technique. Scand J Urol. 2015;49:400–6.
18. Kim SH, Yu A, Jung JH, Lee YJ, Lee ES. Incidence and risk factors of 30-day early and 90-day late morbidity and mortality of radical cystectomy during a 13-year follow-up: a comparative propensity-score matched analysis of complications between neobladder and ileal conduit. Jpn J Clin Oncol. 2014;44:677–85.
19. Eisenberg MS, Thompson RH, Frank I, Kim SP, Cotter KJ, Tollefson MK, et al. Long-term renal function outcomes after radical cystectomy. J Urol. 2014;191:619–25.
20. Harraz AM, Mosbah A, Abdel-Latif M, El-Assmy A, Gad H, Shaaban AA. Impact of the type of ureteroileal anastomosis on renal function measured by diuretic scintigraphy: long-term results of a prospective randomized study. BJU Int. 2014;114:202–9.
21. Choi SY, You D, Hong B, Hong JH, Ahn H, Kim CS. Impact of lymph node dissection in radical cystectomy for bladder cancer: how many vs how far? Surg Oncol. 2019;30:109–16.

19

Tubularized urethral reconstruction using everted saphenous vein graft in a beagle model

Dan Li[1], Zhou Shen[2] and Yujie Xu[3*]

Abstract

Background: A long segment stricture in the anterior urethra is a challenge in urology. We conducted a study to investigate the efficacy of anterior urethral reconstruction using an everted saphenous vein graft (SVG) in a tubular fashion.

Methods: Twelve male beagles were randomly divided into three groups: experimental group (n = 5), control group (n = 5) and normal group (n = 2). A 3 cm defect in the anterior urethra was created. Autologous SVG was harvested. In the experimental group, urethral defect was replaced by an everted SVG in a tubular fashion. In the control group, urethral reconstruction was performed using an uneverted SVG. Beagles in all groups received retrograde urethrography to evaluate urethral patency and were killed for histological examination 6 months after operation.

Results: Four beagles in the experimental group had no voiding difficulty and the other one could not void spontaneously. Retrograde urethrography showed the four beagles in experimental group had wide urethral lumens. Ether urethral stricture or fistula were detected in all animals in the control group. Histological analysis of the four beagles in the experimental group indicated the everted SVG completely integrated into the urethra. The reconstructed urethra contained a wide lumen and was completely covered by urothelium. The periurethral collagen and muscle fibers formed and were highly organized. Everted SVG showed a high ability of neovascularization. In the control group, the reconstructed segment showed a fibrotic urethral lumen where the urothelium was not intact. Only few new capillaries were formed.

Conclusions: Everted SVG demonstrates for a promising strategy for potential urethral stricture repair.

Keywords: Urethral stricture, Saphenous vein graft, Urethral reconstruction, Tubularized urethroplasty

Background

Adult and pediatric disorders of the urethra including hypospadias, trauma, and stricture require substituted urethroplasty to preserve the function of the urinary tract. Reconstruction of the anterior urethra is one of the most challenging problems in urology [1].

Autologous tissues have advantages of excellent biological compatibility as well as rapid and effective neovascularization. Oral mucosa and penile skin flap are preferred substituted materials for urethral reconstruction [2, 3]. Onlay urethroplasty and multi-stage repair are commonly used techniques [4]. In some cases, these methods have problems including stricture recurrence, fistula formation and inadequate donor material. Harvesting oral mucosa is associated with donor site morbidity, such as submucosal scarring, pain, numbness and injury to salivary ducts [5, 6]. These issues highlight a critical need for the development of alternative material and reconstructive strategies for anterior urethral repair.

The saphenous vein is commonly used as vascular substitute material. It is easily harvested, and its associated wound complications were not dramatic, including

*Correspondence: xyj_1213@126.com
[3] Department of Urology, The First Affiliated Hospital of Wannan Medical College (Yijishan Hospital of Wannan Medical College), 2 Zheshan West Road, Wuhu 241000, Anhui Province, China
Full list of author information is available at the end of the article

chronic pain, numbnes and paresthesia/dysesthesia [7]. We previously performed urethroplasty in a rabbit model using everted SVG as an onlay graft and gained encouraging results [8]. The inner wall of blood vessels consist of vascular endothelium. We hypothesized that everting vein graft makes the outside vascular endothelium cling to periurethral tissue. In turn, the endothelium quickly attracts blood supply from the surrounding periurethral tissues including dartos. Here, we compare differences in neovascularization between everted SVG and non-everted SVG.

In addition, saphenous vein has a similar caliber as the urethra in humans. Even though tubularized grafts have not shown to be a preferential form of substitution, it avoids multi-stage surgery of ventral and dorsal onlay urethroplasty. Whether everted SVG can be used for tubularized urethraplasty remains unkown. Thus, we performed anterior urethral reconstruction in a beagle model using everted SVG in the tubular form.

Methods

Urethroplasty using everted SVG

This experimental animal protocol was approved by the Animal Experimentation Ethics Committee of Wannan Medical College in accordance with the Guide for the Care and Use of Laboratory Animals. Twelve male beagle dogs (Animal Research Center of Wannan Medical College. Wuhu, China) weighing 8–10 kg were randomly divided into three groups: experimental group (n = 5), control group (n = 5) and normal group (n = 2).

After general anesthesia with 3% pentobarbital, the beagles in the experimental group and control group were placed on an operating table in supine position. The right thigh and genital organ were shaved and prepared with povidone-iodine solution. A 4-cm incision was performed on the ventral skin of penis. A 3 cm segment of anterior urethra was removed between the external urethral orifice and bulbar urethra, in order to make a urethral defect (Fig. 1a).

A 4-cm incision was carried out on the right thigh skin and a 3-cm SVG was excised (Fig. 1b). In the experimental group, the vein grafts were everted like taking off sleeves,without longitudinally cutting the venous wall, (in order to make the endothelium outside) (Fig. 1c). A 8 F catheter was inserted into the urethra and was used as a stent (Fig. 1d). Urethral defect was repaired by the everted SVG in tubular fashion with 6–0 vicryl separated sutures (Fig. 1e). In the control group, the urethral defect was repaired using uneverted SVG in the same fashion. Nonabsorbable sutures were placed at the anastomosis margins for mark. Muscular tissue around the reconstructed urethra and the skin incision in penis was closed in layers (Fig. 1f). In the normal group, no surgical intervention was performed. The procedures for all animals were performed under sterile conditions by the same surgeon.

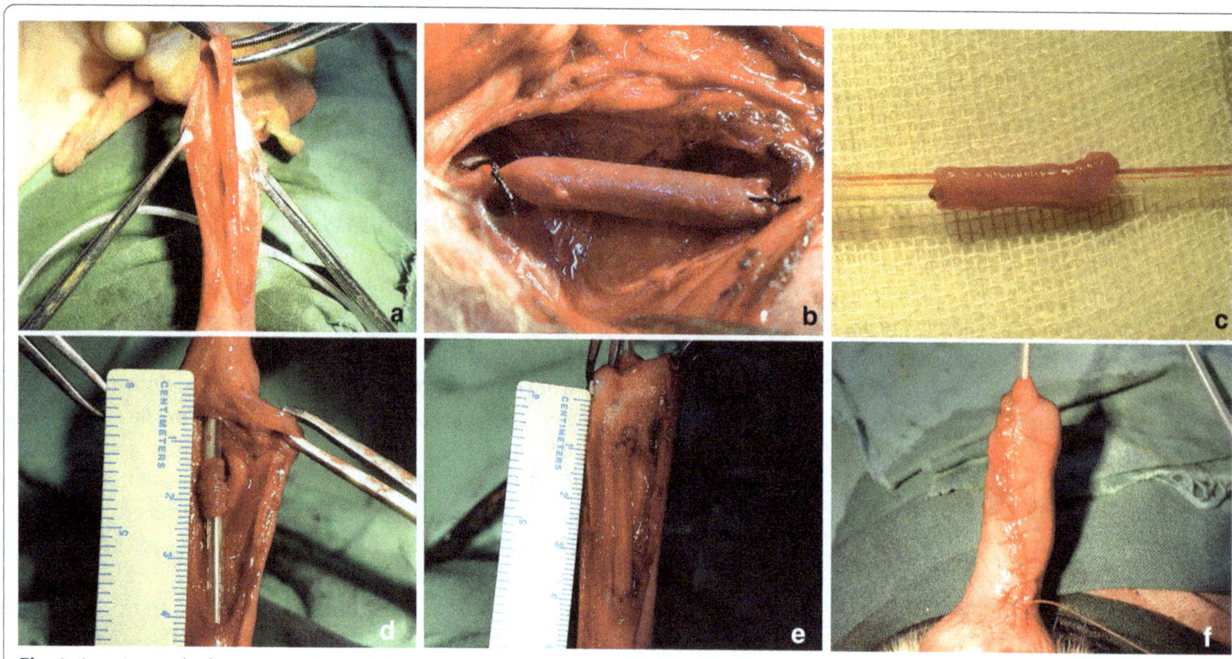

Fig. 1 Anterior urethral reconstruction with SVG. **a** A segment of anterior urethra was separated. **b** A 3-cm SVG was harvested. **c** The SVG was everted in experimental group. **d** The urethral catheter was inserted as a stent. **e** The urethral defect was repaired by SVG in tubular fashion. **f** The subdermal layer in penis and the skin was closed

Postoperative care

An Elizabetan collar was placed around the neck of animal to prevent the catheter removal. The catheter was left indwelling for two weeks. All animals in the experimental group and control group received penicillin 100U/kg/day intramuscularly for 14 days.

Retrograde urethrography

Retrograde urethrography was performed every month after operation. After general anesthesia, the animals were placed obliquely on an examination table. A Foley (6-F) catheter was inserted into the urethra until the balloon entered the urethral orifice. Inflate the balloon with 1 ml sterilized water. X-ray images of urethra were obtained under the fluoroscopy after contrast agent was gently injected through the catheter.

Histological and immunohistochemical analysis

Animals were euthanized by an overdose of 3% pentobarbital and air embolization 6 months after operation. The penises were obtained and the segments of the reconstructed urethra were extracted within the area outlined by the marking sutures. These segments were placed in 10% formalin, dehydrated in graded alcohols, and then embedded in paraffin. Sections (5 mm) were cut and then stained with hematoxylin–eosin (HE) staining, Masson's trichrome(MT) staining, and immunohistochemical(IHC) staining using CD-31 and uroplakin-II(UP-II) antibodies.

IHC staining using CD-31 antibody were quantified to compare neovascularization of the grafts using ImageJ software, in 10 different fields for each tissue sample. Data for these measurements are shown as mean ± SD. Statistical analysis was performed using a t-test through SPSS®, with $p<0.05$ was considered as statistically significant.

Radiologists and pathologists were blinded to the group when they were evaluating.

Results

The surgical procedures were successfully performed on all beagles. There were no major intraoperative complications observed. During the 6 months follow-up period, four beagles in the experimental group showed no voiding difficulty and the other one could not spontaneously void. Two beagles in control group could not spontaneously void and they underwent cystostomy with a suprapubic catheter. Urogenic cutaneous fistula in penis was detected in the other three animals in control group.

Retrograde urethrography

The retrograde urethrograms showed the urethral caliber of four beagles in the experimental group were similar to that of normal beagles (Fig. 2a, b). The contrast agent freely passed through the urethra without any signs of stricture or contrast leak. These indicate that the four beagles in the experimental group maintained wide urethral lumen 6 months postoperatively. The one beagle in the experimental group could not void spontaneously developed urethral stenosis. Ether significant urethral stricture or fistula were detected in all animals in control group (Fig. 2c, d).

Histological and IHC examination

In the experimental group, HE staining indicated the urethral lumen of the reconstructed segment was completely covered by the urothelium (Fig. 3e). There was no obvious difference observed in the normal urethra (Fig. 3a). MT staining showed highly organized collagen fibers and muscle tissue in the reconstructed urethra, but the muscle tissue seemed to be less than what was present in the normal urethra (Fig. 3b, f). The UP-II antibody is a special urothelium marker. IHC staining with UP-II antibody showed positive expression in the urethral inner wall (Fig. 3g).

In the control group, the reconstructed segment showed a narrow urethral lumen and the urothelium was not intact (Fig. 3i). MT staining showed abundant collagen with strong blue staining, indicating severe fibrosis

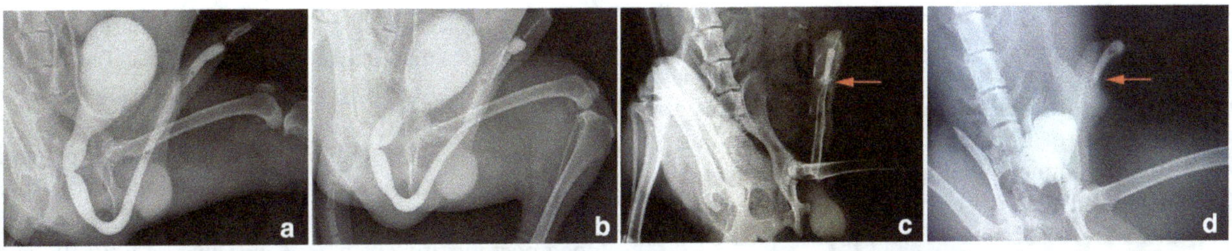

Fig. 2 Retrograde urethrography. **a** Urethrogram in beagle in normal group. **b** Urethrogram in experimental group 6 months postoperatively. **c** Urethral fistula in control group (red arrow point to the contrast leak). **d** Urethral stricture in control group (red arrow point to the stricture)

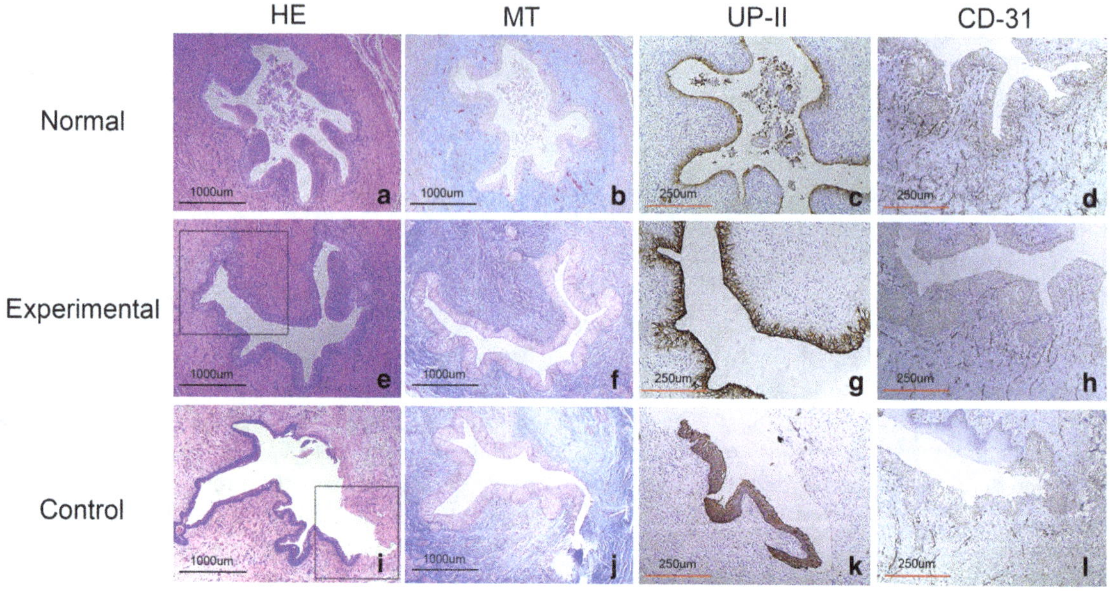

Fig. 3 Histological and IHC analysis. **a–d** HE staining, MT staining, IHC staining with UP-II and CD31 antibodies of the reconstructed urethra in normal group. **e** Wide urethral lumen was completely covered by endothelium in experimental group. **f** MT staining showed highly organized collagen fibers and muscle tissue in subepithelium. **g** IHC staining with UP-II antibody showed expression of uroplakin in the endothelium. **h** IHC staining with the CD31 showed dense capillaries in subepithelium. **i** HE staining showed a narrow urethral lumen and urothelium defect in control group. **j** MT staining showed fibrosis with abundant collagen. **k** IHC staining with the UP-II revealed a fragment of urothelium. **l** Vascular capillaries were sparse in control group

6 months postoperatively (Fig. 3j). IHC staining with UP-II antibody revealed a fragment of urothelium in the urethral inner wall (Fig. 3k).

IHC staining using a CD31 antibody was performed to observe the neovascularization of implanted tissue. In the experimental group, IHC staining with a CD31 antibody showed newly formed dense capillaries after 6 months (Fig. 3h). In the control group, IHC staining using a CD31 antibody indicated sparse vascular capillaries (Fig. 3l). Histomorphometric analysis found that the number of newly formed capillaries in the experimental group was higher than the control group (56.90 ± 1.57 vessels/mm^2 vs 40.30 ± 1.06 vessels/mm^2, $p < 0.01$) (Fig. 4).

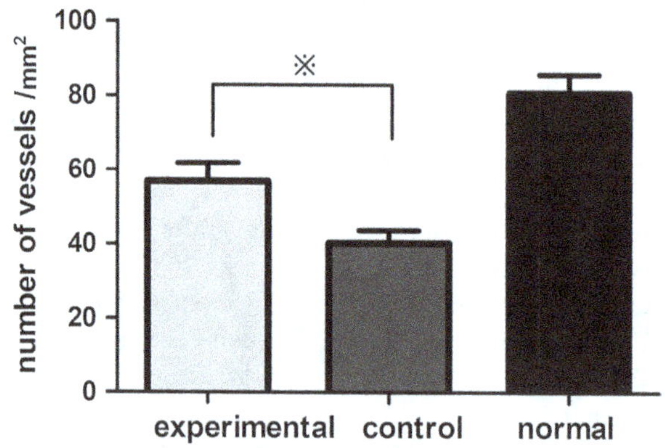

Fig. 4 Histomorphometric analysis of the extent of CD31 + vessels present in the 3 groups. ※Signifificant difference among the experimental and control groups ($P < .01$)

Discussion

Various urethral conditions often require substitute urethral reconstruction including long-segment urethral strictures, traumatic defects, complicated hypospadias and previous failed urethroplasty [9]. Several substituted materials have been adopted for clinical urethroplasty, including full-thickness skin graft, bladder mucosa, oral mucosa (buccal or lingual mucosa) and colonic mucosa [10–12]. Buccal mucosa and preputial skin graft remain the widely used tissues for urethral replacement. However, there are associated complications, such as graft necrosis, hair growth, stricture recurrence, and fistula formation [13, 14]. In addition, harvesting buccal mucosa may also lead to possible morbidities such as intraoperative hemorrhage, submucosal scarring, pain, postoperative infection, and injury to salivary ducts [3, 15]. Wood et al. [16] reported the morbidity of buccal mucosa grafts harvested for urethroplasty in 57 patients. Of these patients, 68% had perioral numbness that persisted after 6 months in 26% of the patients, 83% developed postoperative pain, 67% initially had difficulty with mouth opening that persisted after 6 months in 9% of the patients, and 2% had a mucous retention cyst. When urethral defects are complex, donor tissue extracted from oral cavity or prepuce may be insufficient. For these reasons, many attempts have been made to select alternative tissues that can serve as adequate urethral substitutes. Tissue engineering may be a promising option for the generation of an artificial urethra. However, accompanied techniques are complex containing multi-steps and the results of preliminary clinical applications are not satisfactory [17, 18]. Up to now, tissue engineered urethra is mainly being performed in animal experiments and has not made its way to the clinic [19].

Tuffer et al. performed urethral reconstruction using vein graft for the first time in 1910 [14]. Subsequently, several animal trials have been reported using vein grafts for urethral reconstruction [20–22]. Kahveci et al. [20] suggested that a vein graft mainly acts as a scaffold and the endothelium sloughs off after 3 days. Hubner et al. [22] and Foroutan et al. [23] used everted vein grafts and showed improved outcomes. They believed their modified technique eliminated negative effects on urine stream from the valve inside the venous lumen. We previously performed urethroplasty in a rabbit model with saphenous vein patch as onlay graft and gained encouraging results [8]. Results of everted vs non-everted vein grafts showed more optimal results with the everted graft.

To the best of our knowledge, one of the key factors in reconstructing urethra is adequate blood supply and fast neovascularization of the implanted graft [24, 25]. Insufficient blood supply inevitably results in shrinkage of grafts and the formation of fibrosis. In the study, the saphenous vein was everted and the vascular endothelium became outside. We hypothesized that everting the vein graft making the vascular endothelium on the outside facilitates the everted SVG blood supply gain from surrounding periurethral tissues including dartos. In this study, IHC staining with CD31 antibody showed dense vascular capillaries in the experimental group. Histomorphometric analysis demonstrated that compared to non-everted SVG, everting the vein graft improved its ability of neovascularization.

There is a lack of studies investigating one-stage reconstruction using a tubularized graft. Even though tubularized grafts have not proven to be a preferential substitution, they avoid multi-stage surgery of ventral combined dorsal onlay urethroplasty. The saphenous vein is a hollow tubular structure with a similar diameter of the urethra. The saphenous vein is readily accessible, even for the most extensive urethral reconstruction. Adult male beagles were selected as our experimental model because the urinary tract in beagle resemble the urinary tract in human. Foroutan et al. [23] performed histological study after euthanizing rabbits 7, 10, 14, 22, and 30 days after operation, they found that gradual uroepithelialization occurred within one month and demonstrated that the vein graft functioned as a guide for uroepithelium migration. The histological examination in our previous experiment revealed similar results [8]. The everted vein graft showed full integration in the neourethra. Urethral lumen was completely covered by regenerative uroepithelium 6 months postoperatively. Fistula formation and stenosis at the anastomosis were noted in the animals of control group. The experimental group showed improvement over the control group both in retrograde urethrography and histologic analysis. The MT staining showed that well-formed collagen and muscle fibers in the experimental group. However, abundant collagen fiber, narrow urethral lumen and urothelium defect were observed in control group. The rapid survival of the implant graft contributed to its function, serving as a barrier against urine extravasation, as well as facilitating urothelium cell migration and proliferation in the newly formed urethral tissue [26].

In this study, we create urethral defect models in the healthy urethra of normal animals and cannot fully resemble the exact clinical situation of urethral stricture in humans, which is characterized by the fibrotic urethra bed. Other limitations of this study include a small sample size and a short follow-up time. Further investigations with longer follow-up time are necessary to assess its technical applicability and to translate this technology into clinic.

Conclusion

We first used the everted SVG for tubularized urethral reconstruction in a beagle model. In our study, 80% of the experimental beagles showed no voiding difficulty or urethral fistula. The animals showed wide urethral lumen during the observation period. Everted SVG demonstrates promise for anterior urethral stricture repair. This study provides preclinical evidence and information needed to move toward clinical studies of this technique.

Abbreviations

SVG: Saphenous vein graft; HE: Hematoxylin–eosin; MT: Masson's trichrome; IHC: Immunohistochemical; UP-II: Uroplakin-II.

Acknowledgements

Not applicable

Authors' contributions

Protocol/project development: YX. Data collection or management: DL, ZS. Manuscript writing/editing: YX, DL. All Authors read and approved the final manuscript.

Author details
[1] Department of General Practice, The First Affiliated Hospital of Wannan Medical College (Yijishan Hospital of Wannan Medical College), Wuhu 241000, China. [2] Department of Urology, Anhui Provincial Hospital, Anhui Medical University, Hefei, Anhui, China. [3] Department of Urology, The First Affiliated Hospital of Wannan Medical College (Yijishan Hospital of Wannan Medical College), 2 Zheshan West Road, Wuhu 241000, Anhui Province, China.

References

1. Barbagli G, Palminteri E, Lazzeri M, Guazzoni G. Anterior urethral strictures. BJU Int. 2003;92(5):497–505.
2. Engel O, Fisch M. Urethral reconstruction after failed primary surgery. Urologe A. 2010;49(7):822–6.
3. Bhargava S, Chapple CR. Buccal mucosal urethroplasty: is it the new gold standard? BJU Int. 2004;93(9):1191–3.
4. Lee OT, Durbin-Johnson B, Kurzrock EA. Predictors of secondary surgery after hypospadias repair: a population based analysis of 5,000 patients. J Urol. 2013;190(1):251–5.
5. Sinha RJ, Singh V, Sankhwar SN, Dalela D. Donor site morbidity in oral mucosa graft urethroplasty: implications of tobacco consumption. BMC Urol. 2009;9:15.
6. Soave A, Dahlem R, Pinnschmidt HO, et al. Substitution urethroplasty with closure versus nonclosure of the buccal mucosa graft harvest site: a randomized controlled trial with a detailed analysis of oral pain and morbidity. Eur Urol. 2018;73(6):910–22.
7. Dick F, Hristic A, Roost-Krähenbühl E, et al. Persistent sensitivity disorders at the radial artery and saphenous vein graft harvest sites: a neglected side effect of coronary artery bypass grafting procedures. Eur J Cardiothorac Surg. 2011;40(1):221–6.
8. Xu Y, Shen Z, Liu G, et al. Urethral reconstruction using everted SVG in a rabbit model: one-year outcomes. Urol Int. 2017;99(1):110–7.
9. Peterson AC, Webster GD. Management of urethral stricture disease: developing options for surgical intervention. BJU Int. 2004;94(7):971–6.
10. Liu JS, Han J, Said M, et al. Long-term outcomes of urethroplasty with abdominal wall skin grafts. Urology. 2015;85(1):258–62.
11. O'Riordan A, Narahari R, Kumar V, Pickard R. Outcome of dorsal buccal graft urethroplasty for recurrent bulbar urethral strictures. BJU Int. 2008;102(9):1148–51.
12. Xu Y-M, Qiao Y, Sa Y-L, Zhang J, Fu Q, Song L-J. Urethral reconstruction using colonic mucosa graft for complex strictures. J Urol. 2009;182(3):1040–3.
13. Brannan W, Ochsner MG, Fuselier HA, Goodlet JS. Free full thickness skin graft urethroplasty for urethral stricture: experience with 66 patients. J Urol. 1976;115(6):677–80.
14. Vyas PR, Roth DR, Perlmutter AD. Experience with free grafts in urethral reconstruction. J Urol. 1987;137(3):471–4.
15. Rao AR, Shergill I, Thwaini A, Karim O, Motiwala H. Oral complications after buccal mucosal graft harvest for urethroplasty. BJU Int. 2005;95(4):679.
16. Wood DN, Allen SE, Andrich DE, Greenwell TJ, Mundy AR. The morbidity of buccal mucosal graft harvest for urethroplasty and the effect of nonclosure of the graft harvest site on postoperative pain. J Urol. 2004;172(2):580–3.
17. Mangera A, Chapple CR. Tissue engineering in urethral reconstruction—an update. Asian J Androl. 2013;15(1):89–92.
18. Dorin RP, Pohl HG, De Filippo RE, Yoo JJ, Atala A. Tubularized urethral replacement with unseeded matrices: what is the maximum distance for normal tissue regeneration? World J Urol. 2008;26(4):323–6.
19. Osman NI, Hillary C, Bullock AJ, MacNeil S, Chapple CR. Tissue engineered buccal mucosa for urethroplasty: progress and future directions. Adv Drug Deliv Rev. 2015;82–83:69–76.
20. Kahveci R, Kahveci Z, Sirmali S, Ozcan M. Urethral reconstruction with autologous vein graft: an experimental study. Br J Plast Surg. 1995;48(7):500–3.
21. Kim BS, Kim HT, Kwon SY, et al. Nontransected ventral onlay-augmented urethroplasty using autologous SVG in a rabbit model of urethral stricture. Urology. 2014;83(1):225–31.
22. Hübner W, Rurka I, Porpaczy P, Miko I. Autologous everted vein graft for repairing long-section urethral defects. Urol Res. 1991;19(2):131–4.
23. Foroutan HR, Khalili A, Geramizadeh B, Rasekhi AR, Tanideh N. Urethral reconstruction using autologous and everted vein graft: an experimental study. Pediatr Surg Int. 2006;22(3):259–62.
24. Jia W, Tang H, Wu J, et al. Urethral tissue regeneration using collagen scaffold modified with collagen binding VEGF in a beagle model. Biomaterials. 2015;69:45–55.
25. Niu Y, Liu G, Chen C, et al. Urethral reconstruction using an amphiphilic tissue-engineered autologous polyurethane nanofiber scaffold with rapid vascularization function. Biomater Sci. 2020;8(8):2164–74.
26. Orabi H, AbouShwareb T, Zhang Y, Yoo JJ, Atala A. Cell-seeded tubularized scaffolds for reconstruction of long urethral defects: a preclinical study. Eur Urol. 2013;63(3):531–8.

20

Effects of irrigation fluid temperature during flexible ureteroscopic holmium laser lithotripsy on postoperative fever and shivering

Yue He[1,2*], You-Gang Feng[1], Jun He[1], Bo Liang[1], Ming-Dong Jiang[1], Jun Liu[1], Yong-Ming Kang[1], Li-Ping Ma[3], Qin Zhang[3], Qi-Jia Peng[3], Tao Yang[1], Yao Liu[3], Li Luo[4] and Min Zhang[4]

Abstract

Background: Flexible ureteroscopic holmium laser lithotripsy is used to treat urinary tract calculi, but postoperative complications include shivering, fever and infection. To investigate the effects of irrigation fluid temperature on postoperative complications.

Methods: This randomized controlled trial included 120 consecutive patients undergoing flexible ureteroscopic holmium laser lithotripsy at the Urology Department, Suining Central Hospital, Sichuan, China between January 2017 and July 2019. Patients were randomized 1:1:1 into three groups (17 °C, 27 °C or 37 °C). Primary outcome was fever incidence (body temperature > 37.5 °C) within 48 h after surgery. Secondary outcomes included shivering incidence during recovery from anesthesia, white blood cell count (WBC), serum procalcitonin (PCT) and incidence of suspected infection (temperature > 38.5 °C and PCT > 0.5 μg/L).

Results: There were 108 patients, (17 °C group, n = 36; 27 °C group, n = 35; 37 °C group, n = 37), received flexible ureteroscopic holmium laser lithotripsy and analyzed. Age, gender distribution, body mass index, ASA grade, stone burden, preoperative creatinine, preoperative core temperature and irrigation fluid volume did not differ significantly between groups. 17 °C, 27 °C and 37 °C groups exhibited significant differences in the incidences of postoperative fever (38.9% vs. 17.1% vs. 13.5%) and shivering (22.2% vs. 5.7% vs. 2.7%) ($p < 0.05$ for all pairwise comparisons). There was no significant difference of WBC, PCT and incidence of suspected infection in 37 °C or 27 °C group compared with 17 °C group. One case each of flash pulmonary edema and bleeding occurred in 37 °C group.

Conclusion: Warming the irrigation fluid can reduce the incidence of postoperative fever and shivering, but further studies are needed to determine the optimal temperature.

Keywords: Irrigation fluid, Temperature, Flexible ureteroscopic holmium laser lithotripsy, Calculi, Holmium: YAG laser

Background

Calculi can develop in the urinary tract when the urine becomes supersaturated with a mineral, leading to the formation of crystals comprised of calcium oxalate, calcium phosphate, uric acid or other substances [1]. The

*Correspondence: 330275636@qq.com
[1] Department of Urology, Suining Central Hospital, No. 127 Desheng W. Rd., Chuanshan District, Suining City 629000, Sichuan Province, People's Republic of China
Full list of author information is available at the end of the article

prevalence of urinary calculi is higher in developed countries than in developing countries and has been estimated to be around 9% in the USA and 4% in China [2]. Factors associated with an increased risk of urinary calculi in adulthood include male gender, obesity and diabetes mellitus [1]. Urinary stones often present acutely with pain, infection or hematuria, necessitating treatment. A variety of medical [3] and surgical [4, 5] therapies are available for the treatment of urinary calculi, including stone fragmentation by lithotripsy [6].

The development of endoscopic technology and lithotripsy techniques for the treatment of urinary calculi has led to traditional open surgery being replaced by endoscopic procedures [7]. Ureteroscopes introduced via the urethra can reach upper urinary tract calculi in the ureter, renal pelvis and calyces, permitting holmium laser lithotripsy to be carried out as a treatment [8]. The latest recommendations of the European Association of Urology, which were published in 2019, recommend flexible ureteroscopic lithotripsy as the first-line surgical treatment option for proximal ureteral/renal calculi with a diameter < 20 mm [9]. However, postoperative complications occur in 2.5–6.7% of patients after ureteroscopic stone treatment [10–13], and fever is the most common postoperative complication of ureteroscopic holmium laser lithotripsy [10, 11, 14–18]. Therefore, there is great interest in identifying methods to reduce the incidence of fever after ureteroscopic holmium laser lithotripsy.

The use of irrigation fluid is essential during transurethral endoscopic surgery. Flexible ureteroscopic lithotripsy is often performed with continuous saline irrigation through the working channel to improve the visibility when an instrument is inserted, particularly during stone dusting or when a small venous bleed occurs. Warming the irrigation fluid has been shown to reduce the incidence of hypothermia and shivering during transurethral resection of the prostate (TURP) [19]. Furthermore, the use of isothermic irrigation fluid can help to maintain normal body temperature and avoid hypothermia during percutaneous nephrolithotripsy (PCNL) [20]. However, the effects of irrigation fluid temperature during flexible ureteroscopic holmium laser lithotripsy on body temperature and the postoperative incidences of shivering, fever, infection and other complications remain unknown.

We hypothesized that increasing the temperature of the irrigation fluid during flexible ureteroscopic holmium laser lithotripsy would reduce the incidence of shivering during recovery from anesthesia and fever during the 2-day period after the procedure. Therefore, the aim of this randomized controlled trial was to investigate the effects of irrigation fluid temperature during flexible ureteroscopic holmium laser lithotripsy on the incidence of short-term postoperative complications including fever and shivering.

Methods

Study design

This was a randomized controlled trial conducted at the Department of Urology, Suining Central Hospital, Sichuan, China between January 2017 and July 2019. The Ethics Committee of Suining Central Hospital, Sichuan Province, P.R. China approved the study. All patients read and understood written information describing the study aims and protocol, and all patients signed consent forms agreeing to participate in this clinical research.

Patients

Participants were enrolled using the following inclusion criteria: (1) age 18–70 years; (2) American Society of Anesthesiologists (ASA) grade I or II [21]; (3) diagnosis of unilateral proximal ureteral calculi and/or renal calculi made by computed tomography (CT); (4) diameters of all calculi were < 20 mm; and (5) total stone burden was < 360 mm2. The exclusion criteria were as follows: (1) thyroid disease or dysautonomia; (2) bilateral upper urinary tract stones scheduled to be treated simultaneously during surgery; (3) preoperative fever; (4) urinary tract infection when included in the trial; (5) hydronephrosis > 3 cm on ultrasound; (6) ureteral stenosis.

Randomization and blinding

Patients were randomized 1:1:1 to 37 °C group, 27 °C group or 17 °C group. The random sequence and grouping sequence were generated using the random function in Excel (Microsoft Corp., Redmond, WA, USA), and the generated random sequence was put into sequentially coded, sealed and opaque envelopes. The envelopes were kept by an investigator (TY) who did not participate in the recruitment of patients, intervention or outcome evaluation. The sealed envelope was brought into the operating room with the patient and opened by the anesthesiologist and nurse who were in charge of setting the temperature of the irrigation fluid during surgery.

Intervention

One week before the procedure, a ureteral stent was placed routinely to dilate the ureter. The irrigation fluid used during surgery was sterile physiological saline. The surgical nurse (MLP, ZQ, PQJ), who was responsible for setting the temperature of the irrigation fluid during the operation, placed the irrigation fluid into a medical incubator with a pre-set temperature (37 °C, 27 °C or 17 °C) 6 h before the procedure. The temperature of the irrigation fluid was 37 °C for patients in 37 °C group, 27 °C for patients in 27 °C group, and 17 °C for patients in 17 °C group. Intravenous fluids were given at room temperature to patients in all three groups.

The procedure was carried out under general anesthesia with the patient in the lithotomy position and covered with a single layer of sterile surgical drape. The operating room temperature was adjusted to 24 °C. The intraoperative core (tympanic) temperature was recorded by the anesthesiologist (ZM, LL) every 10 min until the end of the operation. No heating device was used until the core temperature dropped below 34 °C. All procedures were performed by the same surgical team, which was led by a chief surgeon (HJ, HY, FYG) with previous experience of more than 50 ureteroscopic holmium laser lithotripsy procedures.

The Olympus URF-V electronic flexible ureteroscope were used in the operation. For irrigation, a 3-L bag of sterile 0.9% NaCl solution was suspended 70 cm above the kidney. One end of the infusion tube was connected to the fluid bag, and the other end was connected to the water inlet switch of the flexible ureteroscope. The chief surgeon was able to use the water inlet switch to control the fluid inlet flow. In each case, ureteral access sheath (internal and external size: Fr12 and Fr14) was used. The laser fiber was 200 μm, and the basket was COOK (NGE-017115-UDH-MB). Primary technique was dusting to break up the stones. The laser parameters: pulse energy (1 J), frequency (20 Hz). If the diameter is greater than 3 mm, basket was used. A ureteral stent was placed routinely after surgery, about for one month after treatment. Following completion of the operation, the patient was transferred from the operating room to the post-anesthesia care unit (PACU) and returned to the general ward once fully awake. Routine blood tests, measurement of serum procalcitonin (PCT) and renal function tests were performed 24 h after surgery, and body temperature was recorded. The urinary catheter was removed 24 h after the operation, and the patient was discharged 48 h after surgery in the absence of serious complications.

Clinical data and outcomes

Each patient's age, gender, body mass index (BMI), preoperative serum creatinine level, ASA grade, stone location and stone burden were recorded before the intervention. Postoperative parameters including core body temperature at the end of surgery, occurrence of postoperative shivering, maximum body temperature during the 48 h after the operation, white blood cell (WBC) count, serum PCT level, serum creatinine level and duration of hospitalization were also collected for analysis.

Stone burden was defined as the two-dimensional area determined by multiplying the longest diameter by the perpendicular diameter of the stone [22]. In cases of multiple stones, the total (cumulative) stone burden was calculated as the sum of the burden of each stone. Postoperative fever was defined as any temperature reading above 37.5 °C. The combination of body temperature > 38.5 °C and PCT > 0.5 μg/L was considered as suspected infection, necessitating further investigation and the administration of antibiotics and/or delay of discharge, as necessary.

The primary outcome of this study was the incidence of fever (body temperature > 37.5 °C within 48 h after the operation). The secondary outcomes were the incidence of shivering during recovery from anesthesia, WBC count, serum PCT level, incidence of suspected infection and length of hospital stay. Complications were classified according to the modified Clavien-Dindo grading system [23].

Sample size

Calculation of sample size was done on the basis of the formula $n = \frac{1641.6\lambda}{(\sin^{-1}\sqrt{Pmax}-\sin^{-1}\sqrt{Pmin})^2}$, assuming a statistical power (β) of 90% and an α error of 5%. According to the literature, the incidence of fever following ureteroscopy is less than 5%. Using estimated fever rates of Pmin = 5% and Pmax = 35%, the calculated minimum sample size for each group was n = 38. Assuming a rate of exclusion or loss to follow-up of 5%, the study was designed to include 40 patients in each group.

Statistical analysis

The data were analyzed using SPSS 19.0 (IBM Corp., Armonk, NY, USA). Normally-distributed continuous data are described as mean ± standard deviation and were compared between groups using one-way analysis of variance (ANOVA) and the Bonferroni post-hoc test. Non-normally distributed data are described as median (range) and were compared between groups using the Kruskal Wallis H test. Dunnett's test was used to perform multivariate comparisons between 37 °C group and 27 °C group, 17 °C group, respectively. Qualitative data were analyzed using Pearson's chi squared test or Fisher's exact test with Bonferroni correction for multiple comparisons. A p-value < 0.05 was accepted as statistically significant.

Results

Enrolment of the study participants

Among 120 patients initially randomized to the three study groups, a total of 12 patients were subsequently excluded from the analysis due to refusal to participate in the trial (n = 3), refusal of flexible ureteroscopic holmium laser lithotripsy in favor of extracorporeal shock wave lithotripsy or PCNL (n = 3), duration of surgery > 90 min (n = 2), ureteral stenosis (n = 2) or nonideal positioning or displacement of the ureteral stent (n = 2). Therefore, the final analysis included 37 patients in 37 °C group, 35 patients in 27 °C group and 36 patients in 17 °C group (Fig. 1).

Preoperative clinical characteristics

There were no significant differences between the three groups in age, sex distribution, BMI, stone location, stone burden, ASA grade or preoperative serum creatinine level (Table 1).

Intraoperative characteristics

The volume of intraoperative irrigation fluid used and operation time did not differ significantly between groups (Table 2). Core body temperature declined during surgery in all three groups but tended to decrease most rapidly in 17 °C group and most slowly in 37 °C group (Fig. 2). Although preoperative core body temperature did not differ significantly between groups, core body temperature at the end of surgery was significantly lower in 17 °C group than in 27 °C group or 37 °C group ($p < 0.05$; Table 2).

Primary and secondary outcomes

The incidence of postoperative fever (core body temperature > 37.5 °C during the 48 h after surgery) differed significantly between 37 °C group (5/37, 13.5%), 27 °C group (6/35, 17.1%) and 17 °C group (14/36, 38.9%) ($p < 0.05$ for all pairwise comparisons; Table 2). Similarly, the incidence of postoperative shivering differed significantly between 37 °C group (1/37, 2.7%), 27 °C group (2/35, 5.7%) and 17 °C group (8/36, 22.2%) ($p < 0.05$ for all pairwise comparisons; Table 2).

Postoperatively there were no significant differences between groups in the incidence of suspected infection (core body temperature > 38.5 °C and PCT > 0.5 μg/L), WBC count, PCT level or creatinine level, duration of hospital stays (Table 2).

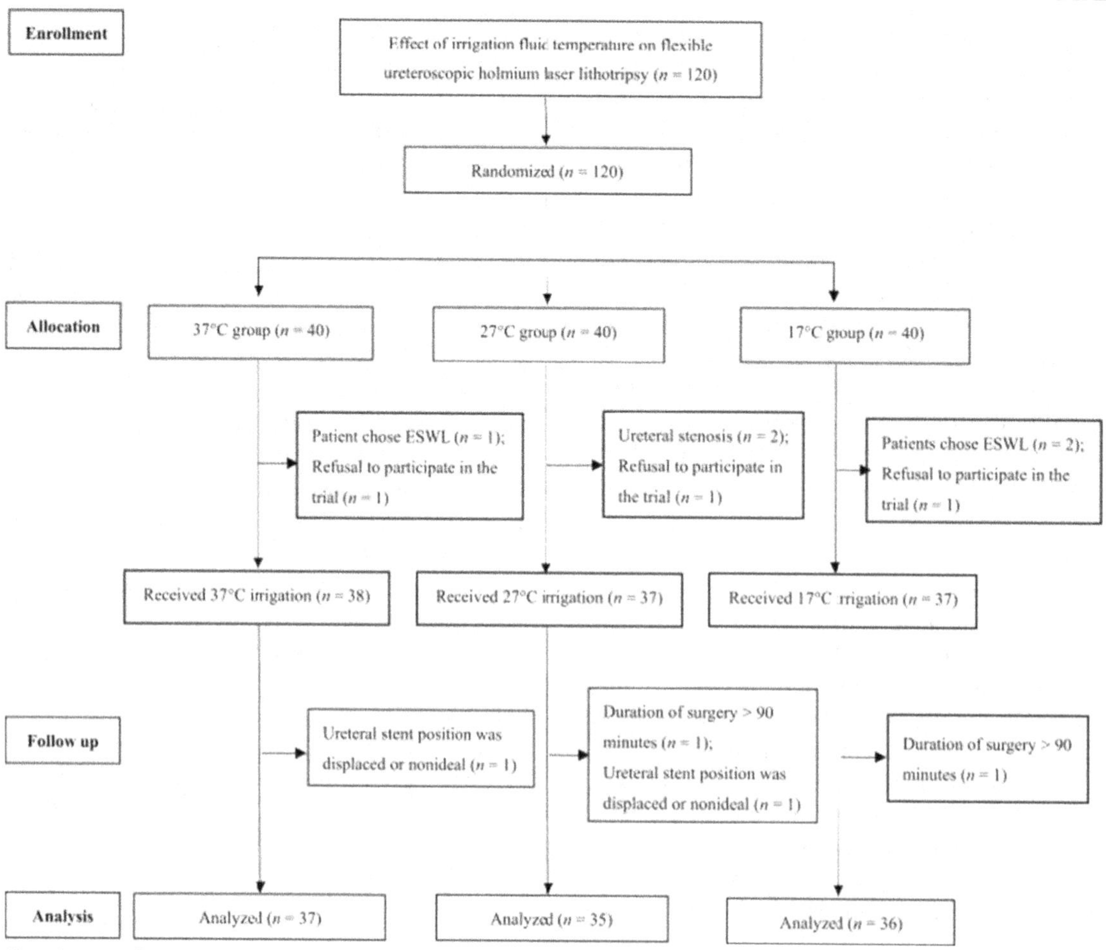

Fig. 1 Flow-diagram of the trial

Table 1 Preoperative clinical characteristics of the study participants

	37 °C (*n* = 37)	27 °C (*n* = 35)	17 °C (*n* = 36)	*p*
Male, n (%)	20 (54.1%)	16 (45.7%)	19 (52.8%)	0.750
Female, n (%)	17 (45.9%)	19 (54.3%)	17 (47.2%)	
Age (years)	42.8 ± 12.3	44.9 ± 13.1	44.3 ± 11.7	0.758
Body mass index (kg/m^2)	24.11 ± 2.88	24.17 ± 2.69	24.26 ± 3.02	0.973
Preoperative creatinine (μ mol/L)	93.0 ± 19.0	92.6 ± 20.0	94.1 ± 18.6	0.942
ASA grade, n (%)				
I	23 (62.2%)	21 (60.0%)	20 (55.6%)	0.843
II	14 (37.8%)	14 (40.0%)	16 (44.4%)	
Stone location, n (%)				
Kidney	9 (24.3%)	7 (20.0%)	11 (30.6%)	0.830
Ureter	9 (24.3%)	8 (22.9%)	6 (16.7%)	
Kidney and ureter	19 (51.4%)	20 (57.1%)	19 (52.7%)	
Stone burden (mm^2)	109 (40–266)	123 (48–304)	140 (45–266)	0.670

Data are presented as n (%), mean ± standard deviation or median (range). ASA, American Society of Anesthesiologists

Table 2 Perioperative and postoperative characteristics

	37 °C (*n* = 37)	27 °C (*n* = 35)	17 °C (*n* = 36)	*p*
Irrigation fluid volume (L)	1.58 ± 0.47	1.69 ± 0.51	1.77 ± 0.56	0.274
Operative time (min)	59.5 ± 14.2	60.7 ± 15.3	63.1 ± 14.6	0.573
Core temperature at start of surgery (°C)	36.59 ± 0.27	36.56 ± 0.25	36.59 ± 0.29	0.858
Core temperature at end of surgery (°C)	35.91 ± 0.36*	35.56 ± 0.32*	35.24 ± 0.36	< 0.001
Shivering during resuscitation from anesthesia	1 (2.7%)*$^{\Delta}$	2 (5.7%)*	8 (22.2%)	0.023
Postoperative creatinine (μmol/L)	96.0 ± 19.7	94.0 ± 20.6	97.0 ± 19.5	0.815
Maximum T (°C)	37.2 (36.6–39.6)*$^{\Delta}$	37.4 (36.9–39.7)	37.45 (36.9–40.0)	0.028
White blood cell count (× 10^9/L)	9.20 ± 2.58	9.43 ± 2.16	10.20 ± 2.43	0.175
Serum procalcitonin (ng/mL)	0.15 (0.03–0.60)	0.15 (0.05–0.95)	0.15 (0.05–0.97)	0.625
Fever	5 (13.5%)*$^{\Delta}$	6 (17.1%)*	14 (38.9%)	0.022
Suspected infection[a]	3 (8.1%)	2 (5.7%)	5 (13.9%)	0.505
Median hospital stays (days)	3 (3–7)	3 (3–7)	3 (3–7)	0.060

Data are presented as n (%), mean ± standard deviation or median (range). T, temperature

* $p < 0.05$ versus 17 °C group; Δ $p < 0.05$ versus 27 °C group

[a] Suspected infection was defined as core body temperature > 38.5 °C and serum procalcitonin level > 0.5 μg/L

Other complications

There was one case of flash pulmonary edema (the patient recovered and was discharged after medical therapy) and one case of postoperative hemorrhage (which stopped 3 days after placement of a three-cavity catheter for bladder irrigation) in 37 °C group. There was one case of urinary retention (the catheter was successfully removed after 1 week) in 37 °C group and one case of ureteral abrasion (the ureteral stent was removed two months later) in 17 °C group. There were no adverse events above grade III (Clavien-Dindo grading system) in this study.

Discussion

Important findings of the present study were that the incidences of postoperative fever and shivering decreased significantly as the temperature of the irrigation fluid was increased from 17 to 37 °C. Postoperative WBC count, serum PCT level and incidence of suspected infection were comparable between groups. Although there was one case of flash pulmonary edema and one case of bleeding in 37 °C group, both complications resolved after therapy. Our novel findings suggest that isothermic irrigation during flexible ureteroscopic holmium laser lithotripsy can reduce the incidence of postoperative fever and shivering. However, further studies are

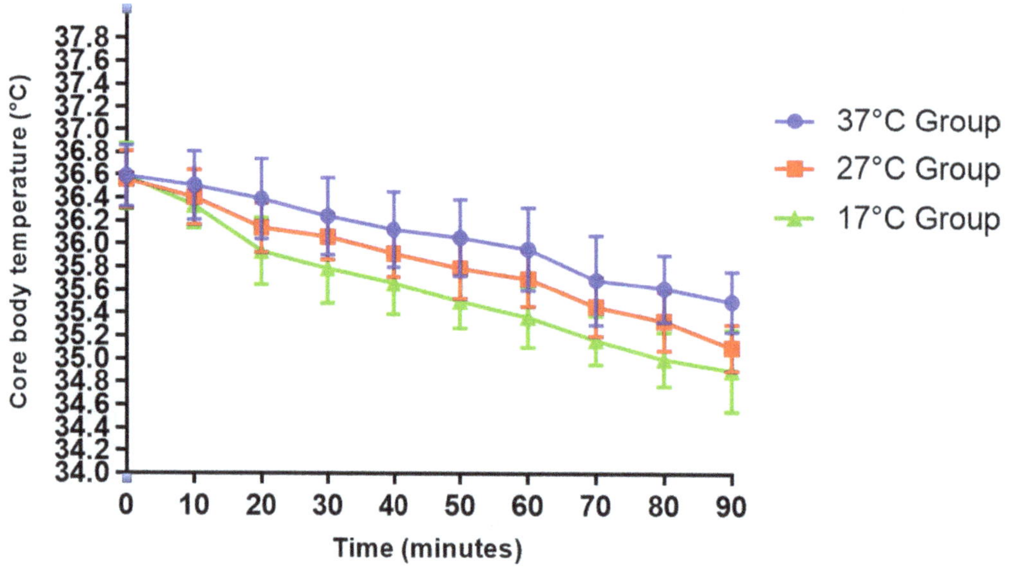

Fig. 2 Intraoperative core body temperature for patients in the three groups

required to establish the optimal temperature for the irrigation fluid.

There are many potential causes of fever after ureteroscopic holmium laser lithotripsy, including ureteral obstruction by stone fragments, urinary tract infection, intraoperative backflow and extravasation of urine due to prolonged high-pressure irrigation, intraoperative and postoperative bleeding, and postoperative backflow of urine in the bladder and ureter due to poor drainage via the catheter [24]. Furthermore, hypothermia and shivering can occur due to the large amounts of intravenous and irrigation fluids administered during surgery and anesthesia [25], particularly given that a substantial amount of irrigation fluid is absorbed by the patient [26, 27]. The present study investigated the effects of varying the temperature of the irrigation fluid on core body temperature during surgery and the incidence of postoperative fever while minimizing the influence of possible confounding factors. For example, all procedures were performed by the same experienced surgical team, irrigation fluid pressure was standardized and maintained below 40 mmHg by suspending the liquid bag at the same height, and patients with preoperative urinary tract infection or postoperative ureteral stent displacement were excluded from the analysis.

In this study, core body temperature at the end of the procedure was significantly lower in 17 °C group than in the other two groups, indicating that the use of irrigation fluid at the lower temperature (17 °C) contributed to the fall in body temperature during surgery. By contrast, core body temperature at the end of the operation did not differ significantly between 37 °C group and 27 °C group, indicating that additional heating of the irrigation fluid from 27 to 37 °C was not beneficial for maintaining body temperature during surgery. This may have been due to the energy generated by the holmium laser during the operation, which increased the local temperature and heated the irrigation fluid [28].

The main finding of this study was that the incidence of postoperative fever (core body temperature > 37.5 °C during the 48 h after surgery) was significantly lower in 27 °C group than in 17 °C group and significantly lower in 37 °C group than in both the other groups. However, there were no significant differences between the three groups in the postoperative WBC count, serum PCT level or incidence of suspected infection (core body temperature > 38.5 °C and PCT > 0.5 μg/L) [29]. The above results suggest that the differences in the incidences of fever between groups were not due to differences in the incidences of infection, further implying that the temperature of the irrigation fluid has little influence on the incidence of postoperative urinary tract infection. The use of hypothermic irrigation fluid can cause intraoperative hypothermia, and the risk of postoperative shivering is increased when core body temperature drops below 36 °C [30]. A recent meta-analysis of 28 randomized controlled trials found that the fall in body temperature during surgical treatment of benign prostatic hypertrophy and the incidence of postoperative shivering were lower for warm irrigation fluid than for room-temperature irrigation fluid [19]. Therefore, our findings are in good agreement with the results of the above meta-analysis [19] and with other studies evaluating the effects of irrigation fluid temperature on body temperature [31, 32]. Our observation that the incidence of postoperative fever increased as the irrigation fluid temperature was decreased (from 37 to 17 °C) might be explained by a compensatory reaction of the body to hypothermia at the end of surgery, with the shivering mechanism possibly contributing to this.

The incidence of postoperative fever in this study was relatively high in comparison to that reported by previous studies, ranging from 13.5 to 38.9%. This may have been due to the wide definition of fever used in this study, since the patient was classified as having fever even if only one temperature reading was above 37.5 °C during the 48 h after surgery. Ten patients (9.2%) had a postoperative body temperature higher than 38.5 °C after the operation: 5 of these patients improved after symptomatic treatment without the use of antibiotics, and the remaining 5 patients were diagnosed with urinary tract infection. The incidence of urinary tract infection in our study (4.6%) was higher than rates of 1–1.8% reported in the literature [10, 11], and we speculate that there may be three reasons for this. First, our study had a small sample size. Second, stone burden was larger in our study than in the previous studies, which may have resulted in more bacteria being released from the stone during the process of laser lithotripsy. Third, our study included more cases with renal calculi, whereas the prior studies mainly included patients with ureteral calculi.

There was one case of flash pulmonary edema in 37 °C group. It has been reported that elevating the temperature of the irrigation fluid increases the amount that is absorbed by the body [26]. Therefore, for the same irrigation pressure and duration of surgery, it would be expected that patients in 37 °C group would have absorbed a greater volume of fluid than patients in the other groups. As a result, high-temperature irrigation fluid is more likely to cause volume overload and lead to pulmonary edema than low-temperature irrigation fluid, especially in elderly patients. However, the risk of irrigation fluid absorption during flexible ureteroscopy is lower than that during TURP or PCNL because flexible ureteroscopy causes far less tissue injury than TURP and uses a smaller perfusion pressure than PCNL [27]. However, there remains a risk of increased fluid absorption for warmed irrigation fluid, which needs further study. Therefore, decisions as to whether or not to warm the irrigation fluid and the degree of warming necessitate full consideration of factors such as the predicted duration of surgery and cardiovascular risk of the patient, among others.

In addition, there was one case of postoperative bleeding in 37 °C group, but the bleeding stopped after irrigation for 24 h using a three-cavity catheter. By contrast, there were no cases of bleeding in the other two groups, raising the possibility that warming the irrigation fluid might increase the risk of bleeding. Cao et al. reported that the amount of blood lost during TURP did not differ significantly between warmed and room-temperature irrigation fluid [19]. However, Kati et al. found that the amount of blood loss during PCNL was significantly lower for patients irrigated with fluid at room temperature [20]. It will be necessary to further study the effects of irrigation fluid temperature on bleeding risk. Although the risk of bleeding is very low for most patients undergoing flexible ureteroscopy, it is higher for patients with coagulation dysfunction or on long-term oral anticoagulants.

One limitation of this study is that there was no calculation of the amount of irrigation fluid absorbed, although it should be noted that the methods used for this are not always very accurate [27]. In addition, patient comfort was not evaluated in our study.

Conclusion

The use of heated irrigation fluid during flexible ureteroscopic lithotripsy can reduce the incidences of postoperative fever and shivering. However, further research is needed to establish the optimal temperature of the irrigation fluid while taking into account local heating effects caused by laser lithotripsy. In addition, decision-making regarding the temperature of the irrigation fluid should also take into consideration the cardiovascular risk of the individual patient and the predicted duration of surgery so as to avoid excessive absorption of irrigation fluid during the operation.

Abbreviations

ASA: American Society of Anesthesiologists; CT: Computed tomography; ESWL: Extracorporeal shock wave lithotripsy; PCNL: Percutaneous nephrolithotomy; PCT: Serum procalcitonin; TURP: Transurethral resection of the prostate; WBC: White blood cell count.

Acknowledgements

We thank the patients and their caregivers for participating in this trial.

Authors' contributions

Study Concept and Design: YH, YGF; Acquisition of Data: LL, MZ, LPM, QJP, QZ; Analysis data: YH, BL, JL; Drafting of the manuscript: YH, MDJ; Substantively revised the work: YH, YMK, YGF, JH, TY, YL. All authors have read and approved the manuscript.

Author details

[1]Department of Urology, Suining Central Hospital, No. 127 Desheng W. Rd., Chuanshan District, Suining City 629000, Sichuan Province, People's Republic of China. [2]Department of Urology, Institute of Urology, West China Hospital, Sichuan University, No. 37 Guoxue Alley, Wuhou District, Chengdu City 610041, Sichuan Province, People's Republic of China. [3]Operation Room, Suining Central Hospital, No. 127 Desheng W. Rd., Chuanshan District, Suining City 629000, Sichuan Province, People's Republic of China. [4]Department of Anesthesiology, Suining Central Hospital, No. 127 Desheng W. Rd., Chuanshan District, Suining City 629000, Sichuan Province, People's Republic of China.

References

1. Khan SR, Pearle MS, Robertson WG, et al. Kidney stones. Nat Rev Dis Primers. 2016;2:16008.
2. Alatab S, Pourmand G, El Howairis MF, et al. National profiles of urinary calculi: a comparison between developing and developed worlds. Iran J Kidney Dis. 2016;10(2):51–61.
3. Skolarikos A. Medical treatment of urinary stones. Curr Opin Urol. 2018;28(5):403–7.
4. Assimos D, Krambeck A, Miller NL, et al. Surgical management of stones: American Urological Association/Endourological Society Guideline. PART I J Urol. 2016;196(4):1153–60.
5. Assimos D, Krambeck A, Miller NL, et al. Surgical management of stones: american urological association/endourological society guideline, PART II. J Urol. 2016;196(4):1161–9.
6. Large T, Krambeck AE. Emerging technologies in lithotripsy. Urol Clin North Am. 2019;46(2):215–23.
7. Li JK, Teoh JY, Ng CF. Updates in endourological management of urolithiasis. Int J Urol. 2019;26(2):172–83.
8. Aldoukhi AH, Roberts WW, Hall TL, Ghani KR. Holmium laser lithotripsy in the new stone age: dust or bust? Front Surg. 2017;4:57.
9. Türk C, Skolarikos A, Neisius A, et al. EAU Guidelines on Urolithiasis. https://uroweb.org/guideline/urolithiasis. Accessed Jan 2019.
10. Perez EC, Osther PJS, Jinga V, et al. Differences in ureteroscopic stone treatment and outcomes for distal, mid-, proximal, or multiple ureteral locations: the Clinical Research Office of the Endourological Society ureteroscopy global study. Eur Urol. 2014;66(1):102–9.
11. Rosette JDL, Denstedt J, Geavlete P, et al. The clinical research office of the endourological society ureteroscopy global study: indications, complications, and outcomes in 11,885 patients. J Endourol. 2014;28(2):131–9.
12. Xu C, Song RJ, Jiang MJ, Qin C, Wang XL, Zhang W. Flexible ureteroscopy with holmium laser lithotripsy: a new choice for intrarenal stone patients. Urol Int. 2015;94(1):93–8.
13. Hyams ES, Munver R, Bird VG, Uberoi J, Shah O. Flexible ureterorenoscopy and holmium laser lithotripsy for the management of renal stone burdens that measure 2 to 3 cm: a multi-institutional experience. J Endourol. 2010;24(10):1583–8.
14. Cohen J, Cohen S, Grasso M. Ureteropyeloscopic treatment of large, complex intrarenal and proximal ureteral calculi. BJU Int. 2013;111(3 Pt B):E127–31.
15. Ma K, Huang XB, Xiong LL, et al. Beijing Da Xue Xue Bao Yi Xue Ban 2015;47(4):615–7
16. Takazawa R, Kitayama S, Tsujii T. Successful outcome of flexible ureteroscopy with holmium laser lithotripsy for renal stones 2 cm or greater. Int J Urol. 2012;19(3):264–7.
17. Ulker V, Cakmak O, Yucel C, Can E, Celik O, Ilbey YO. The efficacy and safety of bilateral same-session ureteroscopy with holmium laser lithotripsy in the treatment of bilateral ureteral stones. Minerva Urol Nefrol. 2019;71(2):174–80.
18. Zhang H, Hong TY, Li G, et al. Comparison of the Efficacy of ultra-mini PCNL, flexible ureteroscopy, and shock wave lithotripsy on the treatment of 1–2 cm lower pole renal calculi. Urol Int. 2019;102(2):153–9.
19. Cao J, Sheng X, Ding Y, et al. Effect of warm bladder irrigation fluid for benign prostatic hyperplasia patients on perioperative hypothermia, blood loss and shiver: a meta-analysis. Asian J Urol. 2019;6(2):183–91.
20. Kati B, Buyukfirat E, Pelit ES, et al. Percutaneous nephrolithotomy with different temperature irrigation and effects on surgical complications and anesthesiology applications. J Endourol. 2018;32(11):1050–3.
21. Doyle DJ, Garmon EH. American Society of Anesthesiologists Classification (ASA Class). In: StatPearls. Treasure Island (FL): StatPearls Publishing; 2020.
22. Lee SH, Kim TH, Myung SC, et al. Effectiveness of flexible ureteroscopic stone removal for treating ureteral and ipsilateral renal stones: a single-center experience. Korean J Urol. 2013;54(6):377–82.
23. Dindo D, Demartines N, Clavien PA. Classification of surgical complications: a new proposal with evaluation in a cohort of 6336 patients and results of a survey. Ann Surg. 2004;240(2):205–13.
24. Doizi S, Traxer O. Flexible ureteroscopy: technique, tips and tricks. Urolithiasis. 2018;46(1):47–58.
25. Singh R, Asthana V, Sharma JP, Lal S. Effect of irrigation fluid temperature on core temperature and hemodynamic changes in transurethral resection of prostate under spinal anesthesia. Anesth Essays Res. 2014;8(2):209–15.
26. de Freitas FM, Andrade CM Jr, de Mello MJ, et al. Effect of temperature on fluidity of irrigation fluids. Br J Anaesth. 2011;106(1):51–6.
27. Guzelburc V, Balasar M, Colakogullari M, et al. Comparison of absorbed irrigation fluid volumes during retrograde intrarenal surgery and percutaneous nephrolithotomy for the treatment of kidney stones larger than 2 cm. Springerplus. 2016;5(1):1707.
28. Aldoukhi AH, Hall TL, Ghani KR, et al. Caliceal fluid temperature during high-power holmium laser lithotripsy in an in vivo porcine model. J Endourol. 2018;32(8):724–9.
29. Miglietta F, Faneschi ML, Lobreglio G, et al. Procalcitonin, C-reactive protein and serum lactate dehydrogenase in the diagnosis of bacterial sepsis. SIRS and systemic candidiasis Infez Med. 2015;23(3):230–7.
30. Kim HY, Lee KC, Lee MJ, et al. Comparison of the efficacy of a forced-air warming system and circulating-water mattress on core temperature and post-anesthesia shivering in elderly patients undergoing total knee arthroplasty under spinal anesthesia. Korean J Anesthesiol. 2014;66(5):352–7.
31. Canturk M, Hakki M, Kocaoglu N. Effects of isothermic irrigation on core body temperature during endoscopic urethral stone treatment surgery under spinal anesthesia: a randomized controlled trial. Urol J. 2020;17(1):1–7.
32. Okeke LI. Effect of warm intravenous and irrigating fluids on body temperature during transurethral resection of the prostate gland. BMC Urol. 2007;7:15.

21

Comparative study of renal drainage with different ureteral stents subject to extrinsic ureteral obstruction using an in vitro ureter-stent model

Yaniv Shilo[1], Jonathan Modai[1], Dan Leibovici[1], Ishai Dror[2] and Brian Berkowitz[2*]

Abstract

Background: To compare the efficacy of different ureteral stents subject to extrinsic ureteral obstruction (EUO), in a controlled in vitro stented ureter experiment.

Methods: We employ an in vitro ureter-stent experimental set-up, with latex tubing simulating flexible ureters attached to vessels simulating renal units and bladders. The flow behavior of five ureteral stents—polymeric 8F, tandem 6F, tandem 7F, endopyelotomy and metal—was tested under a ureteral deformation configuration of 40°, with 2000 g external force over a 3.5 cm length of the ureter. A constant fluid flow was applied through the ureter-stent configurations, and pressure fluctuations in the renal unit were monitored. We considered a renal unit pressure of 10 cmH_2O or flow discontinuation in the bladder as stent failure. Urine containing debris was mimicked by use of a colloidal solution.

Results: Of all assessed ureteral stents, under EUO conditions, only the single 8F stents remained patent throughout the length of the experiment. All other stents—tandem 6F and 7F, single 7F, metal and endopyelotomy—displayed limitations.

Conclusions: Tandem and metal stents show no superiority over large luminal polymeric stents for EUO treatment in this in vitro model. Larger luminal stents offer excellent resistance to external pressure and allow adequate colloidal flow. The need for frequent exchange and bladder irritation should also be considered in the choice of stent configuration for treatment of kidney drainage under EUO.

Keywords: Tandem stents, Metal stents, Endopyelotomy, Stent failure, Colloids

Background

Extrinsic ureteral obstruction (EUO) is a common situation that may be related to different etiologies. EUO is often due to pelvic malignancy—either primary tumor or metastatic disease—while other causes are due to benign etiologies that include ovarian cysts, retroperitoneal fibrosis, benign pelvic masses, surgical complications, and possibly radiation damage [1–3]. As such, patients suffering from EUO usually have poor prognosis and short life expectancy. The main complication of EUO is renal failure due to ureteral obstruction, leading to hydronephrosis; drainage of the relevant kidney with either ureteral stent or nephrostomy tube is imperative.

Double-J ureteral stents generally represent a more appealing drainage option, as nephrostomy tubes carry

*Correspondence: brian.berkowitz@weizmann.ac.il
[2] Department of Earth and Planetary Sciences, Weizmann Institute of Science, 7610001 Rehovot, Israel
Full list of author information is available at the end of the article

the inconvenience of an external urine bag. However, as many as ~ 50% of ureteral stents placed to treat EUO fail (in terms of drainage, leading to renal failure and hydronephrosis), often within weeks [1]. While the exact mechanism(s) for stent failure is unclear, large caliber [2, 3], tandem [4–9] and metal [10–17] stent designs have been suggested to overcome this problem. Several studies—mostly retrospective—have compared the success rates of different stents under EUO, but to date, no clear conclusion defining the stent(s) that offer(s) the best outcome can be drawn.

Here, we examined potential differences in behavior and the likelihood of stent failure among large diameter (8F) and tandem (6F, 7F) polymeric stents, a metal stent, and a polymeric endopyelotomy stent (7F/14F). We employed an in vitro experimental setup [18] to investigate the influence of both ureteral deformation and compression, and the synergistic effect of colloid presence in the fluid, on stent patency.

Materials and methods

In vitro stent-ureter-kidney model

We employed an in vitro ureter-stent experimental setup described in detail elsewhere [18]. Briefly, we used natural latex tubing (inner diameter 4.76 mm, wall thickness 0.79 mm) to simulate flexible ureters attached to glass vessels representing renal units and bladders, and examined flow behavior in ureteral stents. The experimental set-up (single-unit) is shown schematically in Fig. 1; the laboratory system enabled simultaneous running of 12 stent units, housed within a temperature-controlled chamber (37 °C). The ureter-stent configuration simulated external ureteral pressure causing ureteral deformation to $\theta = 40°$ (Fig. 1). EUO was simulated by semi-circular compression of length ~ 3.5 cm located in the region of maximum deformation; the ureter/stent configuration provided an applied force of 2000 g (≈ 19.6 N). In the context of the colloidal fluid experiments considered here, and given our findings ([18] and below) that stent failure is due to colloid accumulation particularly in the region of compression, the EUO location along the ureter (more proximally or distally) is not significant. This was confirmed by a preliminary experiment (not shown), and supported by computational fluid dynamics simulations [19]. Further discussion justifying the choice of materials and applied force appears in the Additional file 1.

Each ureter-stent unit contained double-J stents—either a single 8F stent, tandem (pairs of) 6F or 7F stents (Boston Scientific® Percuflex Plus), a single Resonance® metallic stent (6F, Cook Medical), or a single 7F/14F endopyelotomy stent (Boston Scientific, Retromax Plus).

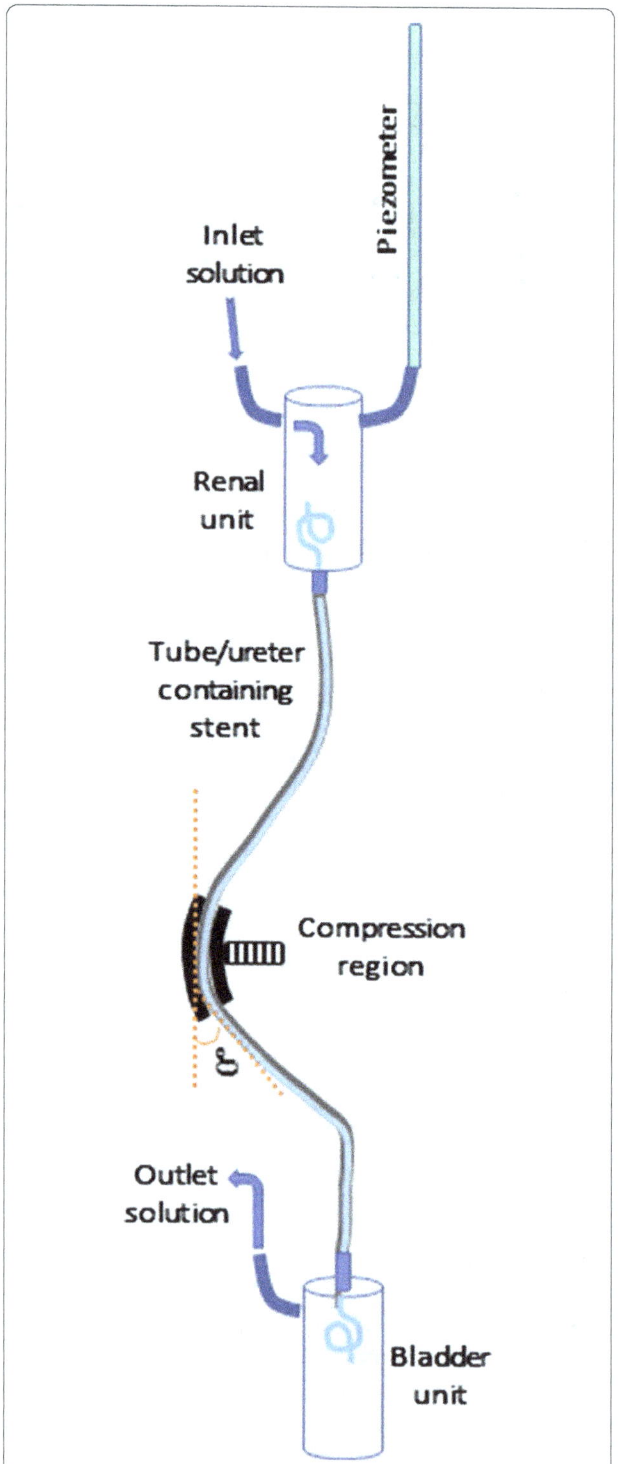

Fig. 1 Schematic showing the experimental setup, with details of a single ureter-stent unit, including of the angle of deformation, $\theta°$

An example of four such ureter-stent units is shown in Fig. 2.

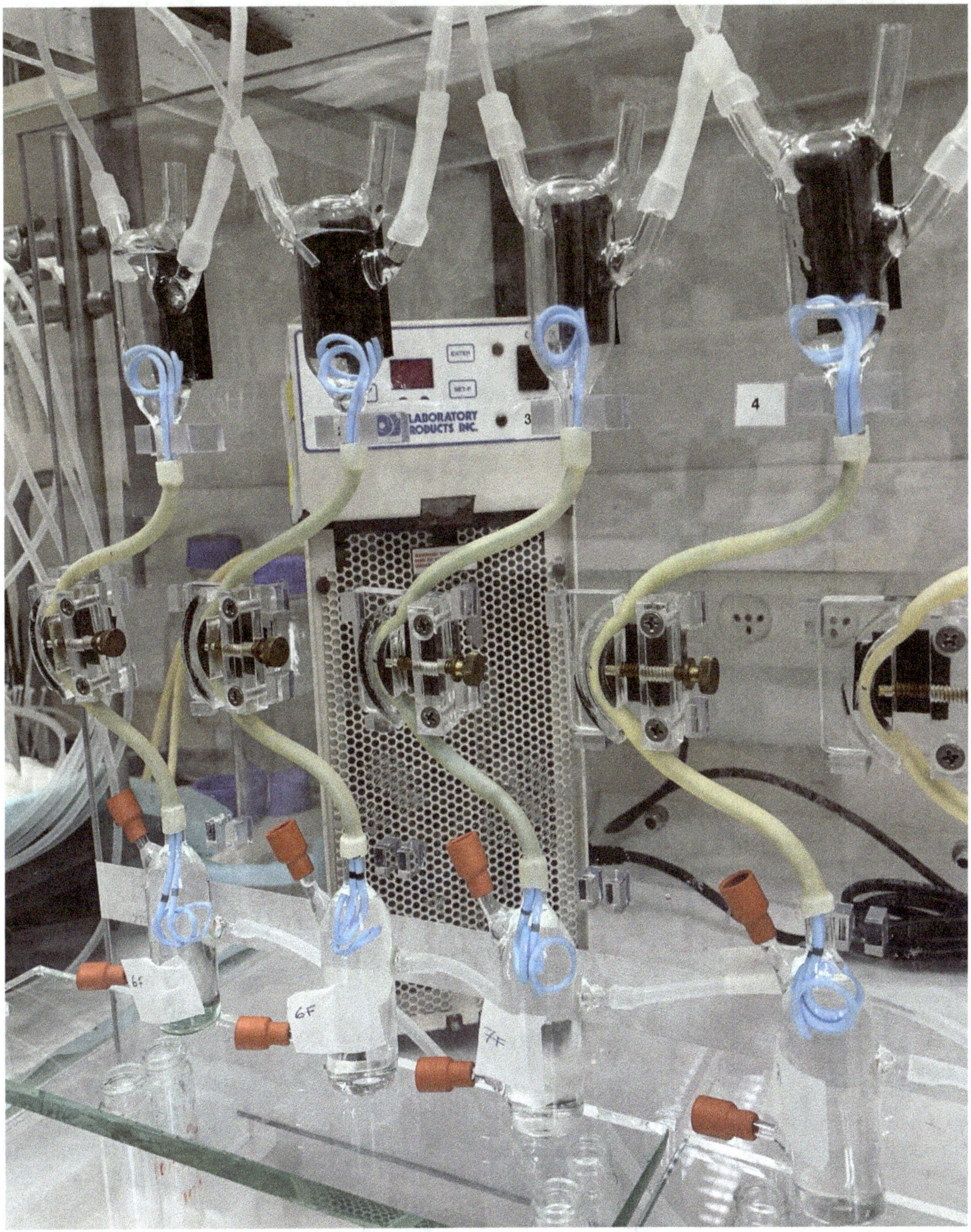

Fig. 2 Photograph of part of the 12-unit experimental systems, showing two tandem 6F and two tandem 7F stent-ureter units, under deformation and compression

In each ureter-stent unit, the proximal and distal pigtails were inserted into renal unit and bladder vessels, respectively. For the endopyelotomy stent, the 14F section was placed at the distal side, with compression acting over part of this region. A constant flow rate was prescribed in each of the 12 units, via a 12-channel peristaltic pump (Ismatec® Model-IPC12-Channel pump); the fluid volume in the renal unit vessel damped small pressure fluctuations induced by the pump. In all experiments, the volumetric flow rate in each renal unit was set

Table 1 Time to stent failure (blockage), in hours, under deformation of 40° and compression of 2000 g in the region of the external ureteral obstruction

Replicate	Stent				
	Tandem 6F (time to blockage, hour)	Tandem 7F (time to blockage, hour)	Resonance® (time to blockage, hour)	Endopyelotomy 14F (time to blockage, hour)	8F† (time to blockage, hour)
1	132	133.5	243.5	300.5	–‡
2	274	103	124.5	235.5	–‡
3	325	329	224		
4	–‡	303.5	–‡		

Entries with "–" indicate no failure. All failure times are rounded to the nearest half hour

† The same result (no blockage) for 4 similar replicates with the 8F stent was reported in [18]

‡ Experiment duration of 348 h

at 30 mL/h, with maximum deviation at the system outlet of 1%; this flow rate is within the general range of flow rates, 25–50 mL/h [20]. Fluid pressure in each renal unit was monitored with a piezometer.

Flow experiments and colloid solution

Fluid flow (saline solution; 9 g NaCl/1 L double distilled water) in each of the five stent configurations (8F, tandem 6F, tandem 7F, Resonance®, endopyelotomy) was first tested over a range of compressive forces up to 2000 g, following tests for single stents [18] (see Additional file 1), to confirm that deformation and pressure do not lead to stent failure. Subsequently, as in Shilo et al. [18], we employed a colloidal solution containing chicken albumin from egg white powder (see Additional file 1).

Here, two sets of (12 ureter-stent unit) experiments (348 h duration; determined by the experimental results presented below) were completed with stented ureters under deformation and compression, together with the colloidal solution. In total, experiments comprised (i) four replicates each of the tandem 6F, tandem 7F and Resonance® stents, (ii) two replicates each of the endopyelotomy (tested for "completeness", though of less clinical interest) and 8F stents (in addition to 4 similar replicates with the 8F stent reported in Shilo et al. [18]), and (iii) two replicates each of the control ureter-stent units, with tandem 6F, tandem 7F, Resonance® and 8F stents, with no deformation or compression. Throughout the experiments, fluid heights in the piezometers varied at ± 1 mm (± 0.1 cmH_2O) due to the action of the peristaltic pump. Fluid heights in each piezometer were monitored over time for stent failure, which was defined as renal unit pressure reaching 10 cm/H_2O (and ultimately complete obstruction of fluid flow).

Results

We showed previously [18, 21] that deformation/compression alone, using a solution without colloids, are not generally sufficient to lead to stent failure under EUO, in tests with 4.8F, 6F, 7F and 8F stents. In particular, we confirmed [18] that the 8F stent shows no decrease in flow (or increase in renal pressure) up to 5000 g compression. In the current experiments, we found, too, in preliminary measurements, that like the single 8F stent, the tandem 6F and 7F stents, the Resonance® metallic stent, and the 7F/14F endopyelotomy stent are similarly unaffected by realistic deformation/compression.

Results of the experiments with the colloidal suspension are summarized in Table 1, with all units, except the controls, kept under deformation/compression. Notably, all control units for the (unperturbed) stented ureters—tandem 6F, tandem 7F, Resonance®, 8F stents—remained open.

The 8F stented ureter was the only system to remain open in all cases. Results for the four replicates of the 8F stent system tested previously [18], using a slightly smaller diameter ureter tube, are relevant here because *in the vicinity of the EUO*, the stent lumen, not the ureter lumen, essentially controls flow; urine flowing within the ureter is likely diverted through the stent, via side holes, to bypass the region of compression (see Additional file 1). Thus, total ureter-stent blockage and pressure buildup are controlled, *ultimately*, by the stent lumen.

From Table 1, the endopyelotomy and tandem 7F stents failed in all replicates, with average times of 268 h (235.5, 300.5 h) and 217 h (103, 133.5, 303.5, 329 h), respectively. The tandem 6F stents failed in three replicates at an average time of 244 h (132, 274, 325 h); one replicate continued to drain freely. Similarly, the Resonance® stents failed in three replicates at an average time of 197 h (124.5, 224, 243.5 h) and one replicate continued to drain. Throughout the experiments, small rises (up to 1–1.5 cm) —and then falls— were observed in many piezometers, including in the control units. The Resonance® and tandem 6F and 7F stents exhibited even broader pressure rises and falls, with some units rising once or twice up to 6 cm before then falling. This behavior was evidently a result of colloid accumulation leading to partial clogging and pressure build-up, and then break-up and release and/or rearrangement of (some of) the accumulated colloids in the stented ureter system (see Discussion below). Once pressure rose above ~ 6 cm, it never decreased and generally continued to rise quickly to > 10 cm.

Discussion

EUO prevalence is growing steadily and continues to be a major treatment challenge for the urologist [3]. Different stent types and configurations have been reported in an effort to adequately drain kidneys and prevent complications. Over recent years, tandem ureteral stents [4–9], metal stents [10–15] or metal-mesh stents [16, 17] have been advocated as the preferred drainage method under EUO. However, few "head-to-head" studies comparing all of these options are available, which can be attributed to limitations that include relatively low numbers of patients with EUO that can be recruited at a single center, different etiologies responsible for EUO, and differences in ideal stent preferences between medical centers. We present here the first comparison of a wide variety of different ureteral stents subjected to EUO in an in vitro model of a stented ureter. Our experiments indicate that neither tandem ureteral stents nor metal stents offer any clear advantage over large luminal polymeric stents in preventing stent failure, although they appear more effective than single, small luminal polymeric stents (comparing failure times to those reported in [18]). In addition, endopyelotomy stents show no superiority over large luminal polymeric stents under EUO conditions of deformation, external ureteral compression and fluids containing colloids.

In a retrospective study, Askawa et al. [13] compared polymeric stents to Resonance® stents in patients with EUO. A total of 54 ureters in 35 patients were drained with polymeric stents, and 72 ureters in 57 patients were treated with Resonance® stents. Overall stent patency for both groups was 70%, while Resonance® stents showed higher patency rates when compared to polymeric stents after one year of follow-up (78% vs. 61%). This difference did not reach statistical significance in multivariate analysis. The authors [13] concluded that the Resonance® stent is superior to polymeric stents as it better resists external compression forces, so that it should be the first choice to drain EUO. Another comparative study by Liu et al. [7] evaluated prospectively, in a non-randomized fashion, 104 patients with EUO using single or tandem 7F polymeric stents based on patient preference. Stent patency duration among 63 renal units drained with tandem stents was 214 days, in comparison to 176 days among 94 patients with single stents. The authors concluded that tandem polymeric stents are superior to single stents.

These authors [7, 13] suggested that a key etiology responsible for stent failure under EUO is external compression forces exerted over the ureter, resulting in deformation, kinking and closure of the stent and ureter lumina. While it may be intuitive to expect that polymeric stents show poor resistance to external ureteral pressure, we showed previously [18, 21] that this is not the case via in vitro experiments. Polymeric stents (4.8F to 8F) were subjected to both ureteral deformation and increasing external forces (compression) of up to 5000 g; the 4.8F stent failed at high compression, while the 6F, 7F and 8F stents remained patent throughout. We concluded [18, 21] that only unrealistic external pressure forces may lead to stent obstruction and therefore external pressure/deformation as sole etiology for stent failure is less reasonable. Two biases should be noted in the two above-mentioned studies [7, 13] comparing polymeric stents to either tandem or metal stents. First, the luminal size of the polymeric stents that were compared to the Resonance® stent was not mentioned; use of a relatively small luminal size might have influenced the results. Second, the tandem and single stents in the comparative study [7] were all 7F. Clearly, the likelihood for a stent to remain patent is higher when comparing two stents of the same size in one ureter to a different ureter drained with only one stent of the same size. A valuable comparison would have been between 7F tandem stents and a single 8F polymeric stent.

In the current experiment, only the 8F stent remained patent consistently throughout the experiment duration, while all other stent configurations—tandem 6F and 7F, Resonance®, endopyelotomy—generally failed. The exact mechanism in which ureteral stents fail under EUO is unclear, although several possible risk factors have been suggested [2, 7], including stent incrustation/encrustation due to mineralization, blockage by debris accumulation, loss of ureteral peristalsis, tissue growth through stent side holes and/or stent buckling. As described previously [21], colloidal fluid can play a critical synergetic role with deformation and compression in the occurrence of stent failure. Assessment of different luminal polymeric sizes stents subjected to EUO in an in vitro model resulted in stent failure of the smaller luminal sizes (4.8F and 6F) as opposed to the larger sizes (7F and 8F) that remained open. We note, too, that tandem stents have been reported to be effective in some clinical settings under EUO [5, 7, 9, 22]. We speculate that this may be due to movement between the stents, which may reduce colloid aggregation and accumulation of colloids, as well as to the possibility that tandem stents maintain a space between the stents to allow urine flow even subject to ureter and stent lumina obstruction.

The time to failure variation of each stent type and configuration is likely related to the "random" nature of colloid accumulation over time. In many cases, we noted steady rising renal pressure and then sudden pressure drops, which were most likely due to accumulation and subsequent release of colloids. Whether mobilization of patients with EUO assists in prevention of colloid accumulation has yet to be proved. We emphasize that we make no claim regarding actual times to stent failure in clinical settings, nor do we consider EUO progression over time. Rather, the experiment was designed to work with a specific colloidal concentration and examine the relative times to failure (or not) among the different stent sizes and configurations.

Existing literature and the results reported here indicate that larger-lumen stents are less likely to become occluded with debris, due to the higher flow rates within them. Because urine flow in a ureter-stent system is generally laminar [18], *illustrative* flow calculations can be derived from Poiseuille's law. We note, too, that while the relative contributions of stent and ureter lumina to overall flow remain poorly understood, the stent lumen likely controls flow behavior particularly in the vicinity of the EUO where the ureter lumen is obstructed, which ultimately affects overall flow through the ureter-stent system; we therefore focus on stent flow in this region. The volumetric flow, Q, through a tube is $Q=(\pi P r^4)/(8\eta l)$, where the dynamic viscosity for urine is [23] $\eta \approx 8.5 \times 10^{-4}$ Pa·s at 37 °C and r is the internal radius. We assume a straight stent length $l=24$ cm (no pigtails), and total stent radii of $r=0.8$, 1.0, 1.17 and 1.33 mm (corresponding to 4.8F, 6F, 7F and 8F stents, respectively). We modify r to account for wall thickness (measured [21] as 0.22 mm for the 4.8F, 0.4 mm for 6F, 7F, 8F stents), and impose a renal unit pressure of 1 cmH_2O ($P=98.0665$ Pa). Calculations of Q in different stent configurations are given in Table 2. Notably, increasing stent luminal diameter, e.g., from 6 to 8F, increases volumetric stent flow by a factor of 5.9. In this context, consideration of tandem stents does not necessarily lead to increased volumetric flow rates. For example, tandem 6F stents have an effective, combined cross-sectional area of 6.28 mm^2, while a single 8F stent has an effective cross-sectional area of 5.55 mm^2; and yet, the volumetric flow in a single 8F stent is still a factor of 2.9 higher than in tandem 6F stents (and a factor of 1.1 higher than tandem 7F stents). These results are controlled by the strong effects of frictional forces on the stent walls, which vary significantly as a function of radius—critically, Q varies with the factor r^4.

The limitations of our study are related to the model design [18, 21]; see Additional file 1 for discussion regarding latex tubing, EUO shape and pressure, and type of colloidal solution (rather than "artificial urine"). Clearly, an in vitro experimental study cannot account for all physiological properties in the human in vivo environment. As such, the findings reported here do not correlate *directly* to clinical findings, particularly in terms of times to stent failure. However, our systematic analysis among ureter-stent configurations yields important relative comparisons of their failure dynamics. The latex tubing simulating a ureter has physical characteristics different than a real ureteral wall, and the lack of (even minimal) peristaltic motion may have some effect on the results (although we note that loss of ureteral peristalsis occurs frequently with stenting [2, 7, 24]). Moreover, dynamic ureteral responses caused by indwelling stents and EUO will likely further affect the flow dynamics over time, such as reflux or retrograde pressure transmission through and/or around the stent. The results here also are a function of the type and concentration of colloid material, and the use of solution containing no other salts, enzymes and organic material. As such, stent mineralization, various colloid aggregation properties, and biological activity remain unaccounted for. Moreover, the occurrence of blockage and the actual times to blockage (and variability among replicate experiments) are

Table 2 Poiseuille flow calculations for flow in stents

–	Stent						
	Single 4.8F	Tandem 4.8F	Single 6F	Tandem 6F	Single 7F	Tandem 7F	Single 8F
Flow rate (mL/h)	77	154	88	176	235	470	516
Internal stent radius (mm)	0.58	–	0.60	–	0.77	–	0.93
Cross-sectional area (mm^2)	2.01	4.02	3.14	6.28	4.30	8.60	5.55

also affected by colloid concentration. Notwithstanding the above, this is the first study to systematically measure effects of colloidal fluid flow in a comparative study of single, tandem, metal, and endopyelotomy stents in stented-ureter systems, both under and without EUO.

Conclusions

With the increased prevalence of EUO and multiple choices of ureteral stent configurations for drainage, comparison of treatment options is important. While tandem and metal stents have been suggested to be superior to single polymeric stents, our results show that large luminal stents offer no inferior patency rates and even better ones, at least in this in vitro model. Larger luminal stents offer excellent resistance to external ureteral pressure and allow adequate urine flow with colloids. In all cases, though, it should be emphasized that "ideal" stent drainage for EUO should take into consideration not only stent patency, but also patient quality of life, frequency of stent exchange, and associated costs that are influenced by stent size and composition.

Abbreviations

EUO: Extrinsic ureteral obstruction; η: Dynamic fluid viscosity; l: Tube length; P: Pressure difference between tube inlet and outlet; Q: Volumetric fluid flow rate; r: Ureter radius.

Supplementary Information

Additional file 1. Ureter, obstruction and colloidal solution set-up for the in vitro experiments.

Acknowledgements

B.B. was supported by a research grant from the Center for Scientific Excellence, Weizmann Institute of Science. B.B. holds the Sam Zuckerberg Professorial Chair in Hydrology.

Authors' contributions

All authors (YS, JM, DL, ID, BB) contributed to the study conception and design. Material preparation, data collection, and analysis were performed by ID, YS and BB. The first draft of the manuscript was written by BB, with key input from YS and ID, and all authors commented on previous versions of the manuscript. All authors read and approved the final manuscript.

Author details

[1]Department of Urology, Kaplan Medical Center, 7661041 Rehovot, Israel. [2]Department of Earth and Planetary Sciences, Weizmann Institute of Science, 7610001 Rehovot, Israel.

References

1. Chung SY, Stein RJ, Landsittel D, Davies BJ, Cuellar DC, Hrebinko RL, Tarin T, Averch TD. 15-year experience with the management of extrinsic ureteral obstruction with indwelling ureteral stents. J Urol. 2004;172:592–5. https://doi.org/10.1097/01.ju.0000130510.28768.f5.
2. Elsamra SE, Leavitt DA, Motato HA, Friedlander JI, Siev M, Keheila M, Hoenig DM, Smith AD, Okeke Z. Stenting for malignant ureteral obstruction: Tandem, metal or metal-mesh stents. Int J Urol. 2015;22:629–36. https://doi.org/10.1111/iju.12795.
3. Haas CR, Shah O, Hyams ES. Temporal trends and practice patterns for inpatient management of malignant extrinsic ureteral obstruction in the United States. J Endourol. 2020;34(8):828–35. https://doi.org/10.1089/end.2020.0053.
4. Hafron J, Ost MC, Tan BJ, Fogarty JD, Hoenig DM, Lee BR, Smith AD. Novel dual-lumen ureteral stents provide better ureteral flow than single ureteral stent in ex vivo porcine kidney model of extrinsic ureteral obstruction. Urology. 2006;68(4):911–5. https://doi.org/10.1016/j.urology.2006.05.025.
5. Varnavas M, Bolgeri M, Mukhtar S, Anson K. The role of tandem double-J ureteral stents in the management of malignant ureteral obstruction. J Endourol. 2016;30(4):465–8. https://doi.org/10.1089/end.2015.0670.
6. Ozyera U, Dirimb A. Tandem ureteral stents in the management of double-J stent dysfunction in gynecological malignancies. Diagn Interv Imaging. 2017;98(9):601–8. https://doi.org/10.1016/j.diii.2017.07.005.
7. Liu K-L, Lee B-C, Ye J-D, Chang Y-H, Chang C-C, Huang K-H, Lee Y-J, Chang Y-C. Comparison of single and tandem ureteral stenting for malignant ureteral obstruction: a prospective study of 104 patients. Eur Radiol. 2019;29:628–35. https://doi.org/10.1007/s00330-018-5560-6.
8. Navetta AF, Durdin TD, Thai K, Wagner KR, Reilly TP, Patel BJ, El Tayeb MM. Tandem Resonance metallic double-J ureteral stents in a single ureter for salvage management of chronic ureteral obstruction. Proc Bayl Univ Med Cent. 2019;32(4):510–3. https://doi.org/10.1080/08998280.2019.1633005.
9. Haifler M, Shvero A, Zilberman D, Ramon J, Winkler H, Margel D, Kleinmann N. Tandem ureteral stents for malignant ureteral obstruction. J Endourol. 2020;34(2):222–6. https://doi.org/10.1016/j.jbiomech.2021.110237.
10. Wang H-J, Lee TY, Luo HL, Chen C-H, Shen Y-C, Chuang Y-C, Chiang PH. Application of resonance metallic stents for ureteral obstruction. BJU Int. 2011;108:428–32. https://doi.org/10.1111/j.1464-410X.2010.09842.x.
11. Abbasi A, Wyre HW, Ogan K. Use of full-length metallic stents in malignant ureteral obstruction. J Endourol. 2013;27(5):640–5. https://doi.org/10.1089/end.2012.0448.
12. Patel C, Loughran D, Jones R, Abdulmajed M, Shergill I. The resonance® metallic ureteric stent in the treatment of chronic ureteric obstruction: a safety and efficacy analysis from a contemporary clinical series. BMC Urol. 2017;17:16. https://doi.org/10.1186/s12894-017-0204-8.
13. Asakawa J, Iguchi T, Tamada S, Ninomiya N, Kato M, Yamasaki T, Nakatani T. Treatment outcomes of ureteral stenting for malignant extrinsic ureteral obstruction: a comparison between polymeric and metallic stents. Cancer Manag Res. 2018;10:2977–82. https://doi.org/10.2147/CMAR.S172283.
14. Hsu J-S, Huang C-Y, Liu K-L, Chow P-M. Risk factors for primary failure of metallic ureteral stents: experience from a tertiary center. J Endourol. 2018. https://doi.org/10.1089/end.2017.0611.
15. Khoo CC, Abboudi H, Cartwright R, El-Husseiny T, Dasgupta R. Metallic ureteric stents in malignant ureteric obstruction: a systematic review. Urology. 2018;118:12–20. https://doi.org/10.1046/j.1464-410x.2000.00401.x.
16. Agrawal S, Brown CT, Bellamy EA, Kulkarni R. The thermo-expandable metallic ureteric stent: an 11-year follow-up. BJU Int. 2008;103:372–6. https://doi.org/10.1111/j.1464-410X.2008.08018.x.
17. Liatsikos EN, Karnabatidis D, Katsanos K, Kallidonis P, Katsakiori P, Kagadis GC, Christeas N, Papathanassiou Z, Perimenis P, Siablis DP. Ureteral metal stents: 10-year experience with malignant ureteral obstruction treatment. J Urol. 2009;182:2613–8. https://doi.org/10.1016/j.juro.2009.08.040.
18. Shilo Y, Modai J, Leibovici D, Dror I, Berkowitz B. Impact of colloidal fluid on stent failure under extrinsic ureteral obstruction: an in vitro experimental study. J Endourol. 2020;34(9):987–92. https://doi.org/10.1089/end.2020.0330.
19. Amitay-Rosen T, Nissan A, Shilo Y, Dror I, Berkowitz B. Failure of ureteral stents subject to extrinsic ureteral obstruction and stent occlusions. Int Urol Nephrol. 2021. https://doi.org/10.1007/s11255-021-02810-0.
20. Peters J, Green J, Hijazi L. Urogenital system. In: Glynn M, Drake WM, editors. Hutchison's clinical methods, chap. 17. 24th ed. Amsterdam: Elsevier; 2018. p. 355–77.
21. Shilo Y, Modai J, Leibovici D, Dror I, Berkowitz B. The impact of ureteral deformation and external ureteral pressure on stent failure in extrinsic ureteral obstruction—an in vitro experimental study. J Endourol. 2020;34(1):68–73. https://doi.org/10.1089/end.2019.0465.

22. Savin Z, Herzberg H, Ben-David R, Dekalo S, Mintz I, Marom R, Barghouthy Y, Mano R, Yossepowitch O, Sofer M. Long-term follow-up of yearly replaced double internal stents for extrinsic malignant ureteral obstruction. J Endourol. 2021;35:71–6. https://doi.org/10.1089/end.2020.0469.
23. Inman BA, Etienne W, Rubin R, Owusu RA, Oliveira TR, Rodriques DB, Maccarini PF, Stauffer PR, Mashal A, Dewhirst MW. The impact of temperature and urinary constituents on urine viscosity and its relevance to bladder hyperthermia treatment. Int J Hyperthermia. 2013;29:206–10. https://doi.org/10.3109/02656736.2013.775355.
24. Kinn AC, Lykkeskov-Andersen H. Impact on ureteral peristalsis in a stented ureter. An experimental study in the pig. Urol Res. 2002;30:213–8. https://doi.org/10.1007/s00240-002-0258-1.

22

Pediatric laparoscopic partial cystectomy for the treatment of benign bladder tumors and urachal cysts

Hongjie Gao[1], Jiawei Chen[2], Guowei Li[2], Xinhai Cui[2] and Fengyin Sun[2*]

Abstract

Objective: To investigate the feasibility and efficacy of carrying out pediatric laparoscopic partial cystectomies (LPC) when treating benign bladder tumors and urachal cysts.

Methods: Retrospectivey analyzing 4 clinical cases involving children with bladder tumors, which were collected from October 2017 to December 2018. In these clinical cases, there were 3 male children and 1 female child, aged from 4.5 to 9.4 years old, with an average age of 6.5 years. An intraperitoneal laparoscopic partial cystectomy was performed in the treatment of 3 of these patients with benign bladder tumors and in 1 patient with an urachal cyst. The surgical procedures included a partial cystectomy and a complete intracavitary bladder suture.

Results: All 4 cases were successful and no operation was transferred to opensurgery. The operation time was 100–120 min, with an average time of 108 min. The intraoperative blood loss was 10–20 ml, with an average loss of 15 ml. 6 h after the operation, the patients still maintained a fluid diet and 1 case of hematuria had occurred, with the catheter removed 12 days after the operation. No postoperative urine leakage, intestinal adhesion or intestinal obstruction occurred, and the average postoperative hospitalization time was 14 days.

Conclusion: Laparoscopic partial cystectomy is a safe and feasible method to be used for the treatment of benign bladder tumors and urachal cysts. It presents the advantages of being minimally invasive, and having a quick recovery and short hospitalization time. It is an alternative surgical method for the treatment of pediatric benign bladder tumors.

Keywords: Laparoscopy, Partial cystectomy, Benign bladder tumor, Urachal cyst

Background

Pediatric bladder tumors are infrequent, with rhabdomyosarcoma (RMS) being the most common. Benign tumors are even less common. They have various pathological types, and usually come to light in case reports. Therefore, clinicians do not know enough about them. In order to improve the diagnosis and treatment of pediatric benign bladder tumors then, we have retrospectively analyzed the clinical data from 4 pediatric benign bladder tumors that were admitted to our hospital from October 2017 to December 2018. From here, we have summarized the surgical experience and the indications.

*Correspondence: 727037502@qq.com
[2] Department of Pediatric Surgery, Qilu Hospital of Shandong University, Jinan, China
Full list of author information is available at the end of the article

Materials and methods

Clinical data

There were 4 cases in this group, including 3 males and 1 female, aged from 4.5 to 9.4 years old, with an average age of 6.5 years. Before the operation, a urinary b-ultrasound, pelvic CT and cystoscopy, as well as other examinations were all performed. The lesions were located in the apical wall in 1 case, the bottom in another case and the lateral wall in the remaining 2 cases, while all patients had symptoms of endless urination and bladder irritation, but no hematuria. In 2 cases, the left lateral wall had significantly thickened and there were rounded nodules on its top part. The CT showed sharp angular tissue shadows above the bladder in 1 case, while the urachus was not closed. Cystoscopy: in 3 cases, semicircular or irregular bulges were observed locally on the bladder wall, but the surface mucosa was smooth and continuous (Table 1, Figs. 1, 2).

Methods

The study was approved by the research ethics committee of Qilu Hospital of Shandong University, shandong, china. All methods were carried out in accordance with the relevant guidelines and regulations. A parent of each participant provided their informed consent for their child to participate in the study. Informed consent for the

Table 1 Perioperative patient data

	Age (yrs)	Gender	Clinical symptom	CT	Cytoscopic examination
Patient 1	4.7	Male	Odynuria 20 days	The left lateral wall is markedly thickened, at top of the left lateral wall are rounded enhanced nodules	There is a 5.2 cm irregular lump on the top of posterior wall, the basilar part is broad, from the ureterostoma 1–2 cm
Patient 2	4.6	Male	Micturition unwell 9 days	The left bladder wall is diffuse thickening, an irregular soft tissue mass protruded into the bladder	There is a 4.32 cm cauliflower-like lump on the left wall, from the ureterostoma about 3 cm
Patient 3	9.5	Male	Ultrasound found space occupying 1 month	The left side wall is thickened with clear boundary and irregular shape	There is a 2 cm cauliflower-like lump on the left of the bottom wall, the basilar part is broad, from the ureterostoma about 3.5 cm
Patient 4	7.3	Female	Paroxysm celialgia half month	A sharp angular shadow of tissue is seen above the bladder, considering urachal duct isn't close	

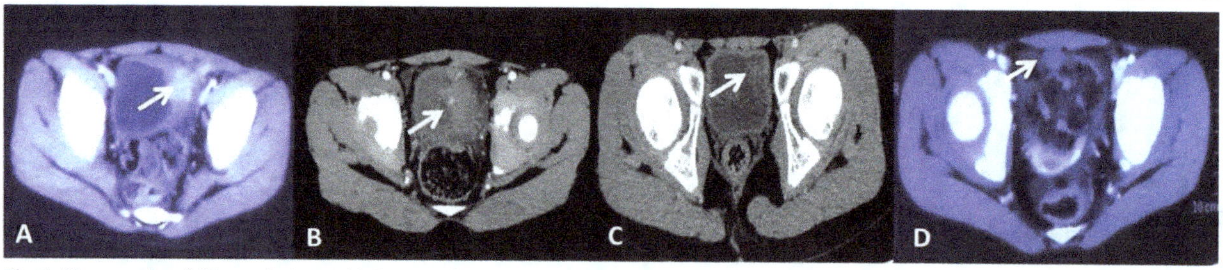

Fig. 1 Photographs of CT scan: Patient 1 (**a**), Patient 2 (**b**), Patient 3 (**c**), Patient 4 (**d**); the arrow points to the tumor

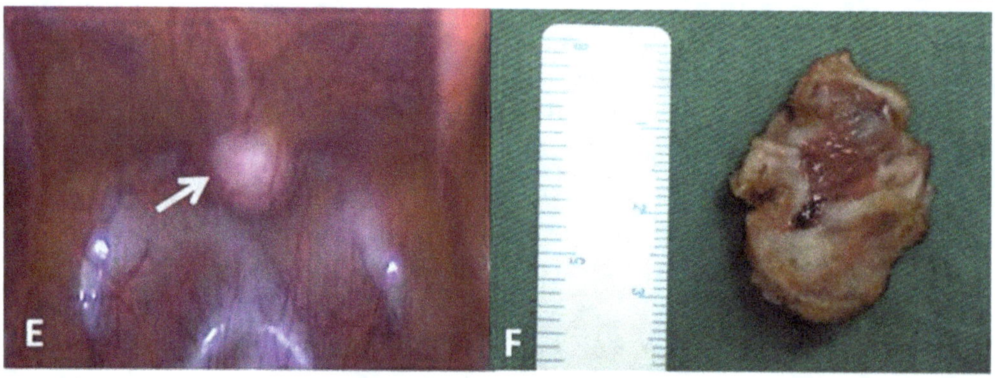

Fig. 2 Photographs of laparoscopic Urachal cyst (**e**), postoperative Urachal cyst (**f**)

publication of this study was also obtained from the parents of all participants in the study.

After administering a satisfactory quantity of anesthesia, place a small pillow under the buttocks and keep the patient in the Trendelenburg position. Routinely disinfect the abdomen and perineum, and after operating, place the inserted urinary tube on the table. Following this, cut open the umbilical region, directly place a 5 mm trocar as the observation hole, fill with CO_2, and maintain the pneumoperitoneum pressure at 8–10 mmHg. Place 5 mm trocars in the left lower abdomen and right lower abdomen under laparoscopy. Through the catheter, the bladder should be filled with an appropriate amount of germfree saline. Following this, through a combination of preoperative imaging and cystoscopy results, the tumor boundaries can be clearly distinguished under laparoscopy. Next, cut open the bladder wall at a position about 0.5 cm from the tumor, and then completely remove the tumor at a position of 0.5 cm around the tumor while under direct vision. Immediately put the specimen into the specimen bag, put it in the iliac fossa, full-thickness suture the incision with 4–0 absorbable suture, and embed it with interrupted seromuscular suture. Place the drainage tube outside the bladder wall at the site of the tumor resection, remove the instruments, suture the incision, and indwell the catheter (Fig. 3).

Tumor location: (1) an exogenous tumor's position can be identified under direct vision. (2) An infiltrative tumor can be located according to the degree of muscle layer thickening, or can be observed by opening the bladder and putting a lens in, whereby the location, size, and the relationship with the bilateral ureteral openings can be directly observed. (3) Using the double lens combination method, whereby a cystoscope is placed through the urethra at a distance of about 0.5 cm from the edge of the tumor. The brightness of the laparoscopic light source is reduced, and the location of the light source of the cystoscope is confirmed, where upon it should be marked with an electric hook (Fig. 4).

Results

All 4 cases were successful and no operation was transferred to open surgery. The operation time was 100–120 min, with an average time of 108 min. The intraoperative blood loss was 10–20 ml, with an average loss of 15 ml. The patients maintained a fluid diet for 6 h after the operation. Hematuria occurred in 1 case. The catheter was removed 12 days after the operation. No postoperative urine leakage, intestinal adhesion or intestinal obstruction occurred, and the average time of postoperative hospitalization was 14 days. Postoperative pathological specimens results: 1 case was inflammatory myofibroblastoma, 1 case was adenomatoid or middle renal metaplasia, 1 case was reepithelialized granulation tissue, and 1 case was an urachal cyst. The 4 patients were followed up with for a period of 3–15 months, with an average follow-up of 10.4 months. There was no infection, recurrence or canceration, and the incision healed well by normosthenuria. (Table 2, Fig. 5).

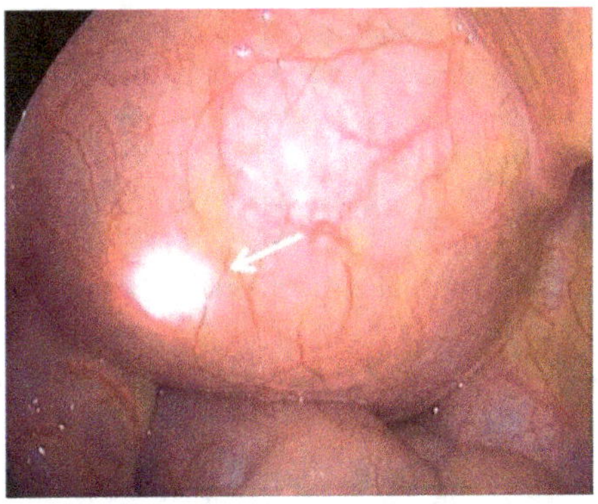

Fig. 4 Double lenses combination method, arrow indicates cystoscope light source

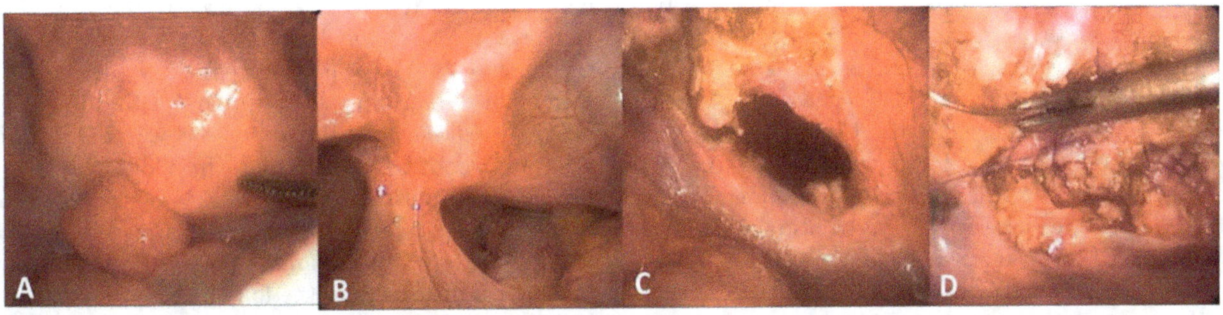

Fig. 3 Photographs of laparoscopic bladder exogenic tumor (**a**), bladder endogenous tumor (**b**), and bladder wound (**c**) and suture of bladder wound (**d**)

Table 2 Postoperative and pathological data

	Operative time (min)	EBL (ml)	Hospital stat (days)	Complications	Bladder biopsy pathology	Postoperative pathology	Follow-up period (mons)
Patient 1	115	45	14	–	Polypoid hyperplasia	Myofibroblastoma	16
Patient 2	125	20	16	Hematuria	Granulation tissue	Adenomatiodmetaplasia	14
Patient 3	120	24	13	–	Inflammatory polyp	Inflammatory granuloma	13
Patient 4	105	15	12	–	–	Urachal cyst	10

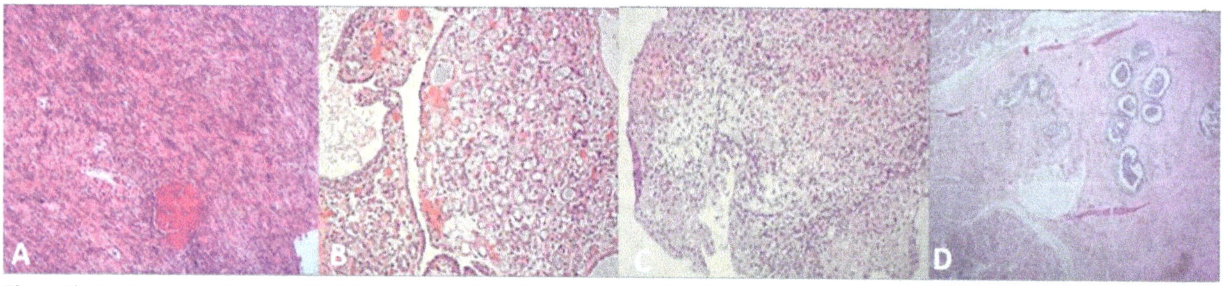

Fig. 5 Photomicrograph of resected bladder lesion showing inflammatory myofibroblastoma (**a**), adenomatoid metaplasia (**b**), inflammatory granuloma (**c**) and urachanl cyst (**d**)

Discussion

In this group, 1 cystoscope biopsy was consistent with the postoperative pathology report, and 2 were inconsistent. Goluboff advocated that preoperative cystoscope biopsies should be performed in order to confirm the diagnosis before treatment. However, due to the deep location of the tumor, it is difficult to obtain ideal lesion specimens for muscular layer and submucosal lesions, which thus results in a low positive rate [1, 2].The pathological bladder tumor types in children are different from those in adults. Most of the tumors in children are non-epithelial in origin,and the bladder surface mucosa is not infiltrated in the early stages. It is difficult to pick up the submucosal tissue using cystoscope biopsy forceps. Despite there being limitations for cystoscopy in children, the size of the lump, its location, and the relationship it has to the ureteral orifice can be intuitively known before surgery, thereby enabling the evaluation of whether a partial resection can be performed and whether the original ureteral orifice can be retained. In addition, rapid pathology can be added during surgery to clarify the pathological type. Ureteral replantation may be necessary during the surgery when the tumor is closely connected to the location of the ureteral orifice detected prior to surgery. However, it also increases the surgical difficulties, and much attention shall be paid to avoid damaging the spermaduct or oviduct.

Rhabdomyosarcoma of the bladder is the main pathological type of pediatric malignant bladder tumor, and it is usually found in the trigone of the bladder, the bladder neck or the prostate urethra. However, most pediatric benign bladder tumors grow outside the trigone of the bladder [3]. In this group, there were 2 cases on the lateralbladder wall, 1 case on the superior wall and 1 case on the inferior wall. Laparoscopic partial cystectomy is suitable for those tumors located at the top or side of the bladder wall but that do not infiltrate the bladder wall. Laparoscopic partial cystectomy is available for only a few patients with localized tumors on the top or lateral wall of the bladder. It is still controversial whether laparoscopic partial cystectomy for the treatment of bladder rhabdomyosarcoma can bring about the risk of intra-abdominal tumor implantation as the surgery is performed through the abdominal cavity and urine is infiltrated into the abdominal cavity after surgery.

The urinary irritation symptoms of the pediatric benign bladder tumor were not obvious, the symptoms appeared late, the tumor infiltrated the muscle layer earlier, and the tumor grew very quickly. The medical history in this group was 7–15 days, with an average time of 10 days, while the tumor size was 2.5–4.5 cm, with an average size of 2.6 cm. In addition, the CT indicated the possibility of a thickening and infiltration of the muscular layer. Due to the size of the tumor and its degree of infiltration, the opportunity of carrying out a transurethral resection was missed. However, laparoscopic partial cystectomy has the advantages of being less traumatic, resulting in less bleeding, being a precise operation, leaving a small scar and having a quick postoperative recovery time. All of which make it suitable for the treatment of pediatric bladder tumors [4–6].Therefore, laparoscopic partial cystectomy was adopted for this group of patients.

The LPC reported in both domestic and foreign literatures is to incise the bladder wall from the top of the bladder, and then incise the bladder in the direction of the tumor slantwise. The operation presents the following problems however: first, when incising the bladder wall, the tumor may also be incised; second, when incising the tumors on the opposite side wall, especially those tumors with a smaller diameter, the bladder incision can come from the middle and becomes large, which then increases the difficulty of suturing in the cavity [7–9]. By performing the 4 cases of laparoscopic partial cystectomy in children, we observed the following techniques and gained this experience:

1. The bladder should be moderately filled, preferably to the pubic symphysis, and the muscle layer of the bladder should be in a certain diastolic state, so as to distinguish the tumor boundary and determine the extent of the surgical resection. Ureteral stents should also be placed bilaterally to protect the ureteral opening.
2. Tumor location: (1) an exogenous tumor's position can be identified under direct vision. (2) An infiltrative tumor can be located according to the degree of muscle layer thickening, or can be observed by opening the bladder and putting a lens in, whereby the location, size, and the relationship with the bilateral ureteral openings can be directly observed. (3) Using the double lens combination method, whereby a cystoscope is placed through the urethra at a distance of about 0.5 cm from the edge of the tumor. The brightness of the laparoscopic light source is reduced, and the location of the light source of the cystoscope is confirmed, whereupon it should be marked with an electric hook.
3. Bladder suturing is difficult in this operation, and the key points to prevent postoperative urinary fistula are as follows: (1) use a reliable suture technique, such as continuous varus suture. The technical difficulty lies in tightening the knot. 4–0 barbed thread can be used, or it can be knotted every 4 needles, and then embedded with an intermittent suture on the seromuscular layer. (2) The outer wall of the bladder at the site of the tumor should be dissociated in an appropriately large area so that the incisal margin can be easily sutured without tension. (3) Check for leakage by injecting water into the bladder.

Robot-assisted laparoscopic cystectomy in children has been reported in a few literatures [10, 11].Compared with conventional laparoscopy, robot-assisted laparoscopes offer wider and clearer 3D surgical fields for both eyes, allowing to more accurate and flexible control capabilities. In particular, the bladder is located in the pelvic floor in a deeper position, and the procedure performed in such a limited space gives full play to the flexible advantages of robot-assisted surgery; The robot is equipped with special surgical instruments, which can perform wrist-like motions, avoiding subtle tremors, thereby realizing precise and stable sutures. Therefore, the requirements of a skilled surgeon who masters the suture technique are lower than those of conventional laparoscopy, and the suture of bladder reconstruction can be easily accomplished. Compared with conventional laparoscopy, the robot-assisted laparoscopy still has some shortcomings. The introduction and application of the Da Vinci system and related devices are high in cost, bringing about a certain economic burden to medical centers and families; The operating system is not configured with stress feedback, and a surgeon must adjust the strength based on vision and experience; Compared with the 5 mm Trocar of conventional laparoscopy, most of the robots require a larger incision for the 8 mm special Trocar, which leaving in longer scars. In general, as the robot-assisted surgery may further improve the surgical effect, we will try such surgery in future cases.

Conclusions

The preliminary experience of these 4 cases of laparoscopic partial cystectomy showed that laparoscopic partial cystectomy is suitable for the treatment of pediatric benign bladder tumors and pediatric urachal cysts, and that it is a safe and feasible method. Laparoscopic partial cystectomy has the advantages of being minimally invasive, resulting in less blood loss, having a rapid recover time, only needing a short hospital stay, and causing less postoperative pain. It is a brilliant surgical procedure, which can be used an improved treatment method for pediatric urachal cysts and pediatric benign bladder tumors.

Abbreviations

RMS: Rhabdomyosarcoma; CT: Computed tomograp.

Acknowledgements

None.

Authors' contributions

HG contributed to the design of the study, and drafting the paper. JC, GL contributed to acquisition of data and revision of the paper. XC contributed to analysis and interpretation of data, and revising the paper critically. FS contributed to design, acquisition, analysis, interpretation of data and revising the paper critically. All authors approved the final version of the paper.

Author details
[1]Department of Pediatrics, Qilu Hospital of Shandong University, Jinan, China.
[2]Department of Pediatric Surgery, Qilu Hospital of Shandong University, Jinan, China.

References

1. Lyons TL, Lee T, Winer WK. Lapamseopie removal of a bladder leiomyoma. J Am Asset Gyneeol Laparom. 1998;5:423–6.
2. Nerli RB, Reddy M, Koura AC, et al. Cystoscopy-assisted laparoscopic partial cystectomy. J Endourol. 2008;22(1):83–6.
3. Diaeonescu S, Burlea M, Miron I, et al. Childhood rhabdomyosarcoma. Anatomo-clinical and therapeutic study on 25 cases. Surgical implications Rom J Morphol Embryol. 2013;54(3):531–7.
4. Ahmed H, Howe AS, Dyer LL, et al. Robot-assisted laparoscopic urachal excision in children. Urology. 2017;106:103–6.
5. Kumar S, Shankaregowda SA, Chandna AA. Rare inflammatory myofibroblastic bladder tumor masquerading urachal carcinoma. Urol Ann. 2018;10(3):336–8.
6. El-Tholoth HS, Al Rasheedi S, Alharbi F, et al. Paraganglioma of urinary bladder managed by laparoscopic partial cystectomy in conjunction with flexible cystoscopy: a case report. J Endourol Case Rep. 2018;4(1):15–7.
7. Cheah PL, Loo LM, Lee GE, Teoh KH, Mun KS, Nazarina AR. Unusual finding of endocervical-like mucinous epithelium in continuity with uroepithelium in endocervicosis of the urinary bladder. Diagn Pathol. 2011;6:56.
8. Olivia Vella JE, Nair N, Ferryman SR, Athavale R, Latthe P, Hirschowitz L. Mullerianosis of the urinary bladder. Intern J Surg Path. 2011;19(4):548–51.
9. Prager M, Wilson T, Krüger K, et al. Laparoscopic extramucosal partial bladder resection in a patient with symptomatic deep-infiltrating endometriosis of the bladder. J Minim Invasive Gynecol. 2012;19(1):113–7.
10. Li P, Zhou H, Cao H, Ma L, et al. Robot-assisted laparoscopic radical cystectomy and sigmoid orthotopic neobladder reconstruction for a bladder rhabdomyosarcoma child: case report and literature review. Urology. 2020;138:144–7.
11. Williams CR, Chavda K. En bloc robot-assisted laparoscopic partial cystectomy, urachal resection, and pelvic lymphadenectomy for urachal adenocarcinoma. Rev Urol. 2015;17(1):46–9.

Localization of external urethral orifice in coronary sulcus during urethroplasty in case of severe hypospadias accompanied by prostatic utricle cyst

Jun Lu[1†], Junjie Cen[1†], Wenwei Wang[1], Hongwei Zhao[2], Pengju Li[1], Jiacong Mo[1], Zhenhua Chen[1], Yiming Tang[1], Jinhuan Wei[1], Junhang Luo[1], Shiying Huang[3*] and Yong Fang[1*]

Abstract

Background: To explore whether opening the external urethral orifice in the coronal sulcus can reduce the incidence of epididymitis after operating on hypospadias with prostatic utricle cyst (PUC) connecting to the vas deferens. Group A consisted of 3 patients with severe hypospadias and PUC undergoing cystostomy, hypospadias correction and urethroplasty, along with the relocation of the external orifice of the urethra to the coronal sulcus. Group B consisted of 4 patients having initial hypospadias repaired with meatus in the orthotopic position in the glans, presenting with multiple epididymitis after hypospadias surgery and unsuccessful conservative treatment. MR confirmed that all the Group B patients had PUC connecting to the vas deferens. Group B patients underwent urethral dilatation along with urethral catheterization, cutting of the original corpus cavernosum that encapsulated the urethra, and extension of the position of the external urethral orifice to the coronal sulcus.

Results: In group A, 3 children underwent bladder fistula removal 2 weeks after the operation. The penis developed normally without any complications. Four children in group B underwent stent removal 12 weeks after operation, and one patient was still stenosed and dilated again. All patients in group B were followed without epididymitis recurrence.

Conclusions: For patients with hypospadias complicating with a PUC, connecting to one side of the vas deferens, the positioning of the external urethral orifice in the coronary sulcus would be helpful to reduce the occurrence of epididymitis.

Keywords: Hypospadias, Prostatic utricle cyst, Urethroplasty, Epididymitis

Introduction

The prostatic utricle cyst (PUC) is a cystic structure located in the anterior rectal bladder and posterior spermatorrhea, which originates from incomplete degeneration of the Mullerian duct. The incidence of simple PUC in children is low, but in children with hypospadias and sex organ abnormalities, the occurrence increases to 11–14%, while in children with severe hypospadias, it can be as high as 57% [1–4]. However, due to the lack of

*Correspondence: daroon@126.com; fymartin@sina.com
†Jun Lu and Junjie Cen have contributed equally to this work
[1] Department of Urology, First Affiliated Hospital of Sun Yat-Sen University, Guangzhou 510080, People's Republic of China
[3] School of Traditional Chinese Medicine, Southern Medical University, Guangzhou 510515, People's Republic of China
Full list of author information is available at the end of the article

systematic examination before hypospadias surgery, the incidence of hypospadias accompanied by PUC is often underestimated [5]. The majority of patients are asymptomatic, but the PUC may be associated with recurrent urinary tract infections, pain, abdominal mass, stone formation, pseudo-incontinence and epididymitis [6, 7]. Especially for patients with PUC and hypospadias, urethroplasty can increase the incidence of epididymitis. The specific reasons are as follows: due to the location of the vas deferens, two types of PUCs can form: one where the vas deferens opens to the PUC and another where the vas deferens is not connected to the PUC. For the first type, urinary pressure increases after urethroplasty, and urine can easily flow back into the vas deferens, leading to epididymitis [4]. In addition to the length of the urinary pathway requiring urethroplasty, another important factor to consider when performing hypospadias surgery is the location of the external urethral orifice. At present, there is an increasing demand for hypospadias surgery, making it necessary to perform more research on this surgery.

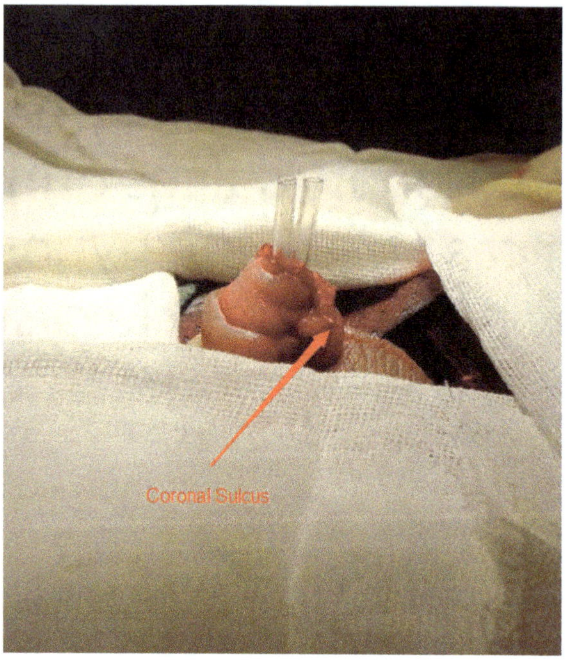

Fig. 1 In patients with hypospadias without PUC, the external orifice of the urethra selected for urethroplasty is located at the front of the glans, surrounded by the glans cavernous body

Materials and methods

The MAGPI (meatal advancement and glanuloplasty incorporated) is an urethroplasty technique, and its key steps include moving the urethra opening to the normal position of the penile glans, surrounded by the glans cavernosum (Fig. 1). However, this method can cause increased pressure on the urethra, which can increase the possibility of developing epididymitis in patients with severe hypospadias and PUC (Group A in our study). Therefore, for these patients,our hospital chose to position the urethral opening, not in the median position of penile glans through the glans cavernosum, but near the coronal sulcus, without enclosure of the glans cavernosum. This is similar to Denis-Browne surgery (Fig. 2), which helps to alleviate the relative urethral pressure, thus reducing the occurrence of epididymitis. For the patients with epididymitis after urethroplasty, whose PUCs connecting to the vas deferens, we dilated the external urethral orifice to the adjacent coronal sulcus and tear the corpus cavernosum, as the corpus cavernosum was made to enclose the urethra in previous operations. Through this method, we were able to achieve successful clinical results. The following report details our methods and results.

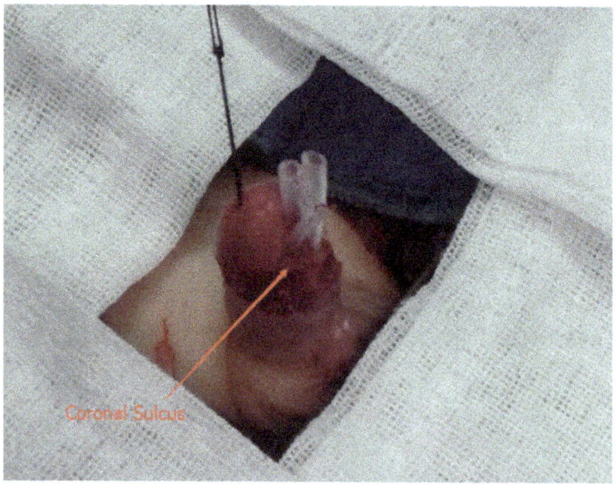

Fig. 2 In patients with severe hypospadias complicated with PUC, the urethral orifice chosen is close to the coronal sulcus without enclosure by the glans cavernosum during urethroplasty

Three cases of hypospadias complicated by the presence of a PUC were operated on for the first time in the group A (Table 1), which accounted for 9.4% of the total corresponding time's cases (32cases). Hospitalization occurred during 2011–2012 and the patients ranged in age from 3.1 to 3.6 years, with an average age of 3.3 years. They all displayed severe hypospadias, with 2 cases of penile-scrotal hypospadias and 1 case of perineal hypospadias. Renal Bladder Ultrasound and MRI showed that the PUC was round or oblong, with an average size of about 2.3 cm × 2.7 cm × 3.2 cm, and one side of vas deferens was connected with PUC in all 3 patients. Four patients (group B) with multiple epididymitis after hypospadias surgery and unsuccessful conservative

Table 1 The individual patient clinic data of group A

Group A	Age (years)	Size of puc (cm)	TH	UOLO	EOO	LFU (years)
Patient 1	3.1	2.5 × 2.3 × 3.0	Penile-scrotal	Coronal sulcus	No	6.5
Patient 2	3.2	2.1 × 2.8 × 3.5	Perineal	Coronal sulcus	No	5
Patient 3	3.6	2.3 × 2.3 × 3.1	Penile-scrotal	Coronal sulcus	No	7

TH: the type of hypospadias; UOLO: urethral orifice location in operation; EOO: epididymitis onset or no; LFU: the length of follow up

Table 2 The individual patient clinic data of group B

Group B	Age (years)	Size of puc (cm)	TH	UOLOO	TEAOO	AIHS (years)	TBEX (years)	LFU (years)
Patient 1	3.5	2.6 × 1.2 × 3.8	Perineal	Top of glan	3	2.0	2.7	5.5
Patient 2	7.3	3.3 × 4.1 × 4.2	Perineal	Top of glan	5	3.2	3.8	2
Patient 3	8.6	1.1 × 2 × 3.5	Penile-scrotal	Top of glan	6	3.5	4.2	10.5
Patient 4	8.2	3.4 × 4.2 × 4.1	Penile	Top of glan	5	2.7	3.5	12

TH: the type of hypospadias; UOLOO: urethral orifice location in original operation; TEAOO: times of epididymitis after original operation; AIHS: the ages at the initial hypospadias surgery; TBEX: times of beginning to experience epididymitis; LFU: the length of follow up

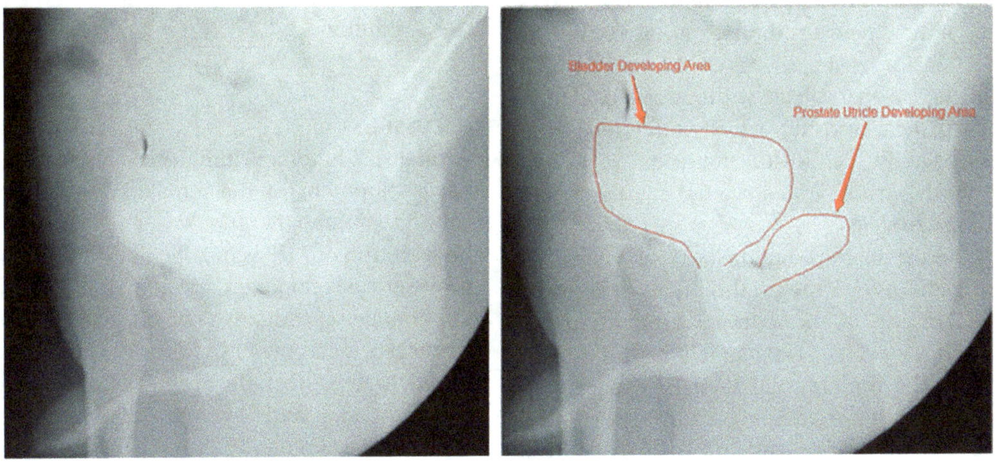

Fig. 3 In group B, the original and enhanced portrait urethrogram of the patients with severe hypospadias and PUC showed1.1 cm × 2 cm × 3.5 cm, PUC posterior to the bladder

treatment were admitted to the hospital from 2006 to 2017 (Table 2), which accounted for 44.4% of the total corresponding time's cases (9 epididymitis after hypospadias cases). The age varied from from 3.5 to 8.6 years, with an average age of 6.9 years. There was no routine examination before hypospadias surgery for these patients with PUC, 1 case of penile hypospadias, 1 case of penile-scrotal hypospadias and 2 cases of perineal hypospadias. Renal Bladder Ultrasound, voiding cystourethrography (VCUG) (Fig. 3) and MRI (Fig. 4) were performed in group B, and MRI showed that the average size of PUC was 2.6 cm × 2.9 cm × 3.5 cm, and one side of vas deferens opened to the PUC in all 4 patients. The study was approved by the ethics committee of the

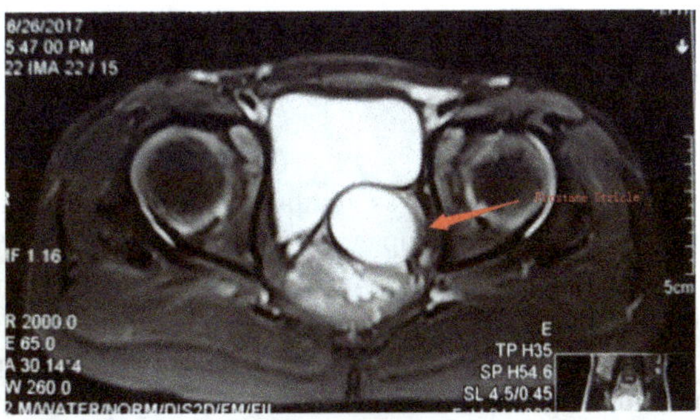

Fig. 4 In group B, magnetic resonance imaging of severe hypospadias with PUC revealed cystic lesions in the left posterior bladder, about 2.6 cm × 1.2 cm × 3.8 cm in size

First Affiliated Hospital of Sun Yat-sen University. The informed consent was obtained from each patient's parents. This study adhered to the guidelines of Chinese diagnosis and treatment of urological diseases. In group A, after filling the bladder with water, a suprapubic tube and drainage were performed 2 cm above the pubic symphysis; the skin was cut under the coronal sulcus, subcutaneous tissue was dissected and subcutaneously separated outside the albuginea. Fibrous bands restricting penile extension were completely separated and released to make the penis straight. After correcting the lower curvature, the average length of the defect urethra was about 5.6 cm in these three cases. Then urethroplasty was performed on the urethral plate and the prepuce was grafted, and the average width of the urethral plate was about 1 cm. The thin prepuce inner plate was transferred to the ventral side of the penis and wrapped around 3–4 stents with side holes. The graft prepuce margin was sutured continuously with 6–0 absorbable sutures. The proximal end was sutured intermittently with the original urethral orifice by varus suture. The distal end was reconstructed with a new urethral external orifice by separating the inferior dermal bridge of the glans, which was located in the coronal sulcus, without encapsulation of the glans corpus cavernosum, which is different from the traditional MAGPI. Penile subcutaneous tissue was sutured. The mesh yarn wrapped around the penis and was fixed with gauze strips.

In group B, the original urethral orifice was located at the top of the glans. When the urethral dilatation probe was inserted, stricture of the external urethral orifice was found in all cases. First, the filamentous probe was inserted through the urethra, and then F8-F18 urinary dilatation strips were inserted sequentially. The ventral margin of the urethral orifice was pulled to the ventral side of the glans, and the original glans cavernosum was torn to the coronal sulcus. In this way, the external orifice of the urethra was no longer surrounded by the glans cavernosum, and there was a gap of about 0.5 cm. After the dilatation, a 5 cm long silica gel stent tube was fixed to the glans (making the urethra about F16 in diameter) (Fig. 5).

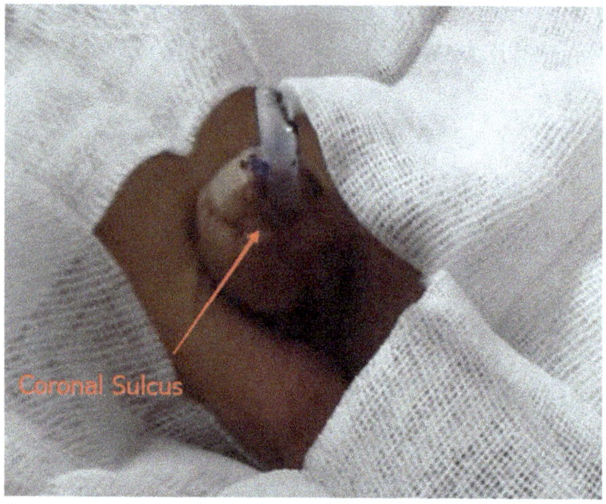

Fig. 5 The original glans, cavernosum was torn to the coronal sulcus and a 5 cm long silica gel stent tube was fixed to the glans

Results

The suprapubic tube was removed 2 weeks after the initial operation in group A, and the internal stent was removed 4 weeks after the operation. The external genitalia developed normally and there were no complications during the follow-up period of 5–7 years. Four children in group B were treated, with stent removal 12 weeks after the operation, and one patient was stenosed and dilated again. All patients in group B were followed up for 2–12 years without epididymitis relapse, and penile erection as well as ejaculation were normal later in adulthood.

Discussion

Normally, Mullerian inhibiting factor (MIF) prevents the development of the female reproductive system in embryos around the 10th week of development. When the secretion of MIF is insufficient or the urogenital sinus is not fully developed in a way that allows for the formation of male reproductive organs, the Mullerian tube can degenerate incompletely and form a cystic dilatation connected to the prostatic urethra, forming PUC or cyst. Cysts are small and asymptomatic and are often found in physical examination. They can also be secondary to infection, stones or obstruction. Additionally, urinary tract infections, epididymitis and scrotal abscesses can occur repeatedly [8], and there are even reports of malignant transformation of prostate cysts [9]. About 90% of PUC cases also display hypospadias or ambiguous external genitalia [10]. The end of the vas deferens (ejaculatory duct), normally opening in the verumontanum, can open into the cyst. According to Monfort [11], in 4 out of 5 cases, the vas deferens entered the cyst. Ritchey et al. [12] explained that the verumontanum originating from the urogenital sinus was affected due to the abnormality of the urogenital sinus and the formation of PUC, where the ejaculatory duct and vas deferens implant ectopically. Postoperative treatment of hypospadias is often complicated by urethral stricture up to 7–12% [13–15]. With the increase of urethral pressure after urethroplasty, epididymitis can often occur after undergoing surgery to remedy hypospadias with a PUC.

PUC is often found in the course of hypospadias surgery when it is difficult to insert a catheter, or when complications such as epididymitis and pelvic inflammatory occur after urethroplasty. Few PUCs are confirmed before urethroplasty. However, if the size and location of cysts are not known before an operation, it can cause difficulties during the operation and affect the success of the operation. Therefore, it is necessary to determine whether there is a PUC before the operation for hypospadias, especially for severe hypospadias. Shima et al. [16] reported that PUCs occurred in 13.9% (21/151) of penile-scrotal and perineal hypospadias patients. Therefore, the incidence of severe hypospadias, especially perineal hypospadias with PUC is high, and relevant imaging examinations should be performed before operating.

For the development of normal penis shape after the operation, the prevalent hypospadias surgery generally places the external urethral orifice in the front of the glans, surrounded by the glans cavernous body. The advantage of this external urethral orifice is that there is a cavernous body in the urethral orifice. The pressure of the cavernous body contraction is conducive to straightening the urethra and making the urine travel distance longer. However, the disadvantage is that it increases the pressure on the urethra during micturition, which is related to the poor compliance of the external urethral orifice in the glans. Compliance means the tendency of an organ to resist deformation by a force [17]; obviously, encapsulation of the external orifice of the urethra by the glans cavernosum reduces urethral compliance. Furthermore, the new external urethral orifice protruded from the glans tends to form scar stricture or even atresia, and the urethral orifice stricture accounts for about 50% of the total urethral stricture after hypospadias surgery [18], Lichen sclerosus may be an important factor in distal urethral stricture [19]. This stricture can also cause increased urethral pressure, therefore, urine can more easily flow back to the testis, causing epididymitis attacks, especially in patients with hypospadias complicated with PUC. For these reasons, we advocate that the external urethral orifice should be placed in the coronal sulcus in these patients. When this method was tried in our hospital, for the 3 patients in group A, the external orifice of the urethra was placed near the coronal sulcus instead of passing through the glans cavernosum in their initial operation, and no epididymitis occurred. The 4 patients in group B suffered from recurrent epididymitis after their initial operation. We performed a second operation in which the urethra was dilated and the external orifice of the urethra was torn to the coronal sulcus. After that, epididymitis did not recur and satisfactory clinical results were achieved. However, the opening of the coronal sulcus has clear drawbacks. First, there is a significant difference between the appearance of the coronal sulcus and the normal penis, which may affect the psychological health and sexual functions of the patients. Second, urination is sprinkled during the passage, which affects the urination process. However, we believe that the advantage of the coronal sulcus opening is greater than the disadvantage of infertility caused by repeated painful attacks of epididymitis and eventual surgical removal of the PUC and blockage of the vas deferens. Of course, there is also a need to clarify why hypospadias patients with PUC are more likely to have epididymitis than ordinary hypospadias patients. We think that there may be the following reasons: first, patients with PUC may also have dysplasia of ejaculatory orifice, and the anti-reflux mechanism is defective; second, the cystic structure is prone to residual more urine, so it is more prone to infection. These theories need further experimental research. Our study confirmed that reducing reflux can reduce the incidence of epididymitis in these patients, which is to deal with only one pathogenic factor to solve this problem. As for improving the anti-reflux effect of the ejaculatory duct or using other mechanisms to fundamentally solve this kind of disease, it is worth further exploring.

Conclusion

The objective of eliminating epididymitis was achieved by locating the urethral orifices in the coronary sulcus in three cases of hypospadias with PUC during urethroplasty and dilatating the urethral orifices to the coronary sulcus in four cases of hypospadias with PUC after repeated epididymitis after urethroplasty. So the patients with hypospadias complicated by the presence of a PUC, especially those with a PUC connects to the vas deferens, we advocate opening the urethral orifice near the coronal sulcus rather than through the glans cavernosum to place it in front of the glans, so that the occurrence of epididymitis after urethroplasty may be reduced.

Abbreviations

PUC: Prostatic utricle cyst; MAGPI: Meatal advancement and glanuloplasty incorporated; MRI: Magnetic resonance imaging; VCUG: Cystourethrography; MIF: Mullerian tube inhibitor.

Acknowledgements

None.

Authors' contributions

JL, JJC and YF collected and analyzed the data, and drafted the manuscript. WWW, HWZ, PJL, ZHC, YMT, JHL and JHW collected the data. JCM, SYH and YF designed the study. All authors read and approved the final manuscript.

Author details

[1]Department of Urology, First Affiliated Hospital of Sun Yat-Sen University, Guangzhou 510080, People's Republic of China. [2]Department of Urology, Affiliated Yantai Yuhuangding Hospital, Qingdao University, Yantai 264000, Shandong, People's Republic of China. [3]School of Traditional Chinese Medicine, Southern Medical University, Guangzhou 510515, People's Republic of China.

References

1. Oh CS, Chung IH, Won HS, et al. Morphologic variations of the prostatic utricle. Clin Anat. 2009;22(3):358–64.
2. Wang W, Wang Y, Zhu D, et al. The prostatic utricle cyst with huge calculus and hypospadias: a case report and a review of the literature. Can Urol Assoc J. 2015;9(5):345–8.
3. Johnson D, Parikh K, Schey W, et al. MRI in diagnosis of a giant prostatic utric. Case Rep Radiol. 2014;2014:217563.
4. Vinod P, Jitendra PS, Shwetank M, et al. prostatic utricle cyst: a clinical dilemma. APSP J Case Rep. 2013;4(2):16.
5. Hester AG, Kogan SJ. The prostatic utricle: An under-recognized condition resulting in significant morbidity in boys with both hypospadias and normal external genitalia. J Pediatr Urol. 2017;13(5):492.e1-492.e5.
6. Farikullah J, Ehtisham S, Nappo S, Patel L, Hennayake S. Persistent Mullerian duct syndrome: lessons learned from managing a series of eight patients over a 10-year period and review of literature regarding malignant risk from the Mullerian remnants. BJU Int. 2012;110(11 Pt C):E1084e9.
7. Goruppi I, Avolio L, Romano P, Raffaele A, Pelizzo G. Roboticassisted surgery for excision of an enlarged prostatic utricle. Int J Surg Case Rep. 2015;10:94e6.
8. Gygi C, Carvajal M. Prostatic utricle: an unusual case report. Eur J Pediatr Surg. 1994;4:211–3.
9. Gualco G, Ortega V, Ardao G, et al. Clear cell adenocarcinoma of the prostatic utricle in an adolescent. Ann Diagn Pathol. 2005;9:153–6.
10. Devine CJ, Gonzalez L, Stecker JF, et al. Utricular configuration in hypospadias and intersex. J Urol. 1980;123:407–11.
11. Monfort G. Transvesical approach to utricular cysts. J Ped Surg. 1982;17:406–8.
12. Ritchey ML, Benson RC, Stephen A, et al. Managementof Mullerian duct remnant in the made patient. J Urol. 1988;140:795–9.
13. Duel BP, Barthold JS, Gonzalez R. Management of urethral strictures after hypospadias repair. J Urol. 1998;160:170–1.
14. Stanasel I, Le HK, Bilgutay A, et al. Complications following staged hypospadias repair using transposed prepucial skin flaps. J Urol. 2015;194:512–6.
15. McNamara ER, Schaeffer AJ, Seager CM, et al. Management of proximal hypospadias with 2-stage repair: 20-year experience. J Urol. 2015;194:1080–5.
16. Shima H, Ikoma F, Terakawa T, et al. Developmental anomalies associated with hypospadias. J Urol. 1979;122:619–21.
17. Jesus LE, Schanaider A, Patterson G, et al. Urethral compliance in hypospadias operated by tubularized incised urethral plate (TIP) with and without a dorsal inlay graft: an experimental controlled study. World J Urol. 2013;31(4):971–5.
18. Wang X, Tang Y, Mao Y, Qin D, Chen S. Reoperation methods and effectiveness of urethral stricture after urethroplasty of hypospadias. Zhongguo Xiu Fu Chong Jian Wai Ke Za Zhi. 2019;33(2):223–6.
19. Hofer MD, Cooley LF, Martins FE. Narrative review of penile distal urethroplasties and suggestions for optimizing outcomes. Transl Androl Urol. 2021;10(6):2609–16.

Study on the correlation between preoperative inflammatory indexes and adhesional perinephric fat before laparoscopic partial nephrectomy

Teng Ma[1†], Lin Cong[2†], Qianli Ma[3], Zhaoqin Huang[1], Qianqian Hua[1], Xiaojiao Li[1], Ximing Wang[1] and Yunchao Chen[1*]

Abstract

Objective: This study was aimed to evaluate the effect of preoperative composite inflammatory index on adhesional perinephric fat (APF), providing a help for preoperative risk assessment of laparoscopic partial nephrectomy (LPN) in patients with renal cell carcinoma.

Materials and methods: A retrospective study was conducted on 231 patients with renal cell carcinoma, who underwent laparoscopic partial nephrectomy. They were divided into two groups according to whether there was APF during operation. Relevant clinical data, laboratory parameters and imaging examination were obtained before operation to calculate the composite inflammatory index and MAP score. The composite inflammatory index was divided into high value group and low value group by ROC curve method. The related predictive factors of APF were analyzed by logistic regression method.

Results: The APF was found in 105 patients (45.5%). In multivariate analysis, systemic immune inflammation index (SII) (high/low), MAP score, tumor size and perirenal fat thickness were independent predictors of APF. The operation time of patients with APF was longer, and the difference of blood loss was not statistically significant.

Conclusion: SII is an independent predictor of APF before laparoscopic partial nephrectomy.

Keywords: Preoperative composite inflammatory index, Adhesional perinephric fat, Laparoscopic partial nephrectomy, Renal cell carcinoma

Introduction

Partial nephrectomy is the preferred choice for cT1a renal tumors [1], including open partial nephrectomy (OPN), laparoscopic partial nephrectomy (LPN) and robotic partial nephrectomy (RPN). Preoperative evaluation of the feasibility and difficulty of partial nephrectomy is a hot topic in clinical research. In addition to the anatomic characteristics of the tumor itself and the thickness of perirenal fat affecting partial nephrectomy,

*Correspondence: drchenyc@126.com
†Teng Ma and Lin Cong have Contribute equally
[1] Department of Radiology, Shandong Provincial Hospital Affiliated to Shandong First Medical University, No.324, Jingwu Road, Jinan 250021, Shandong, China
Full list of author information is available at the end of the article

adhesional perinephric fat (APF) is another important affecting factor [2, 3].

APF is defined as the inflammatory tissue adhering around the kidney [4], which makes the dissociation of the kidney and the exposure of tumor more difficult, increases the difficulty of operation, prolongs the operation time, and may lead to separation bleeding and renal capsule stripping [5]. The mechanism of APF is complex, and chronic systemic inflammation may be one of its potential causes [6, 7]. Studies have found that inflammatory immune response is involved in the occurrence and development of tumor, and many inflammatory indicators have been confirmed as high-risk factors for tumor prognosis [8–10]. In recent years, a number of new composite inflammatory indicators have been used to evaluate the body's inflammatory response, including neutrophil to lymphocyte ratio (NLR), platelet to lymphocyte ratio (PLR), monocyte to lymphocyte ratio (MLR), prognostic nutritional index (PNI), systemic inflammation response index (SIRI), systemic immune inflammation index (SII) and so on. There is no relevant research report on the correlation between the adhesion of fat around the kidney and the above inflammatory indexes.

At present, image and image-based scoring systems are mainly used to evaluate the situation of peripheral fat adhesion. It has been reported that MAP score and perirenal fat thickness could be used as independent predictors of APF [6, 11]. However, the correlation between APF evaluation and composite inflammatory indicators has not been reported.

This study retrospectively analyzed the clinical data of patients with renal cell carcinoma who underwent partial nephrectomy in our hospital in recent years, to explore the correlation between APF and preoperative composite inflammatory indicators.

Materials and methods

Participants

The data of 285 patients with renal cell carcinoma who underwent laparoscopic partial nephrectomy in our hospital from January 2016 to December 2020 were retrospectively analyzed. Fifty-four patients were excluded because of incomplete clinical data. A total of 231 patients were included in the study (Fig. 1), including 156 males and 75 females, with the median age of 55 (IQR 46–63). Laparoscopic partial nephrectomies were all performed by four surgeons with more than five years of surgical experience. According to the operation record by five surgeons with 11 years, 12 years, 12 years, 14 years, and 15 years experiences, respectively, the patients were divided into adhesion group and non-adhesion group according to whether there was APF (perinephric fat showed inflammatory changes and adhesion with renal capsule, renal tumors are difficult to expose). The radiological evaluation of images was independently performed by a radiologist and one of the surgeons. If the score differed between the two observers, a consensus was reached together after discussion.

Inclusive criteria: (1) single renal tumor with normal contralateral renal structure; (2) preoperative computed tomography; (3) no previous history of renal surgery and abdominal surgery; (4) no previous history of malignant tumor; (5) exclusion of preoperative acute urinary tract infection, pulmonary infection, autoimmune diseases and hematological diseases.

Data collection

The general data of patients were collected, including age, gender, past history and personal history.

Operation related data were collected, including operation time, estimated blood loss and adhesion.

Image related data were collected, including R.E.N.A.L score, MAP score and perirenal fat thickness obtaining from preoperative computed tomography. Perinephric fat thickness was evaluated selecting the CT slice of interest at the level of renal hilum. Posterior perirenal fat thickness was measured from the kidney capsule to the posterior abdominal wall. Perinephric fat stranding was defined as follows: absent (0 points), moderate (2 points), severe (3 points). The MAP score was calculated for each subject using measurements of postrenal fat thickness and perirenal fat chain hypothesized by Davidiuk et al. [6].

The routine examination results of peripheral venous blood within 3 days before operation were collected, including neutrophil count, lymphocyte count, monocyte count, platelet count, CRP and eGFR.

The results of SII, SIRI and PNI were calculated according to the following formula.

$$\text{SII} = \text{platelet count}\left(10^9/\text{L}\right) \times \text{neutrophil count}\left(10^9/\text{L}\right) / \text{lymphocyte count}\left(10^9/\text{L}\right)$$

$$\text{SIRI} = \text{monocyte count}\left(10^9/\text{L}\right) \times \text{neutrophil count}\left(10^9/\text{L}\right) / \text{lymphocyte count}\left(10^9/\text{L}\right)$$

$$\text{PNI} = 10 \times \text{serum albumin}(\text{g/dl}) + 0.005 \times \text{lymphocyte count}\left(\text{mm}^3\right)$$

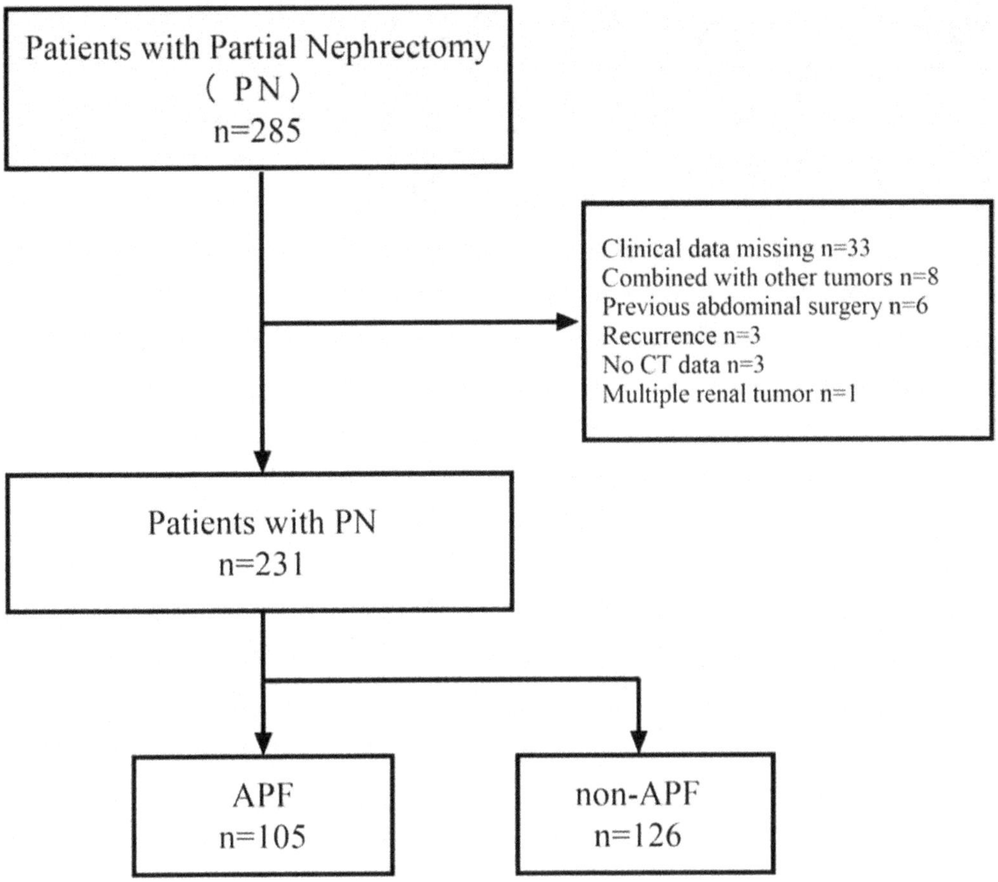

Fig. 1 Patient enrolment process

Statistical method

All analyses were performed with SPSS Statistics, version 23.0 (IBM Corp., Armonk, NY, USA). Descriptive statistics were obtained reporting medians (and interquartile ranges, IQR) for continuous variables, and frequencies and proportions for categorical variables. Univariate and multivariate logistic regression analysis were used to predict the risk factors of APF. $P<0.05$ was considered statistically significant. Independent sample t test was used to compare the measurement data between groups, and chi square test was used to compare the count data between groups.

Results

General information

In this study, 231 patients were collected, including 156 males and 75 females, with the median age of 55 (IQR 46–63). Among them, 45.0% had a history of hypertension, 37.7% had dyslipidemia, 28.1% had a history of smoking, 17.7% had a history of diabetes, and 7.8% had cardiovascular disease (Table 1).

The results showed that there were significant difference in age ($P=0.024$), history of hypertension ($P=0.002$), tumor size ($P<0.001$), MAP score ($P<0.001$) and perirenal fat thickness ($P<0.001$) between patients with APF and patients with non-APF using univariate analysis. Furthermore, the operation time of patients with APF was longer than patients with non-APF (150 min vs 120 min, $P<0.001$). For blood loss, there was no significant difference between groups (50 ml vs 30 ml, $P=0.205$).

Adhesional perinephric fat

The median MAP score was 2 in patients. Patients with APF was observed in 105 patients (45.5%, 105/231), and the corresponding MAP score was higher than patients with non-APF. Among patients with APF, there were 4 patients (5.4%, 4/74) with MAP score of 0–1, 27 patients (45.8% 27/59) with MAP score of 2, and 74 patients (75.5% 74/98) with MAP score of 3–5 (Fig. 2).

Table 1 General information

	All	APF	Non-APF	*P*
Number (%)	231 (100)	105 (45.5)	126 (54.5)	
Age, median (IQR)	55 (46–63)	56 (47–64)	54 (45–60)	0.024
Sex, n (%)				
Male	156 (67.5)	76 (72.4)	80 (63.5)	
Female	75 (32.5)	29 (27.6)	46 (36.5)	
Cardiovascular disease, n (%)	18 (7.8)	8 (7.6)	10 (7.9)	0.929
Hypertension, n (%)	104 (45.0)	59 (56.2)	45 (35.7)	0.002
Diabetes, n (%)	41 (17.7)	18 (17.1)	23 (18.3)	0.826
Dyslipidemia, n (%)	87 (37.7)	39 (37.1)	48 (38.1)	0.882
Smoking, n (%)	65 (28.1)	33 (31.4)	32 (25.4)	0.310
CRP, median (IQR)	1.24 (0.68–2.38)	1.44 (0.79–2.93)	1.14 (0.63–2.19)	0.425
eGFR, median (IQR)	104 (94–111)	104 (93–111)	104 (96–111)	0.425
Creatinine, median (IQR)	65.1 (56.1–74.6)	67.1 (57.3–75.5)	64.1 (54.8–74.5)	0.461
Albumin, mean median (IQR)	42.3 (40.4–44.5)	41.9 (40.0–44.4)	42.8 (40.8–44.7)	0.056
Tumor size, median (IQR)	2.8 (2.0–3.8)	3.0 (2.5–4.2)	2.5 (2.0–3.4)	< 0.001
Location, n (%)				0.754
Left	106 (45.9)	47 (44.8)	59 (46.8)	
Right	125 (54.1)	58 (55.2)	67 (53.2)	
Pathology, n (%)				0.315
Clear cell carcinoma	206 (89.2)	96 (91.4)	110 (87.3)	
Non-clear cell carcinoma	25 (10.8)	9 (8.6)	16 (12.7)	
R.E.N.A.L score, n (%)				0.068
4–6	63 (27.3)	21 (20.0)	42 (33.3)	
7–9	150 (64.9)	76 (72.4)	74 (58.8)	
10–12	18 (7.8)	8 (7.6)	10 (7.9)	
MAP score, median (IQR)	2 (1–3)	3 (2–4)	1 (0–2)	< 0.001
Perirenal fat thickness, median (IQR)	1.1 (0.6–1.7)	1.4 (0.9–2.1)	0.9 (0.5–1.2)	< 0.001
Blood loss, median (IQR)	50 (30–100)	50 (30–100)	30 (30–50)	0.205
Operation time, median (IQR)	130 (110–165)	150 (120–180)	120 (99–150)	< 0.001

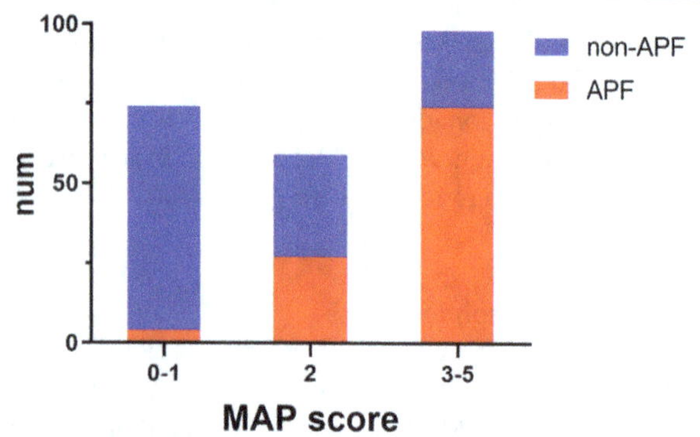

Fig. 2 MAP score distribution in patients

Analysis of inflammatory indexes

The ROC curves of inflammatory indexes were obtained according to the presence or absence of APF. According to the Youden index, the optimal cut-off values of PNI, MLR, PLR, NLR, Siri and SII were 54.9, 0.25, 119.43, 2.14, 0.87 and 523.65, respectively. All patients were divided into high value group and low value group. There were significant differences between groups in NLR ($P=0.002$), MLR ($P=0.007$), SIRI ($P<0.001$) and SII ($P<0.001$) (Table 2).

The independent predictor of APF was analyzed using multivariate analysis (Table 3). The results showed that tumor size (OR = 1.453, $P=0.009$), MAP score (OR = 4.545, $P<0.001$), perirenal fat thickness (OR = 0.503, $P=0.043$), SII (OR = 0.278, $P=0.018$) were independent predictors for patients with APF.

Discussion

With the development of laparoscopy and robot assisted technology, nephron sparing partial nephrectomy has become the preferred treatment for early small renal cell carcinoma [1, 12]. Tumor itself and patient specific variables can increase the complexity of partial nephrectomy

Table 2 Analysis of inflammatory index between groups

	APF	Non-APF	*P*
PNI			
Low	82	86	0.094
High	23	40	
PLR			
Low	37	53	0.290
High	68	73	
NLR			
Low	55	91	0.002
High	50	35	
MLR			
Low	48	80	0.007
High	57	46	
SIRI			
Low	46	90	< 0.001
High	59	36	
SII			
Low	53	95	< 0.001
High	52	31	

[5]. Patient factors refer to the influence of their own physical condition on the operation, including the presence or absence of accessory renal artery and APF, among which APF is the most important factor [4, 13]. APF can cause a series of intraoperative complications. Mibervini et al. studied 1055 patients who underwent PN and found that patients experiencing intraoperative complications had a significantly higher rate of overall postoperative complications (41.6%), surgical postoperative complications (29.2%), Clavien 2 surgical postoperative complications (14.6%) and a significantly longer length of stay (8 days) [14]. Efforts should be made to minimize the risk of intraoperative complications during PN. A recent study showed that assessing the effects of perinephric fat surface density in patients treated with OPN and RPN could help surgeons select the best approach and reduce perioperative complications [15]. However, the mechanism of APF is unclear, which may be related to fibrosis, autoimmunity and inflammatory reaction [3, 16]. In order to further clarify the relationship between the occurrence of APF and systemic inflammatory response in renal cancer patients, 231 patients were collected.

In this study, patients were divided into high value group and low value group according to the best cut-off value of each inflammatory factor. The best cut-off value was obtained from the ROC curve in patients with APF or non-APF. The results showed that there were significant differences in NLR ($P=0.002$), MLR ($P=0.007$), SIRI ($P<0.001$) and SII ($P<0.001$) between groups. Furthermore, the SII was an independent predictors for patients with APF ($P=0.018$).

The levels of neutrophils, lymphocytes and monocytes in peripheral blood reflect the immune function of human peripheral blood and the tumor microenvironment. Neutrophils come from bone marrow, and mature neutrophils are distributed in peripheral blood, which main functions are phagocytosis and killing bacteria. The increase of neutrophils in tumor patients may be due to the secretory function of tumor tissue, which can produce a variety of cytokines to promote bone marrow growth, such as granulocyte colony-stimulating factor (G-CSF) or granulocyte macrophage colony-stimulating factor (GM-CSF) [17, 18]. These growth factors can increase the number of neutrophils in peripheral blood. The increase of neutrophils inhibits the immune activity of lymphocytes, resulting in the decrease of lymphocytes and the decrease of immune function [19]. Under the action of inflammatory chemokines, monocytes in peripheral blood migrate around tumor tissue to form tumor associated macrophages (TAM), which participate in inflammatory immune response and tumor growth

Table 3 Multivariate logistic analysis

Index	Single factor analysis		Multivariate analysis	
	OR (95% CI)	*P*	OR (95% CI)	*P*
Age	1.027 (1.003–1.050)	0.025	–	–
Hypertension	2.309 (1.358–3.924)	0.002	–	–
Tumor size	1.512 (1.205–1.897)	< 0.001	1.453 (1.100–1.023)	0.009
MAP	3.173 (2.346–4.293)	< 0.001	4.545 (2.841–7.273)	< 0.001
Perirenal fat thickness	2.622 (1.770–3.883)	< 0.001	0.503 (0.258–0.978)	0.043
NLR	0.423 (0.245–0.731)	0.002	–	–
MLR	0.484 (0.286–0.821)	0.007	–	–
SIRI	0.312 (0.181–0.538)	< 0.001	–	–
SII	0.333 (0.190–0.581)	< 0.001	0.278 (0.097–0.800)	0.018

[20, 21]. Cytokines produced by systemic inflammatory reaction can also increase the number of platelets, release platelet-derived growth factor, platelet-reactive protein and platelet factor-4, which promote tumor proliferation, invasion and angiogenesis [22, 23]. The increase of neutrophils, platelets and monocytes in the blood often represents the aggravation of inflammation, while the decrease of lymphocyte is the decrease of anti-tumor immune response. The composite inflammatory index composed of inflammatory cells can reflect the relative changes of different blood components, which reflect the host immunity and inflammation more comprehensively compared with single inflammatory index. PLR, MLR and NLR have been proved to be potential prognostic indicators for a variety of malignant tumors [24–26]. SII is a new inflammation index based on neutrophil, platelet and lymphocyte count, which has been proved to be a negative prognostic indicator of small cell lung cancer, hepatocellular carcinoma, esophageal squamous cell carcinoma, and esophagogastric junction tumor [27, 28].

In this study, there were significant differences between high value group and low value group in NLR, MLR, SIRI and SII, which indicated that there was a correlation between APF and systemic inflammatory response. The possible mechanism is that the systemic chronic inflammatory pathway is activated to trigger tissue adhesion. For example, the activated cytokines including interleukin-6 and tumor necrosis factor (TNF-α), chemokines and plasminogen activator inhibitor type 1 (PAI-1) causing the decrease of fibrinolytic activity [29–31]. When this reaction affects the perirenal fat, it will cause fiber adhesion between the fat and renal capsule, leading to the formation of APF, which is manifested as cord like and nodular increased density foci in the perirenal space on CT imaging. Our results were similar to Dariane et al. [32] found that low-level chronic inflammation may eventually lead to renal radiofibrosis.

On the other hand, the role of local inflammatory microenvironment produced by malignant tumor could not be ignored. In this study, the incidence of APF in 231 patients with renal cell carcinoma was 45.5% (105/231), which was close to the results of previous studies [32]. Inflammatory cells, cytokines and chemokines affect tumor growth, differentiation, diffusion and metastasis [33]. Similarly, tumor cells can also react on inflammatory cells. Tumor cells can induce the enhancement of platelet activity and promote the release of platelet granule contents, such as 5-hydroxytryptamine and ADP [34]. Druce et al. [35] found 5-hydroxytryptamine is an important mediator of local and distal fibrosis in small intestinal carcinoid. Therefore, we infer that renal tumor may also indirectly lead to the saponification and adhesion of perirenal fat through the two-way effect of inflammatory microenvironment.

In our study, patients with APF were correlated with age, history of hypertension, tumor size, MAP score and perirenal fat thickness, but not with gender and history of diabetes. Fabrizio et al. showed that metabolic syndrome was the only significant predictor of APF [15]. However, in our study, APF was associated with hypertension, but not with diabetes. The reasons for the differences may be as follows: our study sample size was small, and only patients undergoing LPN were included, but not patients undergoing OPN or RPN. However, it cannot be ruled out that there are a small number of patients who were previously treated for diabetes but did not provide an accurate history of the disease to us. The operation time of patients with APF was longer, but there was no significant difference in blood loss between the two groups. Multivariate logistic regression analysis showed that MAP score (OR = 4.545, $P < 0.001$), tumor size (OR = 1.453, $P = 0.009$), perirenal fat thickness (OR = 0.503, $P = 0.043$) and SII (or 0.278, $P = 0.018$) were independent predictors of perirenal fat adhesion. Previous studies have shown that perirenal fat thickness and MAP score have a strong correlation with APF [6, 36], but our study first reported that SII is one of the independent predictors of APF, further confirmed that systemic inflammatory immune response is involved in the formation of APF. Although MAP score is the strongest predictor of APF (OR = 4.545), we believe that in daily practice, the acquisition process of SII is simpler, and the measurement results are relatively more objective, and the economic cost is lower. Studies by Mari et al. showed that several clinical predictors were associated with postoperative complications [37]. In the future, we will study APF, SII and other factors to verify their influence on postoperative complications.

The limitations of this study are as follows: (1) limited to the retrospective case analysis, we could not further clarify the impact of the dynamic changes of inflammatory indicators on the formation of APF. (2) the critical value of each inflammatory index was determined using ROC curve according to the Youden index. However, there is no consensus on the selection of the critical value at this stage. Therefore, the bias caused by this choice may have a certain impact on the research results. (3) Due to the retrospective nature of the study, there are some missing clinical data of patients that further reduce the reliability of the results. (4) Since all patients underwent LPN, whether the findings of this study can be generalized to patients undergoing OPN or RPN needs further verification. (5) This study is a single center study with a relatively small sample size. Therefore, the exact results need to be confirmed by large-scale prospective multicenter studies in the future.

Conclusions

This study showed that NLR, MLR, SIRI and SII were correlated with APF in patients with renal cell carcinoma, and SII was an independent predictor of APF. Because of the advantages of convenient detection, strong repeatability and low cost, inflammatory markers are expected to play a role in the early prediction of APF, which is helpful for surgeons to assess the operation related risks and make scientific and reasonable preoperative plans.

Acknowledgements
Not application.

Authors' contributions
T.M. and L.C. analyzed and interpreted the patient data regarding patients with renal cell carcinoma who underwent laparoscopic partial nephrectomy. T.M., L.C., Q.M., Z.H., Q.H., X.L., X.W. and Y.C. performed the data collection. T.M. and L.C. were major contributors in writing the manuscript. All authors read and approved the final manuscript.

Author details
[1]Department of Radiology, Shandong Provincial Hospital Affiliated to Shandong First Medical University, No.324, Jingwu Road, Jinan 250021, Shandong, China. [2]Department of Medical Imaging Interventional Therapy, Shandong Provincial Hospital Affiliated to Shandong First Medical University, Jinan 250021, Shandong, China. [3]Department of Radiology, Taian City Central Hospital, Taian 271000, Shandong, China.

References

1. Campbell S, Uzzo RG, Allaf ME, Bass EB, Cadeddu JA, Chang A, Clark PE, Davis BJ, Derweesh IH, Giambarresi L, et al. Renal mass and localized renal cancer: AUA guideline. J Urol. 2017;198(3):520–9.
2. Kawamura N, Saito K, Inoue M, Ito M, Kijima T, Yoshida S, Yokoyama M, Ishioka J, Matsuoka Y, Kihara K, et al. Adherent Perinephric Fat in Asian patients: Predictors and impact on perioperative outcomes of partial nephrectomy. Urol Int. 2018;101(4):437–42.
3. Martin L, Rouviere O, Bezza R, Bailleux J, Abbas F, Schott-Pethelaz AM, Ruffion A, Paparel P. Mayo adhesive probability score is an independent computed tomography scan predictor of adherent Perinephric fat in open partial nephrectomy. Urology. 2017;103:124–8.
4. Bylund JR, Qiong H, Crispen PL, Venkatesh R, Strup SE. Association of clinical and radiographic features with perinephric "sticky" fat. J Endourol. 2013;27(3):370–3.
5. Kocher NJ, Kunchala S, Reynolds C, Lehman E, Nie S, Raman JD. Adherent perinephric fat at minimally invasive partial nephrectomy is associated with adverse peri-operative outcomes and malignant renal histology. BJU Int. 2016;117(4):636–41.
6. Davidiuk AJ, Parker AS, Thomas CS, Leibovich BC, Castle EP, Heckman MG, Custer K, Thiel DD. Mayo adhesive probability score: an accurate image-based scoring system to predict adherent perinephric fat in partial nephrectomy. Eur Urol. 2014;66(6):1165–71.
7. Khene ZE, Peyronnet B, Mathieu R, Fardoun T, Verhoest G, Bensalah K. Analysis of the impact of adherent perirenal fat on peri-operative outcomes of robotic partial nephrectomy. World J Urol. 2015;33(11):1801–6.
8. Aoyama T, Takano M, Miyamoto M, Yoshikawa T, Kato K, Sakamoto T, Takasaki K, Matsuura H, Soyama H, Hirata J, et al. Pretreatment neutrophil-to-lymphocyte ratio was a predictor of lymph node metastasis in endometrial cancer patients. Oncology. 2019;96(5):259–67.
9. Lee SH, Chung MJ, Kim B, Lee HS, Lee HJ, Heo JY, Kim YJ, Park JY, Bang S, Park SW, et al. The significance of the prognostic nutritional index for all stages of pancreatic cancer. Nutr Cancer. 2017;69(3):512–9.
10. Wang L, Wang C, Wang J, Huang X, Cheng Y. A novel systemic immune-inflammation index predicts survival and quality of life of patients after curative resection for esophageal squamous cell carcinoma. J Cancer Res Clin Oncol. 2017;143(10):2077–86.
11. Yang B, Ma LL, Qiu M, Xia HZ, He W, Meng TY, Lu M, Lu J. A novel nephrometry scoring system for predicting peri-operative outcomes of retroperitoneal laparoscopic partial nephrectomy. Chin Med J (Engl). 2020;133(5):577–82.
12. Abou Youssif T, Tanguay S. Natural history and management of small renal masses. Current Oncology. 2009;16:2–7.
13. Yao Y, Gong H, Pang Y, Gu L, Niu S, Xu Y, Li P, Liu K, Tang L, Xuan Y, et al. Risk factors influencing the thickness and stranding of perinephric fat of mayo adhesive probability score in minimally invasive nephrectomy. Med Sci Monit. 2019;25:3825–31.
14. Minervini A, Mari A, Borghesi M, Antonelli A, Bertolo R, Bianchi G, Brunocilla E, Ficarra V, Fiori C, Longo N, et al. The occurrence of intraoperative complications during partial nephrectomy and their impact on postoperative outcome: results from the RECORd1 project. Minerva Urol Nefrol. 2019;71(1):47–54.
15. Fabrizio DIM, Vittori G, Campi R, Mari A, Tellini R, Sforza S, Sessa F, Lucarini S, Miele V, Vignozzi L, et al. Clinical predictors and significance of adherent perinephric fat assessed with Mayo Adhesive Probability (MAP) score and perinephric fat surface density (PnFSD) at the time of partial nephrectomy for localized renal mass. A single high-volume referral center experience. Minerva Urol Nephrol. 2021;73(2):225–32.
16. Gorin MA, Mullins JK, Pierorazio PM, Jayram G, Allaf ME. Increased intra-abdominal fat predicts perioperative complications following minimally invasive partial nephrectomy. Urology. 2013;81(6):1225–30.
17. Balkwill F, Mantovani A. Inflammation and cancer: Back to Virchow? The Lancet. 2001;357(9255):539–45.
18. Asahi Y, Kubonishi I, Imamura J, Kamioka M. Matsushita H: Establishment of a clonal cell line producing granulocyte colony-stimulating factor and parathyroid hormone-related protein from a lung cancer patient with leukocytosis and hypercalcemia. Jpn J Cancer Res. 1996;87(5):451–8.
19. Zhang J, Huang SH, Li H, Li Y, Chen XL, Zhang WQ, Chen HG, Gu LJ. Preoperative lymphocyte count is a favorable prognostic factor of disease-free survival in non-small-cell lung cancer. Med Oncol. 2013;30(1):352.
20. Noy R, Pollard JW. Tumor-associated macrophages: from mechanisms to therapy. Immunity. 2014;41(1):49–61.
21. Wada N, Zaki MA, Hori Y, Hashimoto K, Tsukaguchi M, Tatsumi Y, Ishikawa J, Tominaga N, Sakoda H, Take H, et al. Tumour-associated macrophages in diffuse large B-cell lymphoma: a study of the Osaka Lymphoma Study Group. Histopathology. 2012;60(2):313–9.
22. Nieswandt B, Hafner M, Echtenacher B, Mannel DN. Mannel DN: Lysis of tumor cells by natural killer cells in mice is impeded by platelets. Cancer Res. 1999;59(6):1295–300.
23. Alexandrakis MG, Passam FH, Perisinakis K, Ganotakis E, Margantinis G, Kyriakou DS, Bouros D. Serum proinflammatory cytokines and its relationship to clinical parameters in lung cancer patients with reactive thrombocytosis. Respir Med. 2002;96(8):553–8.
24. Liu J-S, Huang Y, Yang X. Feng J-F: A nomogram to predict prognostic values of various inflammatory biomarkers in patients with esophageal squamous cell carcinoma. Am J Cancer Res. 2015;15(5):2180–9.
25. Krenn-Pilko S, Langsenlehner U, Thurner EM, Stojakovic T, Pichler M, Gerger A, Kapp KS, Langsenlehner T. The elevated preoperative platelet-to-lymphocyte ratio predicts poor prognosis in breast cancer patients. Br J Cancer. 2014;110(10):2524–30.
26. Azab B, Mohammad F, Shah N, Vonfrolio S, Lu W, Kedia S, Bloom SW. The value of the pretreatment neutrophil lymphocyte ratio vs. platelet lymphocyte ratio in predicting the long-term survival in colorectal cancer. Cancer Biomark. 2014;14(5):303–12.
27. Feng JF, Chen S, Yang X. Systemic immune-inflammation index (SII) is a useful prognostic indicator for patients with squamous cell carcinoma of the esophagus. Medicine (Baltimore). 2017;96(4):e5886.
28. Jomrich G, Paireder M, Kristo I, Baierl A, Ilhan-Mutlu A, Preusser M, Asari R, Schoppmann SF. High systemic immune-inflammation index is an adverse prognostic factor for patients with gastroesophageal adenocarcinoma. Ann Surg. 2019;273(3):532–41.
29. Narita S, Kumazawa T, Tsuchiya N, Mingguo H, Saito M, Inoue T, Tsuruta H, Numakura K, Maeno A, Nanjo H, Satoh S. Host-related risk factors for adherent perinephric fat in healthy individuals undergoing laparo-

scopic living-donor nephrectomy. Surg Laparosc Endosc Percutan Tech. 2017;27(4):e69–73.
30. Trayhurn P, Wood IS. Adipokines: inflammation and the pleiotropic role of white adipose tissue. Br J Nutr. 2004;92(3):347–55.
31. Kosaka H, Yoshimoto T, Yoshimoto T, Fujimoto J, Nakanishi K. Interferon-gamma is a therapeutic target molecule for prevention of postoperative adhesion formation. Nat Med. 2008;14(4):437–41.
32. Dariane C, Le Guilchet T, Hurel S, Audenet F, Beaugerie A, Badoual C, Tordjman J, Clement K, Urien S, Pietak M, et al. Prospective assessment and histological analysis of adherent perinephric fat in partial nephrectomies. Urol Oncol. 2017;35(2):e39.
33. Demaria S, Pikarsky E, Karin M, Coussens LM, Chen YC, El-Omar EM, Trinchieri G, Dubinett SM, Mao JT, Szabo E, Krieg A. Cancer and inflammation: Promise for biologic therapy. J Immunother. 2010;33(4):335–51.
34. Kapur R, Semple JW. Platelets as immune-sensing cells. Blood Adv. 2016;22(1):10–4.
35. Druce MR, Bharwani N, Akker SA, Drake WM, Rockall A, Grossman AB. Intra-abdominal fibrosis in a recent cohort of patients with neuroendocrine ('carcinoid') tumours of the small bowel. QJM. 2010;103(3):177–85.
36. Macleod LC, Hsi RS, Gore JL, Wright JL, Harper JD. Perinephric fat thickness is an independent predictor of operative complexity during robot-assisted partial nephrectomy. J Endourol. 2014;28(5):587–91.
37. Mari A, Campi R, Schiavina R, Amparore D, Antonelli A, Artibani W, Barale M, Bertini R, Borghesi M, Bove P, et al. Nomogram for predicting the likelihood of postoperative surgical complications in patients treated with partial nephrectomy: a prospective multicentre observational study (the RECORd 2 project). BJU Int. 2019;124(1):93–102.

25

Diagnosis and treatment of anterior urethral strictures in China: An internet-based survey

Changhao Hou[1,2†], Yubo Gu[1,2†], Wei Yuan[1,2], Zeyu Wang[1,2], Jiahao Lin[1,2], Qiang Fu[1,2*] and Lujie Song[1,2*]

Abstract

Background: To investigate the current diagnostic and therapeutic approaches to anterior urethral strictures of Chinese urologists and to compare with developed countries and the American Urologic Association guidelines.

Methods: Anonymous questionnaires were distributed to members of Official Wechat Account of urology from March 19, 2020 to April 10, 2020. Descriptive and multiple correspondence analysis were used to analyze the data.

Results: A total of 1276 online questionnaires were received. The response rate was 21.7% (1276/5878). The most common diagnostic methods for anterior urethral stricture were urethrography (90.7%) and urethrocystoscopy (85.4%), while urethral dilation (92.3%) and internal urethrotomy (60.1%) were the main therapeutic procedures. End-to-end urethroplasty (45.2%) was the most common open surgery, followed by skin flap urethroplasty (14.9%) and free graft urethroplasty (12.4%). 76.2% of urologists used urethroplasty only after the failure of minimally invasive surgery (reconstructive ladder treatment strategy). Furthermore, middle-aged or elderly urologists who had attended trainings, had senior practice roles, and who utilized a reconstructive ladder treatment approach were most likely to perform urethroplasties.

Conclusions: Anterior urethral stricture treatment in China is still dominated by minimally invasive surgery, with most urologists using the reconstructive ladder treatment strategy. In general, the overall diagnostic and therapeutic strategies were similar between China and developed countries, with some deviations from the American Urologic Association guidelines.

Keywords: Anterior urethral strictures, Practice pattern, Survey, Urethroplasty

Introduction

Although urethral strictures can be traced back to ancient times [1], here is still a poor understanding of this disease. According to recent data, 193–627 out of 100,000 men suffer from urethral strictures [2], with the morbidity and etiology of this disease varying greatly between different countries and regions [3, 4]. Trauma (51.67%), iatrogenic causes (34.49%), infection or inflammation (5.79%), and lichen sclerosus (4.22%) are the main etiologies of male urethral strictures [4]. Anterior urethral strictures are the most common, accounting for more than 90% of cases in the developed world [5, 6].

The clinical symptoms of patients with anterior urethral strictures are varied, however, the most apparent symptom is a weakening of the urinary stream. Although anterior urethral strictures can generally be diagnosed clinically, a stricture's site, length, and scar thickness are more difficult to determine [7]. Therefore, urethroscopy, urethrography, urethral ultrasound, magnetic resonance imaging are used to characterize these lesions [7].

Urethral strictures can be treated surgically using two main approaches: minimally invasive surgery and urethroplasty. The former is generally favored by urologists because of its ease of application and simplicity.

*Correspondence: jamesqfu@aliyun.com; ljsong@sjtu.edu.cn
†Changhao Hou and Yubo Gu have contributed equally to this study.
[1] Department of Urology, Shanghai Jiao Tong University Affiliated Sixth People's Hospital, Shanghai 200233, China
Full list of author information is available at the end of the article

However, this approach has also been found to have an increasing number of complications and a high recurrence rate. Urethroplasty, on the other hand, has a high success rate and low recurrence rate; however, it has not been as widely studied [8]. The clinical management of urethral strictures remains controversial because of its diverse clinical manifestations, numerous surgical methods, various complications, and recent improvements in surgical instrumentation, clinician experience, and postoperative follow-up. Our previous study showed that the rates of endourological urethral surgery decreased significantly and the rates of urethroplasty increased during recent years.

The diagnostic and therapeutic approaches to anterior urethral strictures have been an ongoing focus of research. Investigators in the United States, Germany, Italy, and other developed countries have conducted related studies [9–13]. However, their findings do not necessarily reflect the situation in other regions. Furthermore, studies in developing countries are still lacking. As the largest developing country in the world, China has a vast territory, uneven economic development, and different levels of diagnosis and treatment in different regions. We conducted this study in order to better understand the diagnostic and therapeutic patterns of anterior urethral strictures in Chinese urologists and to explore the differences with developed countries and current guidelines.

Methods

Questionnaire

Based on prior performed surveys in the United States [10], the Netherlands [13] and in Italy [11], we modified a questionnaire suitable for Chinese urologists by referencing relevant literature and consulting experts in the field of urethral reconstruction. This survey queried respondents about demographic information, preoperative evaluations, surgery-related experience, and postoperative management using both single-choice and multiple-choice questions. Before the formal survey, we pilot-tested our survey on a sample of 60 urologists and finalized the 15-question survey (see Additional file 1) based on that feedback (e.g., eliminated outdated options, adjusting terminology).

Next, we use the largest Official Wechat Account of urology in China to distribute the survey. The members of this official account are all urologists. In order to ensure the efficiency of the survey, we set that each urologist can only response in once. One reminder was sent to all urologists. This study was conducted from March 19, 2020 to April 10, 2020 and approved by the ethics committee at our institution. All enrolled urologists signed a digital informed consent form before accessing the questionnaire online.

Statistical analysis

The collected questionnaire data are presented as frequencies and percentages. Statistical analyses were performed using SPSS (version 20.0; SPSS Inc., Chicago, IL, USA). Multiple correspondence analysis (MCA) is a descriptive dimensionality reduction technique that employs categorical variables [14] (respondent demographics, surgery-related experience, and training). The results were explained according to parameters such as the total inertia. The total inertia represents the variability. The explanatory power of the variability provided ranges from 0 to 100% and the greater the variability, the greater the explanatory power. Statistical significance was defined as a P value of < 0.05.

Results

Respondent demographics

The questionnaire was distributed to 5878 urologists. A total of 1276 online questionnaires were received. The response rate was 21.7%. Excluding two incomplete questionnaires and seven respondents who lacked treatment experience with urethral strictures. In the end, 1267 valid questionnaires were obtained. Respondent age, practice role, hospital setting, etc. are shown in Table 1. The distribution of urologists in each province is shown in Additional file 1).

This survey involved urologists in all 31 provinces and municipalities of mainland China. The most common age group of respondents was between 30–39 years old. Attending urologists (31.2%) and associate chief urologists comprised the majority. A majority (54.5%) of urologists worked in grade A tertiary hospitals, while 408 urologists worked in secondary hospitals or those inferior to secondary hospitals. Of all respondents, 53.2% of urologists stated that they had participated in training related to urethral repair and reconstruction.

Preoperative evaluation and surgery related experience

Of all respondents, 52% believed that the maximum length of stricture for internal urethrotomy (IU) was 1 cm or less, while 277 believed that < 2 cm was appropriate, and 25 believed that < 3 cm was appropriate. In addition, 7.9% of urologists stated that stricture length was not the main criterion for IU. Among the types of IU, 57.1% of urologists tended to use cold knife for IU and 20.8% tended to use laser IU. When performing intraoral mucosal urethroplasty, more than half of urologists (687/1267, 54.2%) preferred the buccal mucosa, followed by the lingual mucosa (430/1267, 33.9%), lower lip mucosa (123/1267, 9.8%), and upper lip mucosa (27/1267,

Table 1 Respondent demographics

Characteristics	No. of urologists	Percentage, %
Age (yr)		
<30	70	5.5
30–39	538	42.5
40–49	484	38.2
50–59	164	12.9
≧60	11	0.9
Practice role		
Resident urologist	116	9.2
Attending urologist	471	37.2
Deputy chief urologist	451	35.6
Chief urologist	229	18.1
Hospital setting		
Grade A tertiary hospital	690	54.5
Grade B tertiary hospital	169	13.3
Secondary hospital	394	31.1
Inferior to secondary hospital	14	1.1
*Hospital location**		
Northeast China	96	7.6
Central China	355	28.0
Eastern China	461	36.4
Western China	355	28.0
Attended trainings		
Yes	674	53.2
No	593	46.8

Hospital location: The northeast China* Heilongjiang Province, Jilin Province, Liaoning Province, Neimenggu Province. *The central China* Shanxi Province, Henan Province, Hubei Province, Hunan Province, Jiangxi Province, Anhui Province. *The eastern China* Beijing, Tianjin, Hebei Province, Shandong Province, Jiangsu Province, Shanghai, Zhejiang Province, Fujian Province, Guangdong Province, Hainan Province. *The western China* Chongqing, Sichuan Province, Guangxi Province, Guizhou Province, Yunnan Province, Shaanxi Province, Gansu Province, Ningxia Province, Xinjiang Province, Qinghai Province, Tibet Province

2.1%). When reporting their greatest concern while performing urethroplasty, most urologists were concerned about postoperative complications, such as sexual function and postoperative infection, with the minority of urologists reporting the difficulty of the surgery. Preoperative evaluation and surgery related experience are shown in Table 2.

Postoperative management

After IU, catheters were retained for 2 weeks by 40.1% of urologists, 72 h by 2.6%, 1 week by 12.1%, 3 weeks by 9.7%, 4 weeks by 27.5%, and more than 4 weeks by 9.9%. After urethral reconstruction, 32.6% of urologists indwelled catheters for 2 weeks, 15% indwelled for 3 weeks, 32% indwelled for 4 weeks, and 13% indwelled for more than 4 weeks, with 5% removing the catheter after 1 week. Six urologists believed that catheters could be removed after 72 h.

Correspondence of respondent demographics, surgery related experience and training

Based on the above survey results, we identified variables with statistical differences, including age ($P<0.01$), practice role ($P<0.01$), hospital location ($P<0.01$), treatment strategy ($P<0.01$), management ($P<0.01$) and number of urethroplasties ($P<0.01$). Hospital setting ($P=0.129$) was excluded. We then used the MCA technique to show correlations between categorical variables. MCA is a descriptive dimensionality reduction technique that employs categorical variables. The positions of the categories of each variable in the multidimensional plane can be used to determine groups with similar patterns through graphical representation [15]. Then, a hierarchical cluster analysis was performed from the coordinates obtained in the MCA to confirm the verified groups by proximity in the visual inspection. Next, a hierarchical cluster analysis was performed from the coordinates obtained in the MCA map according to the proximity in the visual inspection [16]. The closer the distance between the two variables is, the stronger the correlation between the two variables is.

In the MCA of respondent demographics and training, the inertia for all variables in the two dimensions were 0.300 and 0.411, respectively (Fig. 1A). The total inertia corresponding to the two dimensions in the MCA explained for 71.1% of the total data variability. The MCA map (Fig. 1B) for urologists who did not attend training showed that the following characteristics were associated with this group: performed 0 or 1–5 cases, 30–39 years of age, attending urologist, and the reconstructive ladder treatment strategy. In contrast, the group of urologists who had attended training were associated with the following characteristics: performed 6–10, 11–20, or ≧20 cases; 40–49, 50–59, or ≧60 years of age; associate chief or chief urologist; and a non-reconstructive ladder treatment strategy.

In the MCA of surgery-related experience and training, the inertia for all variables in the two dimensions were 0.596 and 0.500, respectively (Fig. 1C). Urethral dilation, urethral realignment, and IU were associated with urologists who had not attended training, while perineal urethrostomy, skin flap urethroplasty, and free graft urethroplasty were associated with urologists who had attended training (Fig. 1D). There was a strong correlation between these factors, demonstrating that urologists who had attended training were significantly more likely to perform open surgeries.

Table 2 Approach to preoperative evaluations for anterior urethral strictures and surgery-related experience of Chinese urologists

		No. of urologists	Percentage, %
Treatment strategy	Reconstructive ladder treatment strategy[a]	965	76.2
	Performance of a primary Urethroplasty[b] if indicated	302	23.8
What methods do you usually use to diagnose anterior urethral strictures? (multiple choice)	Uroflowmetry	680	53.7
	Postvoid residual urine	548	43.3
	Urethroscopy	1076	84.9
	Urethrography	1143	90.2
	Urethral ultrasound	127	10.0
	Trial catheterization	699	55.2
	Trial urethral dilation	762	60.1
	Other	23	1.8
Which of the following procedures have you performed in the last year? (multiple-choice)	Urethral dilation	1170	92.3
	Internal urethrotomy	762	60.1
	Urethral anastomosis	573	45.2
	Skin-flap urethroplasty	189	14.9
	Free-graft urethroplasty	157	12.4
	Endourethral stent	136	10.7
	Perineal urethrostomy	142	11.2
	Urethral realignment	548	43.3
	Urethral meatotomy	427	33.7
	Other	11	0.9
No. of urethroplasties	0	384	30.3
	1–5	595	47.0
	6–10	175	13.8
	11–20	53	4.2
	>20	60	4.7
Greatest concern when performing urethroplasty	Major hemorrhage during the operation	187	14.8
	Difficulty obtaining samples from the oral mucosa	281	22.2
	Trauma during oral mucous membrane sampling	135	10.7
	Difficulty obtaining genital skin flap from an	260	20.5
	unclear dissection	614	48.5
	Influencing sexual function	306	24.2
	Postoperative infection	632	49.9
	Urethral restenosis	1167	92.1
	Other	36	2.8

[a] *Reconstructive ladder strategy* Starting with minimally invasive procedures (including dilatation/urethrotomy) and only considering open urethroplasty after failure of the initial approach

[b] *Urethroplasty* Urethral anastomosis, skin-flap urethroplasty, free-graft urethroplasty, urethral traction, perineal urethrostomy, urethral realignment, urethral meatotomy

Discussion

To the best of our knowledge, this survey included the largest number of participants of any existing survey related to anterior urethral strictures and was the first survey of anterior urethral strictures conducted in China, Asia, or any developing country. It was also the first internet-based anterior urethral stricture survey. Internet-based surveys can overcome the limitations of traditional questionnaires, allowing for the collection of more samples at a lower cost over less time. It is worth mentioning that the urologists who participated in our survey were not limited to specialists in the field of urethral repair and reconstruction, since, in China, both general urologists and specialists participate in the diagnosis and treatment of this disease. Therefore, our study better reflects the contemporary characteristics of the diagnosis and treatment of anterior urethral strictures in China.

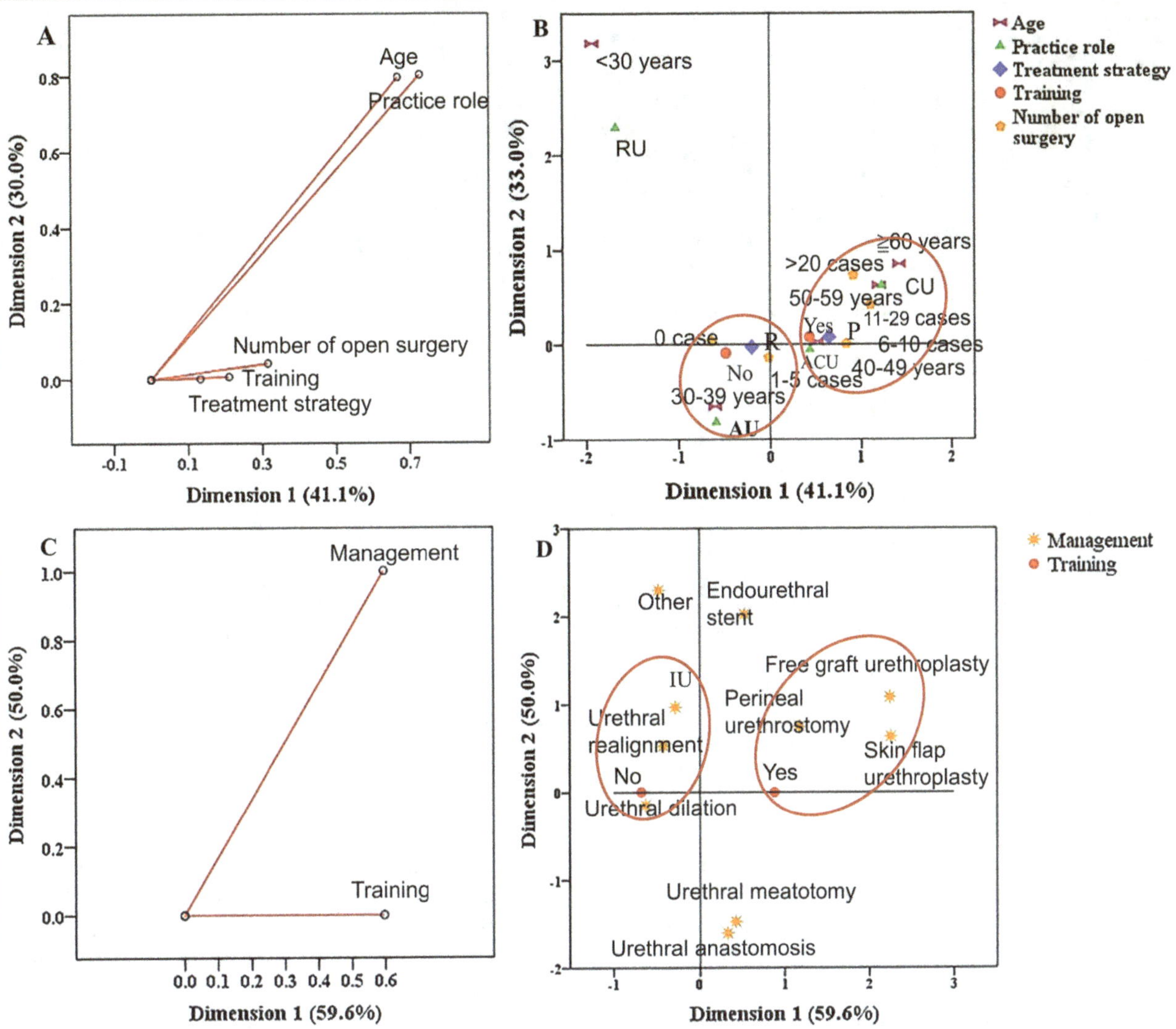

Fig. 1 Correspondence of respondent demographics, surgery related experience and training. **A** Discrimination measures graph: training and respondent demographics. **B** MCA map between training and respondent demographics. **C** Discrimination measures graph: training and management. **D** MCA map between training and management. MCA was used to explore the correspondence of respondent demographics, surgery related experience and training. These figures show the correlations between the scattered points of each variable in each category. The closer the distance between the scattered points, the more obvious the correlation. (*RU* resident urologist, *CU* chief urologist, *AU* attending urologist)

Although it has been 13 years since the first related survey in the USA [10], our results found that the overall diagnostic and therapeutic approaches to anterior urethral strictures in China have not changed much in comparison to developed countries [9–13]. There were, however, some discrepancies with American Urologic Association (AUA) guidelines [17]. In terms of the preoperative diagnosis, 78% of Chinese urologists did not rely on a single diagnostic procedure but rather used multiple methods, which is consistent with the AUA guidelines that one individual test cannot make a definitive diagnosis and that retrograde urethrography should be the primary choice [17]. Urethrography was the most common diagnostic method (90.7%) reported in this survey, which was higher than has been reported in other countries, including the Netherlands (72%), Turkey (55%), and Italy (22%). The percentage of urologists utilizing urethroscopy was similar to what has been reported in prior studies. Compared with the Netherlands (93.8%) and Turkey (69.7%), the utilization rate of uroflowmetry (53.7%) was low (Fig. 2A), perhaps because, in patients with typical symptoms of

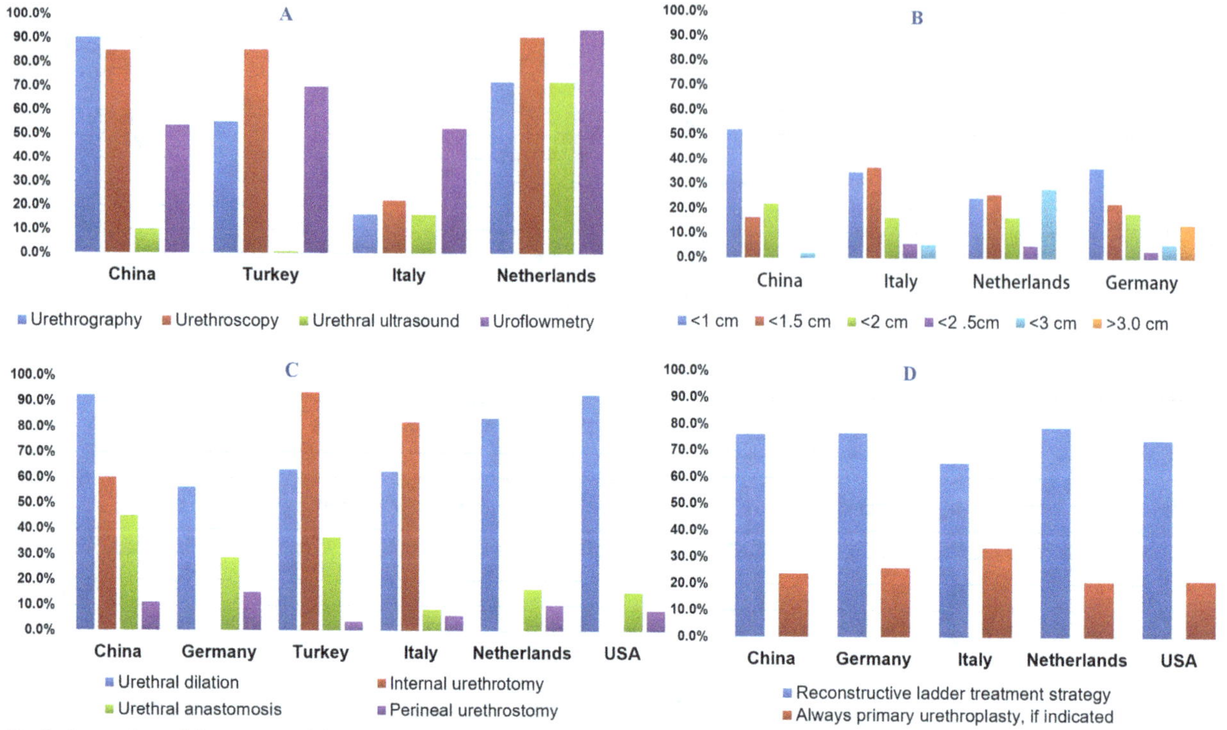

Fig. 2 Comparison of diagnostic and therapeutic approaches to anterior urethral strictures in different countries. **A** Comparison of diagnostic methods for anterior urethral strictures in different countries. **B** Maximum stricture lengths for IU in different countries. **C** Surgical procedures performed for anterior urethral strictures in the last year; and **D** treatment strategies in different countries

an anterior urethral stricture (e.g., dysuria) some urologists may not think a uroflowmetry examination is necessary. Additionally, 10.1% of urologists used urethral ultrasonography. Furthermore, a considerable number of urologists adopted invasive approaches during evaluations, such as trail urethral dilation and trail catheterization, which has not been mentioned in previous surveys or AUA guidelines.

Increasing evidence demonstrates that urethroplasty is the gold standard for treatment of urethral strictures [18]. However, our survey results showed that urethral dilation (92.3%) and IU (60.1%) were still the most commonly used procedures by Chinese urologists, which is consistent with all previous surveys. While Chinese urologists most commonly used urethral dilation, previous studies have shown a tendency to use IU (Germany, 87.2%; Turkey, 93.5%; China, 60.1%) (Fig. 2C). More than half of urologists preferred to use cold-knife IU, which is in accordance with our clinical practice. Also, only about one-fifth of respondents followed the AUA guideline [17] that the maximum suitable length for IU is less than 2 cm (Fig. 2B), which was higher than in developed countries, such as the Netherlands (16.6%), Germany (18.4%), and Italy (16.4%). AUA guidelines also recommend removing the urethral catheter within 72 h following a dilation or direct visual internal urethrotomy [17]. However, only 2.6% of our respondents followed this recommendation.

An article about learning curves of urologists pointed out that the average number of anterior urethroplasties required to reach proficiency (defined as a success rate of > 90%) is approximately 100 cases [19]. To our surprise, 33.3% of respondents stated that they had not performed urethroplasties, compared with 77% in the Netherlands, 73.2% in Germany, 60.8% in Italy, and 57.8% in the USA. However, the majority of respondents (77.3%) had performed less than five urethroplasties in the prior year, with only eight (8.9%) performing more than 10 cases. Therefore, most respondents were likely unfamiliar with urethroplasty. The rate of urethroplasty may also have been low because of financial factors, with some urologists believing that the cost of IU is less than that of urethroplasty. Although our survey did not address this problem, existing models have proven that urethroplasty is economically advantageous [19]. Santucci [20] stated that, if urethroplasty is not performed, patients with urethral stricture should be referred to urologists with expertise, instead of being treated with futile repeated dilation, which is similar to the expert opinions in the AUA guidelines. Furthermore, about two-thirds of urologists have performed urethroplastyies, but some still prefer minimally invasive surgery, such as urethral dilatation or IU. In fact, this is consistent with the treatment strategy of anterior urethral stricture that we learn from our survey.

In our survey, 72.2% of urologists considered urethroplasty only after failure of minimally invasive surgical approaches, with 23.8% believing that urethroplasty should be performed first if the indication is appropriate, which was almost identical to the rates in Germany, Italy, the Netherlands, and the USA (Fig. 2D). In addition, the practice role, hospital location, and participation in training were significantly different based on the treatment strategy ($P < 0.01$). Bullock et al. [10] considered that the "reconstructive ladder" strategy is erroneous, educating urologists to understand the high reference rate of successive IU and the myth of the reconstructive ladder is critical. But Clemens [12] argued that this treatment strategy is justifiable and the most cost-effective approach for short bulbar strictures. Topakta et al. [21] analyzed 133 patients who underwent urethroplasty for bulbar urethral strictures and evaluated the effects of a previous IU, demonstrating that the success rates for urethroplasties could be affected by a previous history of any endoscopic procedures, which suggests that a non-reconstructive ladder treatment approach may be more appropriate.

The MCA technique is a multivariate statistical analysis that can describe the correlation between different variables or between different categories of the same variable [15]. An MCA map can intuitively reflect the relationship between variables, especially for categorical variables. Based on the MCA results, there were significant differences in respondent demographics and surgery-related experience between urologists who had attended training and those who had not. Urologists were more likely to perform urethroplasties if they had attended training were in senior practice roles, were middle-aged or elderly, or if they utilized the reconstructive ladder treatment approach. Michael et al. [22] conducted an anonymous survey about barriers to accessing urethroplasty, with the results suggesting that the best predictor of a urethroplasty recommendation was formal training in urethroplasty. Therefore, we speculate that strengthening training may help to improve the diagnostic and therapeutic level to anterior urethral strictures. As the largest urethral repair referral center in China, our institution plays an important role in this task.

It should, however, be noted that our study has some limitations. First, our survey does not cover all the questions about the diagnosis and treatment of anterior urethral stricture, because we have to consider the answer time of the questionnaire. Second, the content chosen by urologists represents their main views on the diagnosis and treatment of anterior urethral stricture, but many factors in clinical practice may affect their final decision. Therefore, there may be differences in the actual treatment measures adopted by urologists and the choice of questionnaires. In addition, our response rate was low (21.7%). It is worth mentioning that the urologists who participated in our survey were general urologists. A certain percentage of urologists are not familiar with the field of urethral repair and reconstruction. This is the main reason why the response rate is not high. Our survey cannot guarantee that the respondents who participated in this survey were representative of general urologists in China in terms of age, practice role, hospital setting, etc., which may be related to our use of online surveys.

Conclusions

In China, anterior urethral strictures are primarily managed by minimally invasive surgery and the majority of urologists use the reconstructive ladder treatment strategy. The overall diagnostic and therapeutic strategies for anterior urethral strictures were similar between China and developed countries, with some deviations from the AUA guidelines. The standard of care should be in line with guidelines in managing urethral stricture disease. Finally, strengthening relevant training for urologists may help to improve the diagnostic and therapeutic approaches to anterior urethral strictures.

Abbreviations

AUA: American Urologic Association; IU: Internal urethrotomy; MCA: Multiple correspondence analysis; RUG: Retrograde urethrography.

Supplementary Information

Additional file 1. The questionnaire and the distribution of urologists in each province.

Acknowledgements

The Official Wechat Account of the Learning Alliance provided technical support for this survey. We thank Breyer, Benjamin for his valuable comments on draft manuscripts.

Authors' contributions

CH, QF and LS were responsible for the study design, planning and data collection. CH, YG and WY were responsible for data analysis and interpretation. ZW and JL were responsible for the collection and assembly of data. All authors was responsible for writing the initial draft of the manuscript, and subsequent drafts were reviewed by all authors listed. All authors had input on interpretation and reporting of study findings. All authors provided approval for the published version of this manuscript.

Author details
[1]Department of Urology, Shanghai Jiao Tong University Affiliated Sixth People's Hospital, Shanghai 200233, China. [2]Shanghai Eastern Institute of Urologic Reconstruction, Shanghai 200233, China.

References

1. Webster GDKR, Sihelnik SA. Urethroplasty management in 100 cases of urethral stricture: a rationale for procedure selection. J Urol. 1985;134(5):892–8.
2. Santucci RAJG, Wise M. Male urethral stricture disease. J Urol. 2007;177(5):1667–74.
3. Ansari MSYP, Srivastava A, et al. Etiology and characteristics of pediatric urethral strictures in a developing country in the 21st century. J Pediatr Urol. 2019;15(4):403.e401-403.e408.
4. Xu YMSL, Wang KJ, et al. Changing trends in the causes and management of male urethral stricture disease in China: an observational descriptive study from 13 centres. BJU Int. 2015;116(6):938–44.
5. Palminteri EBE, Verze P, et al. Contemporary urethral stricture characteristics in the developed world. Urology. 2013;81(1):191–6.
6. Stein DMTD, Barbagli G, et al. A geographic analysis of male urethral stricture aetiology and location. BJU Int. 2013;112(6):830–4.
7. Heidenreich ADW, Bonfig R, et al. Ultrasound in the evaluation of urethral stricture disease: a prospective study in 175 patients. Br J Urol. 1994;74(1):93–8.
8. Pickard RGB, Carnell S, Shen J, et al. Open urethroplasty versus endoscopic urethrotomy for recurrent urethral stricture in men: the OPEN RCT. Health Technol Assess. 2020;24(61):1–110.
9. Akyuz MSZ, Koca O, et al. Adult urethral stricture: practice of Turkish urologists. Int Braz J Urol. 2016;42(2):339–45.
10. Bullock TLBS. Adult anterior urethral strictures: a national practice patterns survey of board certified urologists in the United States. J Urol. 2007;177(2):685–90.
11. Palminteri EMS, Berdondini E, et al. Male urethral strictures: a national survey among urologists in Italy. Urology. 2014;83(2):477–84.
12. Rosenbaum CMRC, Borgmann H, et al. Management of anterior urethral strictures in adults: a survey of contemporary practice in Germany. Urol Int. 2017;99(1):43–50.
13. van Leeuwen MA, Brandenburg JJ, Kok ET, et al. Management of adult anterior urethral stricture disease: nationwide survey among urologists in the Netherlands. Eur Urol. 2011;60(1):159–66.
14. Nenadic OGM. Correspondence analysis in R, with two- and three-dimensional graphics: the ca package. J Stat Softw. 2007;20(1):1–13.
15. Sivasankaran SK, Balasubramanian V. Investigation of pedestrian crashes using multiple correspondence analysis in India. Int J Inj Contr Saf Promot. 2020;27(2):144–55.
16. Silva MD, de Oliveira RD, Braga JU, et al. Breastfeeding patterns in cohort infants at a high-risk fetal, neonatal and child referral center in Brazil: a correspondence analysis. BMC Pediatr. 2020;20(1):372.
17. Wessells HAK, Elliott S, et al. Male urethral stricture: American Urological Association Guideline. J Urol. 2017;197(1):182–90.
18. Rourke KFWB, Kodama R, et al. Canadian Urological Association guideline on male urethral stricture. Can Urol Assoc J. 2020;14(10):305–16.
19. Rourke KF, Jordan G. Primary urethral reconstruction: the cost minimized approach to the bulbous urethral stricture. J Urol. 2005;175(4):1206–10.
20. Santucci RA. Should we centralize referrals for repair of urethral stricture? J Urol. 2009;182(4):1259–60.
21. Topaktas RAMKM, Kanberoglu H, et al. Is minimal invasive technique harmful in treatment of urethral stricture? Niger J Clin Pract. 2019;22(3):406–9.
22. Consolo MJSK, Robison C, et al. Barriers to accessing urethroplasty. Rev Urol. 2016;18(4):188–93.

26

A systematic review of penile prosthesis infection and meta-analysis of diabetes mellitus role

Lucas Mira Gon*, Caio César Citatini de Campos, Brunno Raphael Iamashita Voris, Luís Augusto Passeri, Adriano Fregonesi and Cássio Luís Zanettini Riccetto

Abstract

Background: Infection is the most feared complication of a penile prosthesis. Diabetes mellitus (DM) is widely known to increase the risk of several infections, but its role in the penile prosthesis is still controversial. This systematic review aims to show the contemporary scenario of penile prosthesis infection and present a meta-analysis about DM contribution to penile prosthesis infection.

Methods: The review was performed with no language or time limitation, including ten databases. The included articles were about the male population who received a penile prosthesis with no model restriction, with a minimum follow up of 1 year, and outcomes adequately reported.

Results: The mean infection incidence of penile prosthesis ranged from 0.33 to 11.4%. In early 2000, the general incidence of infection was 3 to 5%, then, the introduction of coated materials decreased it to 0.3 to 2.7%. The meta-analysis showed that diabetes mellitus is related to an increased risk of penile prosthesis infection with an *odds ratio* of 1.53 (95% CI 1.15–2.04).

Conclusions: Penile prosthesis infection decreased in the last decades but remains a significant cause of reoperation, and it is related to lower prosthesis survival. Meta-analysis concludes that diabetes mellitus is related to a higher risk of penile prosthesis infection.

Keywords: Penile prosthesis, Penile implants, Infection, Review, Meta-analysis, Diabetes mellitus

Background

The penile prosthesis was introduced in the 1970s and remained the most effective treatment to erectile dysfunction refractory to oral and injectable drugs [1, 2]. In the last 40 years, several improvements in materials and surgical techniques led to high satisfaction rates of 80 to 90% [3, 4]. However, complications do exist and range from 7 to 20% [5], mostly related to mechanical malfunction, infection, and erosion. The estimated cost of penile prosthesis removal is about 10 thousand dollars, which is six-fold higher than the initial implantation [6].

Surgical site infection is the most feared complication. It causes pain, local abscess, and even sepsis that requires prompt hospitalization and reoperation [7]. The prosthesis removal leads to fibrosis of the cavernosum corpus and reduction of penile length and girth, making a new prosthesis insertion much more difficult [8].

Diabetes mellitus (DM) impairs microcirculation and causes neuropathy, and approximately 50% of diabetic patients have some degree of erectile dysfunction. The corpus cavernosum of diabetic patients are less responsive to relaxation due to the superoxide radicals production, impairing nitrous oxide and cyclic-GMP

*Correspondence: lucasmgon@gmail.com
Division of Urology of Department of Surgery, Faculty of Medical Sciences, Hospital de Clinicas, University of Campinas – UNICAMP, Rua Vital Brazil, 250, Campinas, SP 13083-590, Brazil

production. Thus, diabetic patients are less responsive to oral therapy [9]. Patients with diabetes are more prone to infection because of leucocyte dysfunction and micro-angiopathy. There is evidence of a three-fold higher risk of penile prosthesis infection in DM compared to non-diabetic patients. However, other studies show no difference, and there is still controversy about whether DM increases the risk of penile prosthesis infection [10, 11].

Several device improvements reduced mechanical failures of penile prosthesis, but infection remained an important cause of reoperation. Therefore, the efforts were directed to reduce infection in the past years [8, 12]. This study aims to gather information about penile prosthesis evolution regarding infections and to present a meta-analysis of diabetes mellitus contribution to penile prosthesis infection.

Methods

This review was performed with no language or time limitation, to gather all available data about penile prosthesis, in ten databases: Medline, PubMed, LILACS, IBECS, MEdCarib, CINAHL, Scopus, Web of Science, Embase and Cochrane Library. The search strategy included the terms: "*penile prosthesis*" or "*penile implantation*" and "*postoperative complications*" or "*prosthesis-related infections*" or "*treatment outcome*". It followed the PRISMA statement, was registered at PROSPERO with number CRD 42019117734, and had no founding resources.

All the articles had the title and abstract evaluated by two independent authors who selected relevant studies blinded from each other. A third and more experienced author resolved conflicting selection. The included articles were about the male population who received a penile prosthesis with no model restriction, with a minimum follow up of 1 year, outcomes and complications adequately reported. The studies had quality assessed using "Grading of Recommendations, Assessment, Development and Evaluations" (GRADE) framework [13]. The evaluated outcomes were surgical site infection, prosthesis infection, prosthesis revision, and removal. The outcomes were compared with time, techniques, prosthesis types, and diabetes mellitus presence.

The exclusion criteria were case reports, articles about surgical technique, and in vitro tests. All studies about transgender patients were excluded, as they assess a specific population and different surgical procedures. The studies focused on the quality of life without outcomes assessment, and those that stated to have no complications were excluded either. Considering infection incidence, studies that started with less than a hundred patients were excluded due to the risk of underestimation of complications.

Each study had data extracted including author, publication year, study design, penile prosthesis type, the number of patients, mean age, follow-up, infection, reoperation, prosthesis removal, or replacement. The data are presented as incidence ratio, with mean and standard deviation when available. The relation between diabetes mellitus and penile prosthesis infection is presented with a meta-analysis, and *odds ratio* calculated with Open Meta for Macintosh version 12.11.14. Significance was adopted as $p < 0.05$ and 95% confidence interval (95% CI).

Results

Literature overview

The research strategy was completed in January 2018 and turned out 4164 articles. After excluding 2012 duplicates, the 2152 articles had titles analyzed by two authors, who excluded yet 464 duplicates. The remaining had the abstract analyzed to exclude case reports, experimental studies, retrospective, and small series. In the end, 80 articles were fully assessed for eligibility, and 41 included in the analysis. The study selection is shown in a flow diagram (Fig. 1), while Table 1 presents the characteristics of the included studies and the infection rates.

The literature about penile prosthesis relies on prospective cohorts, retrospective studies, and case series; the majority of studies do not present controls, or use historical data as controls. There is only one randomized trial available about the AMS 700 (*American Medical Systems, Minneapolis, MN, USA*) and the Titan (*Coloplast, Minneapolis, MN, USA*), presented in 2013 [14]. Both are inflatable and coated penile prosthesis, and were evaluated for satisfaction, curvature correction for Peyronie's disease and mechanical survival. There were only 2 cases of infection from 138 patients with no report of group or time. The authors state that there was no statistical difference between groups, and the study was not designed to assess infection. Table 1 shows all the included studies with the infection incidence in each one.

Diabetes mellitus and penile prosthesis infections

Diabetes mellitus is a well-established risk factor for several infections; however, the relation with penile prosthesis infection is still controversial. Diabetic patients are more susceptible to infections because of impaired defense mechanisms, including leukocyte dysfunction and impaired mobilization to the infection site due to angiopathy [10].

We summarized the available evidence about penile prosthesis infection and DM in a meta-analysis, including 9041 diabetic patients and 36,517 non-diabetics. The meta-analysis shows that DM increases the incidence of penile prosthesis infection with an *odds ratio* of 1.53 (95% CI 1.15–2.04; $p = 0.004$), as shown in Fig. 2.

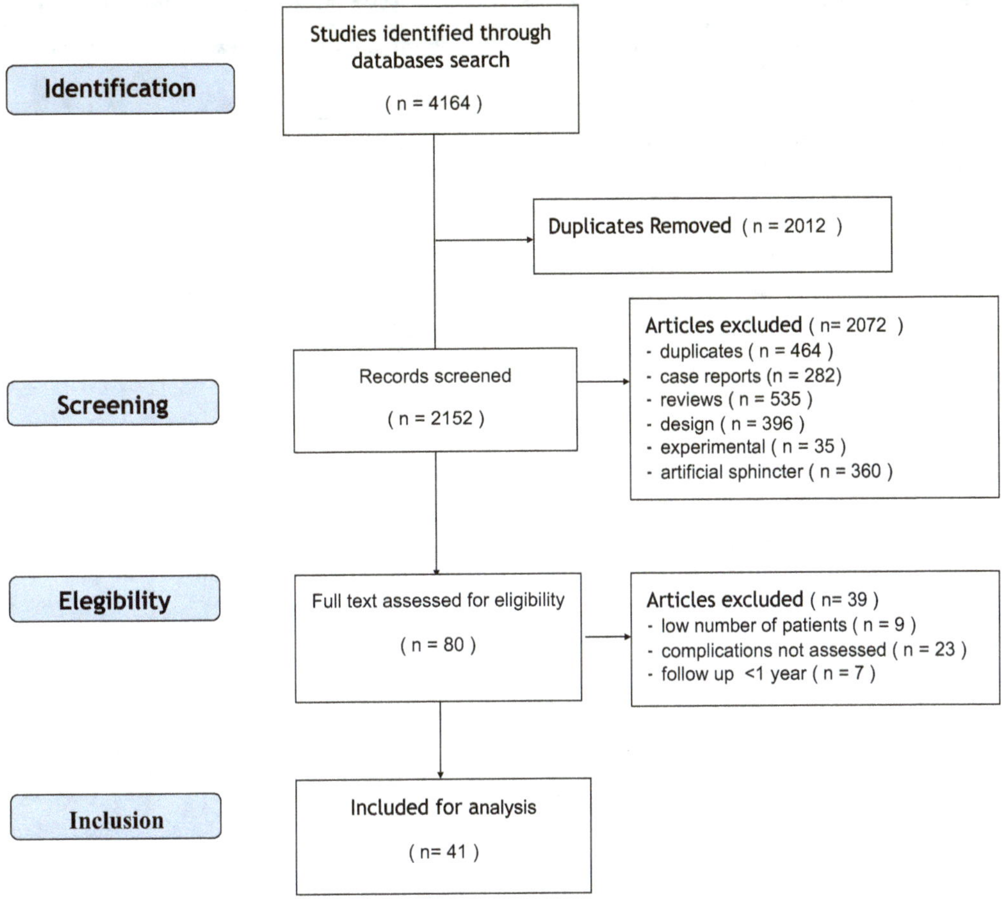

Fig. 1 Study flow diagram. The diagram shows methodological steps of the systematic review

Fallon and Ghanen reported a three-fold higher risk of infection in diabetic patients, while Bishop et al. [15] suggested glycosylated hemoglobin as an infection predictor in the early 1990s. On the other hand, Wilson and Delk [16] found no relation between diabetes mellitus and infection in a retrospective study with 823 patients. However, three years later, the same authors presented a prospective study with 114 diabetic patients and 275 non-diabetics and found a trend toward more infection in the diabetic group (8.8% vs. 4%; $p = 0.06$) [10]. Mulcahy and Carson [11], in a review of the manufacturer's database, including 31,341 men using a coated penile prosthesis, reported that the general revision rate was significantly higher in patients with diabetes: 1.72% versus 1.26% ($p = 0.005$).

Decreasing infection strategies

The mean incidence of penile prosthesis infection decreased over time. Around the 1980s and 1990s, the incidence was about 8 to 11%, and in early 2000 it was 3 to 5%. The introduction of the coated prosthesis and technique improvements decreased the infection incidence to a current rate of about 0.3 to 2.7%. The incidence of infection in the included studies is shown in Table 1.

In 2000, the American Medical Systems (AMS) introduced a prosthesis coated with the InhibiZone™, which consists of an antibiotic coating using minocycline and rifampicin that elutes in tissues around the device and inhibit the bacterial growth. In 2004, Carson described results from the manufacturer's database, showing 0.28% rate of infection in prosthesis with InhibiZone™, while regular uncoated ones had 1.59% at 60 days after surgery (p 0.003). At 6 months, the incidence was 0.68% in the coated group and 1.61% in the control one (p 0.005) [17].

In 2002 Mentor (now Coloplast) introduced the Titan, which has a hydrophilic coating that reduces bacterial adherence and can diffuse antibiotics when immersed into an antibiotic solution during surgery [18]. In 2004, Wolter and Hellstrom published data about infection from Mentor's database and FDA explantation reports. At 1 year follow-up, the infection rate in Titan prosthesis

Table 1 Included articles. The list of studies included as results of the systematic review, and infection rates

	Study	Year	Design	Level of evidence grade	Period	Prosthesis type	Patient *n*	Infection *n*	Infectionrate (%)
1	Carson et al. [34]	1983	Prospective	Low quality	1979–1982	Inflatable	100	1	1.00
2	Furlow et al. [35]	1987	Prospective	Low quality	1985–1987	Inflatable	120	1	0.83
3	Kabalin and Kessler [36]	1988	Prospective	Low quality	1975–1985	Scott reoperation	153	4	2.61
						Scott naive	264	5	1.89
4	Cumming and Pryor [37]	1991	Prospective	Low quality	1983–1987	Inflatable and malleable	280	32	11.43
5	Radomski and Herschorn [38]	1992	Prospective	Low quality	1979–1989	Inflatable and semi-rigid	269	6	2.23
6	Bishop et al. [15]	1992	Prospective	Low quality	1987–1988	Not sppecified	90	5	5.56
7	Goldstein et al. [39]	1993	Prospective	Low quality	1989–1991	Alfa 1—Mentor	112	3	2.68
8	Choi et al. [40]	1994	Retrospective	Low quality	1983–1993	Variable	295	3	1.02
9	Fein et al. [41]	1994	Prospective	Low quality	1988–1991	GFS II—Mentor	122	5	4.10
10	Wilson and Delk [16]	1995	Prospective	Low quality	1986–1993	Inflatable reoperation	428	43	10.05
						Inflatable naive	823	24	2.92
11	Holloway and Farah [42]	1997	Prospective	Low quality	1989–1994	Inflatable	145	3	2.07
12	Anafarta et al. [43]	1998	Prospective	Low quality	1989–1998	AMS Dynaflex	120	5	4.17
13	Wilson et al. [10]	1998	Prospective	Low quality	1994–1996	Inflatable	389	21	5.40
14	Garber and Marcus[44]	1998	Prospective	Low quality	7 years	Mentor A1 (3piece IPP)	360	6	1.67
15	Kabalin and Kessler [45]	1998	Prospective	Low quality	1975–1980	Scott; Small-carion	145	5	3.45
16	Montague et al. [46]	2001	Retrospective	Low quality	1986–1999	3 piece inflatable; database	491	10	2.04
17	Cakan et al. [47]	2003	Retrospective	Low quality	1993–2000	Malleable 2 piece	135	12	8.89
18	Ferguson and Cespedes [48]	2003	Prospective	Low quality	1992–1996	Malleable	94	1	1.06
19	Carson [17]	2004	Database	Low quality	2001–2003	AMS 700 InhibiZone™	2261	15	0.66
						AMS 700 no coating	1944	32	1.65
20	Wolter and Hellstrom [12]	2004	Database	Low quality	2002–2003	Titan coated	2357	25	1.06
						Alpha 1—no coating	482	10	2.07
21	Minervini et al. [49]	2005	Prospective	Low quality	1975–2000	Malleable—variable	504	40	7.94
22	Wilson et al. [23]	2007	Database	Low quality	2001–2004	AMS 700 InhibiZone™ naive	306	1	0.33
						AMS 700 InhibiZone™ reoperations	161	8	4.97
23	Kim et al. [50]	2010	Prospective	Low quality	1991–2009	AMS 700	397	8	2.02
24	DiBlasio et al. [51]	2010	Retrospective	Low quality	1997–2007	Inflatable	79	5	6.33
25	Carson et al. [19]	2011	Database	Low quality	2001–2008	AMS 700 no coating	3527	81	2.30
						AMS 700 inhibiZone™	34,556	408	1.18
26	Mulcahy and Carson [11]	2011	Database	Low quality	2001–2008	Inflatable coated	35,737	394	1.10
						Inflatable no coating	3268	82	2.51
27	Caire et al. [52]	2011	Retrospective	Low quality	2005–2007	Variable; reoperation	105	7	6.67
28	Dhabuwala et al. [20]	2011	Retrospective	Low quality	2002–2010	Titan; AMS InhibiZone™	497	10	2.01
29	Chung et al. [14]	2013	Prospective	Low quality	2006–2010	AMS 700; Titan (both coated)	138	3	2.17
30	Eid et al. [26]	2012	Prospective	Low quality	8.5y	AMS 700 InhibiZone™	704	14	1.99
						AMS 700 InhibiZone™ +"no touch"	1511	7	0.46

Table 1 (continued)

	Study	Year	Design	Level of evidence grade	Period	Prosthesis type	Patient *n*	Infection *n*	Infectionrate (%)
						AMS no coating	132	7	5.30
31	Omarbasha et al. [53]	2012	Retrospective	Low quality	2001–2011	Variable no coating	74	2	2.70
						InhibiZone™ and Titan	118	5	4.24
32	Henry et al. [54]	2012	Prospective	Low quality	2000–2007	Variable reoperation	214	12	5.61
33	Henry et al. [55]	2011	Prospective	Low quality	2000–2011	Variable; salvage surgeries	148	10	6.76
34	Chung et al. [2]	2012	Prospective	Low quality	1981–2010	Variable	955	14	1.47
35	Cohen and Eid [56]	2013	Prospective	Low quality	2003–2013	Variable coated reoperation	120	4	3.33
						Reoperation and "no touch"	283	1	0.35
36	Pozza et al. [57]	2015	Prospective	Low quality	1984–2013	Variable	500	15	3.00
37	Mohamed et al. [29]	2016	Retrospective	Low quality	2008–2015	Malleable	128	7	5.47
38	Chiang et al. [7]	2016	Prospective	Low quality	2004–2008	Variable	91	6	6.59
39	Antonini et al. [58]	2016	Prospective	Low quality	2011–2013	AMS 700 e Titan both coated	180	5	2.78
40	Katz and Love [59]	2017	Prospective	Low quality	2012–2015	Inflatable coated + "no touch"	150	1	0.67
41	Sevinc et al. [60]	2017	Prospective	Low quality	1998–2012	Malleable and inflatable	181	4	2.21

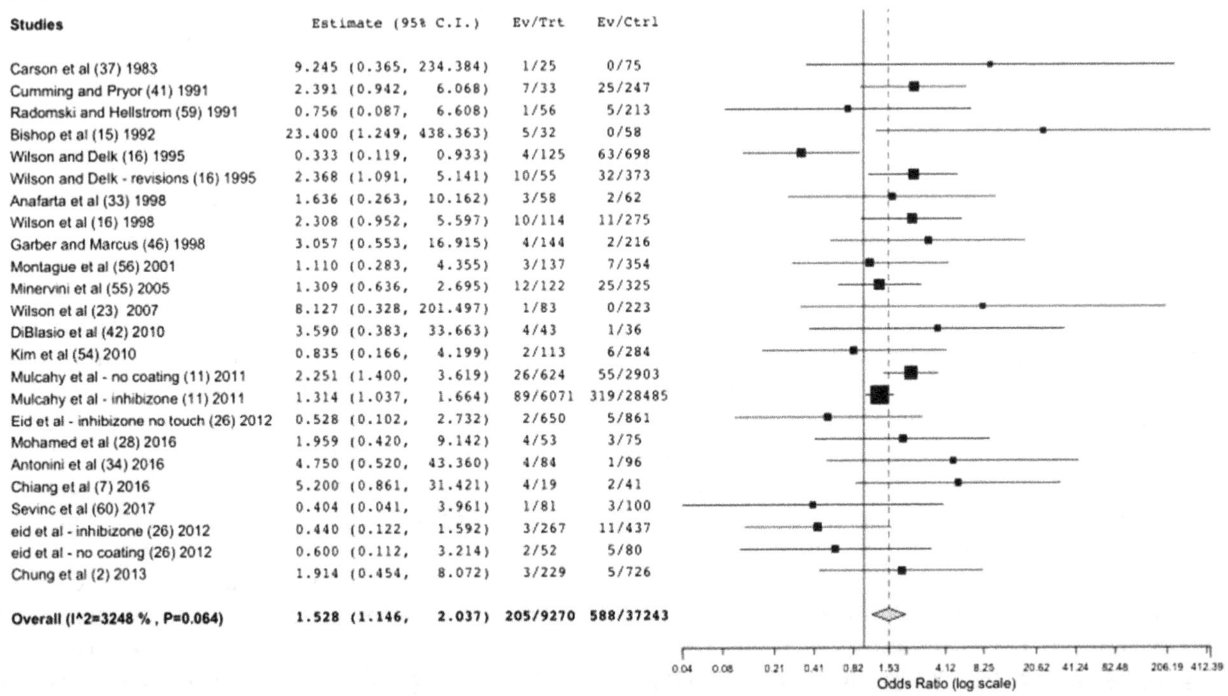

Fig. 2 Forest plot diagram showing articles included in meta-analysis. The overall result shows that diabetic patients have more infections of penile prosthesis than non-diabetics, with an *odds ratio* of 1.53 (95% CI 1.15–2.04; $p = 0.004$)

implants was 1.06% (25/2357), while in non-coated prosthesis it was 2.07% (10/482) (p 0.033) [12].

In 2011, Carson et al. published an extensive manufacturer's database review, including more than 39 thousand implants, with 90% of them with InhibiZone™; implanted between 2001 and 2008 and followed up to 7.7 years. They found that the revision rate for all causes (not only due to infection) was significantly lower on coated implants (6.7% vs. 12.5%, log-rank $p=0.002$) [19]. Dhabuwala et al. compared the Titan immersed in rifampicin 10 mg/ml and gentamicin 1 mg/ml or vancomycin and gentamicin to AMS with InhibiZone™. There was no difference in infection rates between InhibiZone™ (1/77) and Titan with rifampicin and gentamicin (0/81). However, the vancomicyn + gentamicin group had 4.4% of infection (8/181), which was significantly higher than the other two groups ($p<0.05$) [20]. Coated implants also had better results than regular ones regarding infection when used in reoperations [21–23].

The concept of "center of excellence" is widely used for heart and oncologic surgeries, based on the evidence that surgeons with a high volume of a specific surgery trend to have superior outcomes. In 2009, Henry et al. introduced this concept to the urological field, comparing the results of penile prosthesis implants of a high volume urologist with ten general urologists. The single urologist had more than 50 cases per year, had shorter operative time (34 min versus 94 min, $p<0.0001$), and eight-fold fewer reoperations (p 0.028). The concept was adopted and included as a recommended strategy to reduce infection [24, 25].

The most recent strategy was a technical improvement, presented by Eid in 2011, called the "*no-touch*" technique. It includes an antibiotic coated drape over the skin to reduce contact of hands and materials with the patient's skin [26]. In 2012, the same authors achieved an infection incidence of 0.4% using coated prosthesis and the "*no-touch*" technique [26].

Discussion

This review presents essential information from a wide variety of available articles in ten databases and brings contemporary data about penile prosthesis infections. It summarizes device and technique improvements that contributed to reduction of infection and reoperations. Although penile prosthesis infection has decreased over the last decades, it is still a feared complication once it leads to reoperation, loss of function, and increases costs [8, 27].

For the first time, we present a meta-analysis about diabetes mellitus role in penile prosthesis infection, which brings light to a long controversy. The meta-analysis suggests that DM is related to a higher risk of penile prosthesis infection, with an *odds ratio* of 1.53. There is a considerable heterogeneity, which comes from the different studies' designs, and significant disparity in the number of subjects. The results at both sides of the forest plot show the controversy in the literature.

While older studies, from the 1990s, started to suggest the higher infection rates in diabetic patients, subsequent studies did not confirm it [28]. However, it is crucial to notice that most of the studies were not designed to evaluate DM properly, and most of them lack information about diabetes treatments and glucose control. For example, Mohamed et al. [29] reported that all patients in his study had glycosylated hemoglobin inferior to 7.0%. Thus, one may consider the contemporary practice to achieve good glycemic control before elective surgeries, and the lack of information about glycemic control on the databases. That may limit the evaluation of the glycosylated hemoglobin (Hb1Ac) role in most studies and contribute to the controversy regarding diabetes mellitus relation with infection.

In this scenario, it is essential to look at a prospective study designed to predict the importance of Hb1Ac levels at penile prosthesis infection. Habous et al. [30] recently analyzed 902 patients, who received different types of penile prosthesis, and found that Hb1Ac was significantly related to a higher incidence of infection. They had 80 implants with infection, which means an infection rate of 8.9%. The mean Hb1Ac in patients with infection was 9.5%, and it was significantly higher than in patients with no infection, with a mean Hb1Ac of 7.8% ($p<0.001$). They constructed a ROC curve and proposed the Hb1Ac level of 8.5% as the threshold to predict infection with 80% sensitivity and 65% specificity.

Li et al. [6] also in 2018 reported diabetes mellitus, HIV, and Charles Comorbidity Index as factors associated with prosthesis removal. On the other hand, a recent retrospective study performed by Canguven et al. [31] included 300 patients and had only 2 cases of prosthesis infection, and both of them on non-diabetic patients. A superficial comparison could easily trick with the conflicting results, but one needs caution to interpret the studies' designs. A retrospective cohort may present biases, mainly due to the lack of information provided by patient charts or data loss, which invariably interfere with the results. The recent studies focused on penile prosthesis complications confirm our meta-analysis finding.

Our review is limited by the quality of the available evidence, the lack of controls, and studies based on the manufacturer's database and FDA reports, which may have standardization and selection biases. However, it is crucial to consider the low incidence of infection, which requires a very high number of patients to show a decrease of incidence. Considering a baseline infection rate of 3%, it is estimated that a prospective study would require about 3 thousand patients to show a 50% reduction on infection rate or 34 thousand patients to show a 25% reduction [32]. It is also difficult to propose a trial to compare coated and uncoated implants when the available evidence suggest the superiority of the coated ones, which could bring ethical issues to the trial [33].

This is the most extensive review about penile prosthesis infection to our knowledge, including references from 10 databases, which brings information from the current scenario of penile prosthesis infection and gathers enough data to perform the first meta-analysis about the role of DM in penile prosthesis infection. The results encourage further studies focused on diabetic patients, which will be interesting to evaluate glycosylated hemoglobin levels, treatments in use, and the time elapsed from DM diagnosis to surgery.

Conclusions

Penile prosthesis infection decreased in the last decades due to several improvements in materials and techniques. It remains a significant complication, and the meta-analysis indicates that diabetes mellitus is related to a higher risk of penile prosthesis infection.

Acknowledgements
Special thanks to Ana Paula de Morais e Oliveira and all the staff from the Library of the Faculty of Medical Sciences—University of Campinas for supporting data acquisition.

Authors' contributions
LG and LP did the project conception and development. CC and BV have collected and analyzed data. LG and CR had supervised the data management and analysis. LG drafted the manuscript, while CC, BV and CR edited and revised it. AF gave intelectual contributions and critical revision of the manuscript. All authors read and approved the final manuscript.

References

1. Scott FB, Bradley WE, Timm GW. Management of erectile impotence. Use of implantable inflatable prosthesis. Urology. 1973;2(1):80–2.
2. Chung E, Van CT, Wilson I, Cartmill RA. Penile prosthesis implantation for the treatment for male erectile dysfunction: clinical outcomes and lessons learnt after 955 procedures. World J Urol. 2013;31(3):591–5.
3. Rajpurkar A, Dhabuwala CB. Comparison of satisfaction rates and erectile function in patients treated with sildenafil, intracavernous prostaglandin E1 and penile implant surgery for erectile dysfunction in urology practice. J Urol. 2003;170(1):159–63.
4. Bennett N, Huang IS. Inflatable penile prosthesis in the radical prostatectomy patient: a review. F1000Res. 2018;7:770.
5. Natali A, Olianas R, Fisch M. Penile implantation in Europe: successes and complications with 253 implants in Italy and Germany. J Sex Med. 2008;5(6):1503–12.
6. Li K, Brandes ER, Chang SL, Leow JJ, Chung BI, Wang Y, et al. Trends in penile prosthesis implantation and analysis of predictive factors for removal. World J Urol. 2018;37:639–46.
7. Chiang HS, Liao CH, Chang ML. Benefits of antibiotic-impregnated inflatable penile prosthesis (InhibiZone®) in patients at high risk of infection in Taiwan. Urol Sci. 2016;27(3):144–7.
8. Carson C. Antibiotic impregnation of inflatable penile prostheses: effect on perioperative infection. Expert Rev Med Devices. 2004;1(2):165–7.
9. Angulo J, Gonzalez-Corrochano R, Cuevas P, Fernandez A, La Fuente JM, Rolo F, et al. Diabetes exacerbates the functional deficiency of NO/cGMP pathway associated with erectile dysfunction in human corpus cavernosum and penile arteries. J Sex Med. 2010;7(2 Pt 1):758–68.
10. Wilson SK, Carson CC, Cleves MA, Delk 2nd JR. Quantifying risk of penile prosthesis infection with elevated glycosylated hemoglobin. J Urol. 1998;159(5):1537–9 (discussion 9-40).
11. Mulcahy JJ, Carson CC 3rd. Long-term infection rates in diabetic patients implanted with antibiotic-impregnated versus nonimpregnated inflatable penile prostheses: 7-year outcomes. Eur Urol. 2011;60(1):167–72.
12. Wolter CE, Hellstrom WJ. The hydrophilic-coated inflatable penile prosthesis: 1-year experience. J Sex Med. 2004;1(2):221–4.
13. Atkins D, Eccles M, Flottorp S, Guyatt GH, Henry D, Hill S, et al. Systems for grading the quality of evidence and the strength of recommendations I: critical appraisal of existing approaches The GRADE Working Group. BMC Health Serv Res. 2004;4(1):38.
14. Chung E, Solomon M, Deyoung L, Brock GB. Comparison between AMS 700™ CX and Coloplast™ titan inflatable penile prosthesis for Peyronie's disease treatment and remodeling: clinical outcomes and patient satisfaction. J Sex Med. 2013;10(11):2855–60.
15. Bishop JR, Moul JW, Sihelnik SA, Peppas DS, Gormley TS, McLeod DG. Use of glycosylated hemoglobin to identify diabetics at high risk for penile periprosthetic infections. J Urol. 1992;147(2):386–8.
16. Wilson SK, Delk JR 2nd. Inflatable penile implant infection: predisposing factors and treatment suggestions. J Urol. 1995;153(3 Pt 1):659–61.
17. Carson CC 3rd. Efficacy of antibiotic impregnation of inflatable penile prostheses in decreasing infection in original implants. J Urol. 2004;171(4):1611–4.
18. Henry GD. Historical review of penile prosthesis design and surgical techniques: part 1 of a three-part review series on penile prosthetic surgery. J Sex Med. 2009;6(3):675–81.
19. Carson CC 3rd, Mulcahy JJ, Harsch MR. Long-term infection outcomes after original antibiotic impregnated inflatable penile prosthesis implants: up to 7.7 years of followup. J Urol. 2011;185(2):614–8.
20. Dhabuwala C, Sheth S, Zamzow B. Infection rates of rifampin/gentamicin-coated Titan Coloplast penile implants, Comparison with Inhibizone-impregnated AMS penile implants. J Sex Med. 2011;8(1):315–20.
21. Brant MD, Ludlow JK, Mulcahy JJ. The prosthesis salvage operation: immediate replacement of the infected penile prosthesis. J Urol. 1996;155(1):155–7.
22. Mulcahy JJ. Long-term experience with salvage of infected penile implants. J Urol. 2000;163(2):481–2.
23. Wilson SK, Zumbe J, Henry GD, Salem EA, Delk JR, Cleves MA. Infection reduction using antibiotic-coated inflatable penile prosthesis. Urology. 2007;70(2):337–40.
24. Henry GD, Kansal NS, Callaway M, Grigsby T, Henderson J, Noble J, et al. Centers of excellence concept and penile prostheses: an outcome analysis. J Urol. 2009;181(3):1264–8.
25. Levine LA, Becher EF, Bella AJ, Brant WO, Kohler TS, Martinez-Salamanca JI, et al. Penile prosthesis surgery: current recommendations from the international consultation on sexual medicine. J Sex Med. 2016;13(4):489–518.
26. Eid JF, Wilson SK, Cleves M, Salem EA. Coated implants and "no touch" surgical technique decreases risk of infection in inflatable penile prosthesis implantation to 0.46%. Urology. 2012;79(6):1310–5.
27. Mulcahy JJ. Penile prosthesis infection: progress in prevention and treatment. Curr Urol Rep. 2010;11(6):400–4.
28. Christodoulidou M, Pearce I. Infection of penile prostheses in patients with diabetes mellitus. Surg Infect (Larchmt). 2016;17(1):2–8.
29. Mohamed ER, Hammady AR, Eldahshoury MZ, Elsharkawi AM, Riad AM, Elmogazy HM, et al. Surgical outcomes and complications of Tube(R) (Promedon) malleable penile prostheses in diabetic versus non-diabetic patients with erectile dysfunction. Arab J Urol. 2016;14(4):305–11.
30. Habous M, Tal R, Tealab A, Soliman T, Nassar M, Mekawi Z, et al. Defining a glycated haemoglobin (HbA1c) level that predicts increased risk of penile implant infection. BJU Int. 2018;121(2):293–300.
31. Canguven O, Talib R, El Ansari W, Khalafalla K, Al Ansari A. Is Hba1c level of diabetic patients associated with penile prosthesis implantation infections? Aging Male. 2019;22(1):28–33. https://doi.org/10.1080/13685538.2018.1448059.
32. Darouiche RO. Antimicrobial approaches for preventing infections associated with surgical implants. Clin Infect Dis. 2003;36(10):1284–9.
33. Al Mohajer M, Darouiche RO. Infections associated with inflatable penile prostheses. Sex Med Rev. 2014;2(3–4):134–40.

34. Carson CC. Inflatable penile prosthesis: experience with 100 patients. South Med J. 1983;76(9):1139–41.
35. Furlow WL, Goldwasser B, Gundian JC. Implantation of model AMS 700 penile prosthesis: long-term results. J Urol. 1988;139(4):741–2.
36. Kabalin JN, Kessler R. Five-year followup of the Scott inflatable penile prosthesis and comparison with semirigid penile prosthesis. J Urol. 1988a;140(6):1428–30.
37. Cumming J, Pryor JP. Treatment of organic impotence. Br J Urol. 1991;67(6):640–3.
38. Radomski SB, Herschorn S. Risk factors associated with penile prosthesis infection. J Urol. 1992;147(2):383–5.
39. Goldstein I, Bertero EB, Kaufman JM, Witten FR, Hubbard JG, Fitch WP, et al. Early experience with the first pre-connected 3-piece inflatable penile prosthesis: the Mentor Alpha-1. J Urol. 1993;150(6):1814–8.
40. Choi HK, Cho IR, Xin ZC. Ten years of experience with various penile prosthesis in Korean. Yonsei Med J. 1994;35(2):209–17.
41. Fein RL. GFS Mark II inflatable penile prosthesis: four-year clinical study. Urology. 1994;43(2):209–13.
42. Holloway FB, Farah RN. Intermediate term assessment of the reliability, function and patient satisfaction with the AMS700 Ultrex penile prosthesis. J Urol. 1997;157(5):1687–91.
43. Anafarta K, Yaman O, Aydos K. Clinical experience with Dynaflex penile prostheses in 120 patients. Urology. 1998;52(6):1098–100.
44. Garber BB, Marcus SM. Does surgical approach affect the incidence of inflatable penile prosthesis infection? Urology. 1998;52(2):291–3.
45. Kabalin JN, Kessler R. Infectious complications of penile prosthesis surgery. J Urol. 1988b;139(5):953–5.
46. Montague DK, Angermeier KW, Lakin MM. Penile prosthesis infections. Int J Impot Res. 2001;13(6):326–8.
47. Cakan M, Demirel F, Karabacak O, Yalcinkaya F, Altug U. Risk factors for penile prosthetic infection. Int Urol Nephrol. 2003;35(2):209–13.
48. Ferguson KH, Cespedes RD. Prospective long-term results and quality-of-life assessment after Dura-II penile prosthesis placement. Urology. 2003;61(2):437–41.
49. Minervini A, Ralph DJ, Pryor JP. Outcome of penile prosthesis implantation for treating erectile dysfunction: experience with 504 procedures. BJU Int. 2006;97(1):129–33.
50. Kim DS, Yang KM, Chung HJ, Choi HM, Choi YD, Choi HK. AMS 700CX/CXM inflatable penile prosthesis has high mechanical reliability at long-term follow-up. J Sex Med. 2010;7(7):2602–7.
51. DiBlasio CJ, Kurta JM, Botta S, Malcolm JB, Wan JY, Derweesh IH, et al. Peyronie's disease compromises the durability and component-malfunction rates in patients implanted with an inflatable penile prosthesis. BJU Int. 2010;106(5):691–4.
52. Caire A, Boonjindasup A, Richardson B, Hellstrom W. Does the need for a replacement inflatable penile prosthesis lead to decreased patient satisfaction? J Urol. 2011;185(4):e369.
53. Omarbasha B, Basso AC, Howland L, Wilson S. Penile implant infections experienced in a community practice during the ERA of the coated implant. J Sex Med. 2012;9:7–8.
54. Henry G, Wilson SK, Donatucci C, Delk J, Lentz A, McNamara E, et al. Single component exchange during penile prosthesis revision appears to have higher infection rates and lower overall device survival rates than complete component replacement: a multicenter analysis. J Urol. 2012;187(4):e752–3.
55. Henry G, Carson C, Delk J, McKim S, McNamara E, Cleves M, et al. Positive culture growths from infection retardant-coated penile prostheses at the time of revision/savlage surgery: a multicenter study. J Urol. 2011;185(4):e723.
56. Cohen SD, Eid JF. The "no touch" technique decreases the risk of infection after removal and replacement of malfunctioned penile prosthesis to 0.35%. J Urol. 2013;189(4):e685–6.
57. Pozza D, Pozza M, Musy M, Pozza C. 500 penile prostheses implanted by a surgeon in Italy in the last 30 years. Arch Ital Urol Androl. 2015;87(3):216–21.
58. Antonini G, Busetto GM, De Berardinis E, Giovannone R, Vicini P, Del Giudice F, et al. Minimally invasive infrapubic inflatable penile prosthesis implant for erectile dysfunction: evaluation of efficacy, satisfaction profile and complications. Int J Impot Res. 2016;28(1):4–8.
59. Katz DJ, Love C. The minimally invasive no touch (MINT) penile implant, the first 150 consecutive cases. J Sex Med. 2017;14(1):S18–9.
60. Sevinc C, Ozkaptan O, Balaban M, Yucetas U, Karadeniz T. Outcome of penile prosthesis implantation: are malleable prostheses an appropriate treatment option in patients with erectile dysfunction caused by prior radical surgery? Asian J Androl. 2017;19(4):477–81.

27

Serologic and urinary characteristics of laboratory-confirmed genitourinary tuberculosis at a tertiary hospital in the Philippines

Paolo Nikolai H. So* and Anthony Russell T. Villanueva

Abstract

Background: Genitourinary tuberculosis (GUTB) is known to cause high rates of structural organ damage, however, literature on its biochemical manifestations is limited. Additionally, local studies in the Philippine setting, where cases are rampant, are few and dated. This study aimed to determine the serologic and urinary profile of patients with GUTB admitted at a tertiary hospital within January 2009 to March 2020 and their association with short-term outcomes.

Methods: This retrospective study included 112 patients with laboratory-confirmed GUTB (i.e., positivity in acid-fast smear, polymerase chain reaction, culture, or histology). Demographic data, clinical characteristics, laboratory and radiologic findings, histopathology reports, treatment, and short-term outcomes were recorded.

Results: Bladder (54.5%) and kidney (36.4%) were the most affected organs. The male:female ratio was 1:1.15, and the mean age was 35.79 ± 18.29 years. Weakness (14.29%) was the most common chief complaint. A majority presented with anemia (83.04%), while several had leukocytosis (41.96%) and thrombocytosis (26.79%). Hypoalbuminemia (58.10%), impairment of renal function (36.94%), and electrolyte abnormalities such as hyponatremia (50.93%), hypercalcemia (20.19%), and hypokalemia (21.82%) were common. Proteinuria (67.96%) and pyuria (67.96%) were the most frequent abnormal findings, followed by hematuria (51.46%), acidic urine (45.63%) and low specific gravity (31.07%). Age, leukocytosis, and the need for pressors were all significantly associated with mortality (p values of <0.001, 0.010, and <0.001, respectively).

Conclusions: The young age at presentation with severe clinical and laboratory manifestations may reflect local epidemiology as TB continues to be widespread in the country. Apart from the more commonly cited abnormalities in literature, multiple electrolyte imbalances and urinary concentration defects were also observed in many cases, possibly indicating tubulointerstitial involvement—a complication increasingly mentioned in case reports. As several patient characteristics were found to be associated with the high mortality rates observed in the study, further research is recommended to explore predictive modeling.

Keywords: Genitourinary tuberculosis, Electrolytes, Urinalysis, Association

Introduction

Tuberculosis (TB) remains an important global epidemic, with latest estimates of disease burden amounting to 10.0 (range, 9.0–11.1) million people in 2018 [1]. Extrapulmonary TB (EPTB) is reported to comprise

*Correspondence: paolonikolaiso@gmail.com
Division of Nephrology, Department of Medicine, University of the Philippines Manila – Philippine General Hospital, Taft Avenue, Ermita, 1000 Manila, Philippines

around 16.5–25% of all cases, attributing 4.5–27% to genitourinary TB (GUTB) [2–4]. GUTB historically pertains to the infection of the urogenital system organs in any combination by *Mycobacterium tuberculosis* (MTB) or *Mycobacterium bovis* [5–8]. It presents with insidious and late-onset symptoms, making its diagnosis and treatment difficult and delayed, and consequently leading to high rates of structural organ damage and kidney failure [9, 10]. Some physicians advocate the term *urogenital TB* (UGTB) as kidney TB is the most relevant infection and is more frequently diagnosed than genital TB [5, 6, 11].

Philippines ranked 4th among the countries with high TB burden in 2018, accounting 6% of the global total. It has a TB incidence rate of 554 (311–866) per 100,000 population, and a mortality rate of 24.57 (20–32) per 100,000 population [1]. This high disease prevalence in the country is multifactorial, attributing to high poverty rate, marked social inequities, and rise in slum housing and crowded living conditions from rapid urbanization [12]. In the Filipino pediatric population, GUTB is found to cause 3% of extrapulmonary TB cases admitted in a tertiary hospital [13].

Despite these figures, there is paucity in literature regarding local experience on GUTB, especially with regards to serologic and urinary findings [14–16]. The last available reference was published 25 years ago, which also needs to be updated. The study aims to determine the serologic and urinary profile of patients with genitourinary TB admitted at a tertiary government hospital in Philippines and their association with short-term outcomes.

Methods

Study design and population

This is a single-center, retrospective study performed at the Philippine General Hospital (PGH; 1500 beds). This study included GUTB patients diagnosed from January 2009 to March 2020 through positivity in at least one of the following: (1) urine acid-fast bacilli (AFB) staining, (2) urine or tissue polymerase chain reaction (PCR) for *Mycobacterium tuberculosis*, (3) urine or tissue *M. tuberculosis* culture, and (4) histologic findings of granulomatous inflammation (granulomas composed of epithelioid cells and Langhans giant cells with or without caseous necrosis) [14, 15, 17–19]. Culture-positive samples solely involving the female genital tract without urologic involvement, out-patients, in-patients without baseline serologic and urinary tests, and those who got discharged against medical advice were excluded. This study was approved by the University of the Philippines Manila Research Ethics Board and the requirement for informed consent was waived since the investigators evaluated anonymized data.

Data collection and definition of variables

Data collection was done through chart review of patient medical records. This included patient demographics; comorbidities; clinical symptoms; complete blood counts; serum chemistries; urinalysis; results of microbial smears and cultures, diagnostics, and histopathology; treatment; and short-term outcomes. Organ involvement was distinguished in those with tissue samples obtained from biopsies or operations.

Serologic abnormalities were defined as follows: (1) anemia as hemoglobin of < 150 g/L in neonates 0–30 days old, < 105 g/L in 1–23 months of age, < 115 g/L in children 2–9 years of age, < 125 g/L in males 10–17 years of age, < 120 g/L in non-pregnant females 10 years of age and above, < 110 g/L in pregnant women, and < 130 g/L in men 15 years of age and above [20, 21]; (2) thrombocytopenia as platelets < 84,000/μL in newborns ≤ 1 week old, and < 150,000/μL for the rest of the age groups [21, 22]; (3) thrombocytosis as platelets > 450,000/μL [22]; (4) leukocytosis as white blood cells > 34,000/μL in neonates 0–30 days, > 14,000/μL in infants 1–23 months of age, > 12,000/μL in 2–9 years of age, > 10,500/μL in 10–18 years of age, and > 11,000/μL in adults [21, 23]; (5) leukopenia as white blood cells < 9100/μL in neonates 0–30 days, < 6000/μL in infants 1–23 months of age, < 4000/μL in 2–18 years of age, and < 4400/μL in adults [21, 23]; (6) hypoalbuminemia as serum albumin < 18 g/L in premature neonates 1 day old, < 25 g/L in full term neonates < 6 days old, < 19 g/L in 8 days-1 year old, < 34 g/L in 1–3 years of age, < 35 g/L in 4–19 years of age, and < 34 g/L in adults [21]; (7) impaired renal function as estimated glomerular filtration rate < 60 mL/min/1.73 m [2]; (8) hyperkalemia as plasma K^+ concentration ≥ 5.5 mM [22], (2) hypokalemia as plasma K^+ concentration < 3.5 mM [22], (9) hyponatremia as plasma Na^+ concentration < 135 mM [22], and (10) hypercalcemia as total serum calcium concentration ≥ 10.4 mg/dL [24].

Urinary findings were defined as: (1) acidic urine as urine pH ≤ 5.5 [24], (2) low specific gravity as urine specific gravity ≤ 1.010, (3) hematuria as three or more erythrocytes per high-power field [24], (4) proteinuria as detection of proteinuria by dipstick examination [22], and (5) pyuria as detection of more than 5 white blood cells per high-power field in urine microscopy or positive leukocyte esterase dipstick testing [15, 24].

Table 1 Proportion of patients with GUTB

Diagnosis	No. of patients (%) (n = 112)
Urine AFB smear-positive	56 (50.00%)
Urine PCR-positive	16 (14.29%)
Urine culture-confirmed	18 (16.07%)
Histopathology	22 (19.64%)
Bladder	12
Kidney	6
Kidney and ureter	2
Ureter	2

Table 2 Laterality of organ involvement in GUTB patients confirmed by histopathology

Organ	No. of patients (%) (n = 10)		
	Right	Left	Unspecified
Kidney	1	4	1
Kidney and ureter	0	2	0
Ureter	1	0	1
Total	2 (20.0%)	6 (60.0%)	2 (20.0%)

Statistical analysis

Descriptive statistics were used in the analysis of this study. Frequency and percentage were used to describe categorical variables and proportions of patients who improved, expired, or developed short-term outcomes such as the need for pressors or renal replacement therapy. Continuous variables were expressed as median.

Associations were determined by bivariate analysis using Fisher's exact test for characteristics involving 2 categories or Chi-square test for those with > 2

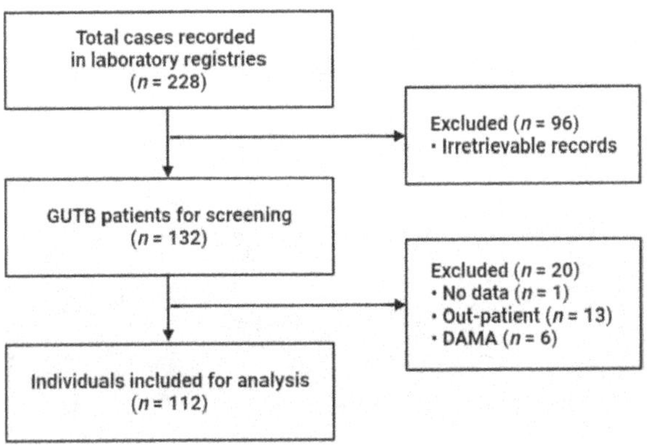

Fig. 1 Flow diagram of study selection. *DAMA* discharged against medical advice

Table 3 Clinical characteristics of patients with GUTB

Clinical characteristics	No. of patients (%) (n = 112)
Gender	
M	52 (46.43%)
F	60 (53.57%)
Age	
0 months–1 year	1 (0.89%)
1 year–5 years	2 (1.79%)
6 years–10 years	4 (3.57%)
11 years–18 years	18 (16.07%)
19 years–29 years	21 (18.75%)
30 years–49 years	35 (31.25%)
50 years–69 years	27 (24.11%)
70 years or older	4 (3.57%)
Marital status	
Single/widowed	69 (61.61%)
Married	43 (38.39%)
Occupation	
Employed	19 (16.96%)
Unemployed	58 (51.79%)
Not applicable (i.e., pediatric)	26 (23.21%)
Unspecified	9 (8.04%)
Location	
Urban	60 (53.57%)
Rural	48 (42.86%)
Unspecified	4 (3.57%)
Co-morbidity	
Previous TB	14 (12.50%)
Diabetes mellitus	5 (4.46%)
HIV/AIDS	12 (10.71%)
Steroid use (e.g., SLE, NS)	9 (8.04%)
Malignancy	1 (0.89%)
Chronic kidney disease	5 (4.46%)
History of urolithiasis	8 (7.14%)
RTA Type 1	1 (0.89%)
COPD	2 (1.79%)
Bronchial asthma	2 (1.79%)
Hypertension	13 (11.61%)
Heart failure	2 (1.79%)
Cerebrovascular disease	1 (0.89%)
Other organ involvement	64 (57.14%)
Pulmonary	57 (50.89%)
Gastrointestinal	28 (25.00%)
Abdominopelvic	11 (9.82%)
Central nervous system	7 (6.25%)
Bone	4 (3.57%)
Lymph node	8 (7.14%)
Ear	2 (1.79%)
Psoas	2 (1.79%)
Cutaneous/wound	3 (2.68%)

Table 3 (continued)

Clinical characteristics	No. of patients (%) (n = 112)
Chief complaint	
Weakness	16 (14.29%)
Difficulty of breathing	14 (12.50%)
Flank pain	13 (11.61%)
Abdominal pain	11(9.82%)
Hematuria	9 (8.04%)
Dysuria	9 (8.04%)
Fever	8 (7.14%)
Abdominal/pelvic mass on diagnostic	5 (4.46%)
Pedal edema	4 (3.57%)
Umbilical discharge	3 (2.68%)
Gluteal pain	2 (1.79%)
Vaginal bleeding	2 (1.79%)
Cough	2 (1.79%)
Seizure	2 (1.79%)
Urinary retention	1 (0.89%)
Inguinal pain	1 (0.89%)
Fistula formation (ureterocutaneous)	1 (0.89%)
Scrotal discharge	1 (0.89%)
Double J stent reinsertion	1 (0.89%)
Decrease in sensorium	1 (0.89%)
Vomiting	1 (0.89%)
Others	5 (4.46%)

COPD chronic obstructive pulmonary disease, *F* female, *HIV/AIDS* human immunodeficiency virus or acquired immunodeficiency syndrome, *M* male, *NS* nephrotic syndrome, *RTA Type 1* renal tubular acidosis Type 1, *SLE* systemic lupus erythematosus, *TB* tuberculosis

categories. Mean lengths of hospital stay between those with and without the identified clinical, serologic, and urinary characteristics were compared using Mann–Whitney U-test for characteristics involving 2 categories or Kruskal–Wallis test for those with >2 categories. For all tests, *p* value of at most 0.05 indicate significance.

Results

A total of 228 patients with laboratory-confirmed GUTB were identified. Ninety-six charts were irretrievable due to institutional limitations in records retention, while 20 cases met the exclusion criteria (Fig. 1). Among the 112 patients included in the study, half (50.0%) had positive smears for urine AFB (Table 1). In those with histopathologic evidence of infection, bladder (n = 12, 54.5%) and kidney (n = 8, 36.4%) were the most involved genitourinary organs. Among those with kidney and ureter involvement, left laterality was observed in 60% (Table 2).

Patient characteristics

Baseline clinical characteristics of the patients with GUTB are shown in Table 3. The mean age (±SD) was 35.79 ± 18.29 years (range, 1–82 years) and the male-to-female ratio was 1:1.15 (52:60). Most patients were single or widowed (61.61%) and lived in urban areas (53.57%). Fourteen patients (12.5%) had a previous history of tuberculosis, while 64 patients (57.14%) had present

Table 4 Serologic characteristics of patients with GUTB

Serologic abnormalities	No. of patients (%)
Anemia	93 (83.04%, n = 112)
Thrombocytopenia	6 (5.36%, n = 112)
Thrombocytosis	30 (26.79%, n = 112)
Leukocytosis	47 (41.96%, n = 112)
Leukopenia	6 (5.36%, n = 112)
Hypoalbuminemia	61 (58.10%, n = 105)
Renal function impairment	41 (36.94%, n = 111)
Hyperkalemia	9 (8.18%, n = 110)
Hypokalemia	24 (21.82%, n = 110)
Hyponatremia	55 (50.93%, n = 108)
Hypercalcemia	21 (20.19%, n = 104)

Table 5 Urinary characteristics of patients with GUTB

Urinary abnormalities	No. of patients (%) (n = 103)
Acidic pH	47 (45.63%)
Low specific gravity	32 (31.07%)
Proteinuria	70 (67.96%)
Negative	33 (32.04%)
Trace	15 (14.56%)
1+	36 (34.95%)
2+	16 (15.53%)
3+	3 (2.91%)
Hematuria	53 (51.46%)
Pyuria	70 (67.96%)
Pyuria + hematuria	50 (48.54%)
Casts	17 (16.50%)
Crystals	4 (3.88%)

Table 6 Imaging findings associated with GUTB

Intravenous pyelography
Unilateral renal parenchymal disease
Non-functioning kidney
Calcification of the urinary tract: medullary nephrocalcinosis, nephrolithiasis, ureterolithiasis, cystolithiasis
Bladder wall thickening
CT scan
Hypodense renal foci with or without internal septations or peripheral calcifications
Renal cysts, Bosniak I and II
Renal mass
Calcification of the urinary tract: nephrolithiasis, ureteropelvic junction lithiases
Urinary tract dilatation: hydronephrosis, ureteropelvocaliectasia with possible distal ureteral stricture
Ureteral wall thickening
Bladder wall thickening
Vesicocutaneous fistulous tract
Evidence of extra-renal TB infection:
Pulmonary tuberculosis with or without endobrochial spread
Distal ileal and ileocecal wall thickening with multiple abscess formation (intraabdominal, pelvic, and prostatic regions) and lymphadenopathies
Multilevel vertebral lesions with disc destruction (Pott's disease) with abscess formation involving adjacent muscles (psoas, iliopsoas and gluteus maximus)
Ultrasound
Unilateral or bilateral renal parenchymal disease with or without signs of chronicity
Echogenic renal walls with or without internal echoes suggestive of pyelitis or pyelonephritis
Pyonephrosis
Renal cysts or mass
Calcification of the urinary tract: nephrocalcinosis, nonspecific parenchymal/perinephric/periureteral calcifications, nephrolithiasis, urolithiases,
Urinary tract dilatation: hydronephrosis, focal caliectasia, pelvocaliectasia, ureteropelvocaliectasia
Irregular, diffuse, or heterogeneous bladder wall thickening
Bladder wall foci or mass
Evidence of abdominopelvic Koch's infection: tobacco pouch appearance of fallopian tube, thickening of uterine serosa and peritoneum, palisading bowel loops, and massive ascites

Table 7 Management of admitted patients with GUTB

Intervention	No. of patients (%) (n = 112)
Anti-Koch's therapy	71 (63.39%)
Operation	29 (25.89%)
Percutaneous tube nephrostomy	10 (8.93%)
Double J stent insertion	11 (9.82%)
Nephrectomy	2 (1.79%)
Subcapsular nephrectomy	5 (4.46%)
Cytoreductive nephrectomy	1 (0.89%)
Aspiration of renal abscess	1 (0.89%)
Radial nephrolithotomy	1 (0.89%)
Pelvolithotomy	1 (0.89%)
Ureterotomy	1 (0.89%)
Ureteroneocystostomy	1 (0.89%)
Bladder mass excision	3 (2.68%)
Transurethral resection of bladder tumor	1 (0.89%)

Table 8 Short-term outcomes of admitted patients with GUTB

Length of hospital stay in days, median (min–max)	11 (0.67–90)
Improved, n (%)	103 (91.96%)
Expired, n (%)	9 (8.04%)
Need for pressors, n (%)	15 (13.39%)
Need for renal replacement therapy, n (%)	1 (0.89%)

evidence of other organ involvement, with lungs (50.89%) being the most concomitantly involved organ. Twenty-four patients (21.43%) exhibited systemic symptoms such as weakness (14.29%) and fever (7.14%), while 57 patients (50.89%) had genitourinary manifestations as their chief complaint. Flank or abdominal pain was the most common presenting genitourinary symptom (21.43%).

Table 9 Bivariate analysis: clinical characteristics and mortality

Characteristic	Category	Mortality				*p* value
		Survived		Expired		
		Count	Row %	Count	Row %	
Gender	Male	48	92.3	4	7.7	1.000
	Female	55	91.7	5	8.3	
Age	0 months to 1 year	0	0.0	1	100.0	**<0.001**
	1–5 years	0	0.0	2	100.0	
	6–10 years	4	100.0	0	0.0	
	11–18 years	17	94.4	1	5.6	
	19–29 years	19	90.5	2	9.5	
	30–49 years	33	94.3	2	5.7	
	50–69 years	26	96.3	1	3.7	
	≥ 70 years	4	100.0	0	0.0	
Marital status	Single/widowed	63	91.3	6	8.7	1.000
	Married	40	93.0	3	7.0	
Occupation	Employed	18	94.7	1	5.3	0.394
	Unemployed	54	93.1	4	6.9	
	Not applicable	22	84.6	4	15.4	
	Unspecified	9	100.0	0	0.0	
Location	City	55	91.7	5	8.3	0.834
	Province	44	91.7	4	8.3	
	Unspecified	4	100.0	0	0.0	
Co-morbidity	Yes	50	94.3	3	5.7	0.495
	No	53	89.8	6	10.2	
Diabetes mellitus	Yes	5	100.0	0	0.0	1.000
	No	98	91.6	9	8.4	
Hypertension	Yes	13	100.0	0	0.0	0.595
	No	90	90.9	9	9.1	
Chronic kidney disease	Yes	4	80.0	1	20.0	0.347
	No	99	92.5	8	7.5	
History of urolithiasis	Yes	8	100.0	0	0.0	1.000
	No	95	91.3	9	8.7	
Malignancy	Yes	1	100.0	0	0.0	1.000
	No	102	91.9	9	8.1	
HIV/AIDS	Yes	10	83.3	2	16.7	0.247
	No	93	93.0	7	7.0	
Steroid use	Yes	9	100.0	0	0.0	1.000
	No	94	91.3	9	8.7	
Systemic lupus erythematosus	Yes	8	100.0	0	0.0	1.000
	No	95	91.3	9	8.7	
Nephrotic syndrome	Yes	1	100.0	0	0.0	1.000
	No	102	91.9	9	8.1	
Cerebrovascular disease	Yes	1	100.0	0	0.0	1.000
	No	102	91.9	9	8.1	
Coronary artery disease	No	103	92.0	9	8.0	No test*
Heart failure	Yes	2	100.0	0	0.0	1.000
	No	101	91.8	9	8.2	
COPD	Yes	1	100.0	0	0.0	1.000
	No	102	91.9	9	8.1	
Bronchial asthma	Yes	2	100.0	0	0.0	1.000
	No	101	91.8	9	8.2	

Table 9 (continued)

Characteristic	Category	Mortality				p value
		Survived		Expired		
		Count	Row %	Count	Row %	
Spina bifida	No	103	92.0	9	8.0	No test*
RTA Type 1	Yes	1	100.0	0	0.0	1.000
	No	102	91.9	9	8.1	
Previous TB	Yes	14	100.0	0	0.0	0.599
	No	89	90.8	9	9.2	
Other organ involvement of TB	Yes	57	89.1	7	10.9	0.296
	No	46	95.8	2	4.2	
Pulmonary TB	Yes	50	87.7	7	12.3	0.162
	No	53	96.4	2	3.6	
Gastrointestinal TB	Yes	24	85.7	4	14.3	0.224
	No	79	94.0	5	6.0	
Abdominopelvic TB	Yes	11	100.0	0	0.0	0.595
	No	92	91.1	9	8.9	
CNS TB	Yes	6	85.7	1	14.3	0.453
	No	97	92.4	8	7.6	
Bone TB	Yes	3	75.0	1	25.0	0.288
	No	100	92.6	8	7.4	
Cutaneous/Wound TB	Yes	3	100.0	0	0.0	1.000
	No	100	91.7	9	8.3	
TB Adenitis	Yes	7	87.5	1	12.5	0.500
	No	96	92.3	8	7.7	
Ear TB	Yes	1	50.0	1	50.0	0.155
	No	102	92.7	8	7.3	
Psoas TB	Yes	1	50.0	1	50.0	0.155
	No	102	92.7	8	7.3	
Dysuria	Yes	7	100.0	0	0.0	1.000
	No	82	90.1	9	9.9	
Hematuria	Yes	7	77.8	2	22.2	0.192
	No	82	92.1	7	7.9	
Urinary retention	Yes	1	100.0	0	0.0	1.000
	No	88	90.7	9	9.3	
Flank pain	Yes	11	100.0	0	0.0	0.592
	No	78	89.7	9	10.3	
Inguinal pain	Yes	1	100.0	0	0.0	1.000
	No	88	90.7	9	9.3	
Umbilical discharge	Yes	3	100.0	0	0.0	1.000
	No	86	90.5	9	9.5	
Fistula (uretero-cutaneous fistula)	Yes	1	100.0	0	0.0	1.000
	No	88	90.7	9	9.3	
Scrotal discharge	Yes	1	100.0	0	0.0	1.000
	No	88	90.7	9	9.3	
Double J stent reinsertion	Yes	1	100.0	0	0.0	1.000
	No	88	90.7	9	9.3	
Pedal edema	Yes	4	100.0	0	0.0	1.000
	No	85	90.4	9	9.6	
Fever	Yes	7	100.0	0	0.0	1.000
	No	82	90.1	9	9.9	

Table 9 (continued)

Characteristic	Category	Mortality				p value
		Survived		Expired		
		Count	Row %	Count	Row %	
Weakness	Yes	14	93.3	1	6.7	1.000
	No	75	90.4	8	9.6	
Abdominal pain	Yes	6	75.0	2	25.0	0.157
	No	83	92.2	7	7.8	
Abdominal/pelvic mass on diagnostic	Yes	4	100.0	0	0.0	1.000
	No	85	90.4	9	9.6	
Vaginal bleeding	Yes	2	100.0	0	0.0	1.000
	No	87	90.6	9	9.4	
Difficulty of breathing	Yes	10	83.3	2	16.7	0.303
	No	79	91.9	7	8.1	
Others	Yes	9	81.8	2	18.2	0.266
	No	80	92.0	7	8.0	

Bold values indicate statistically significant differences

*No test was done since all patients were classified under the *No* category

COPD chronic obstructive pulmonary disease, *HIV/AIDS* human immunodeficiency virus or acquired immunodeficiency syndrome, *RTA Type 1* renal tubular acidosis Type 1, *TB* tuberculosis, *y* year

Table 10 Bivariate analysis: serologic characteristics and mortality

Characteristics	Category	Mortality				p value
		Survived		Expired		
		Count	Row %	Count	Row %	
Anemia	Yes	84	90.3	9	9.7	0.353
	No	19	100.0	0	0.0	
Thrombocytopenia	Yes	6	100.0	0	0.0	1.000
	No	97	91.5	9	8.5	
Thrombocytosis	Yes	28	93.3	2	6.7	1.000
	No	75	91.5	7	8.5	
Leukocytosis	Yes	47	100.0	0	0.0	**0.010**
	No	56	86.2	9	13.8	
Leukopenia	Yes	5	83.3	1	16.7	0.402
	No	98	92.5	8	7.5	
Hypoalbuminemia	Yes	54	88.5	7	11.5	0.298
	No	42	95.5	2	4.5	
Renal function impairment	Yes	39	95.1	2	4.9	0.481
	No	63	90.0	7	10.0	
Hyperkalemia	Yes	8	88.9	1	11.1	0.550
	No	93	92.1	8	7.9	
Hypokalemia	Yes	23	95.8	1	4.2	0.681
	No	78	90.7	8	9.3	
Hyponatremia	Yes	48	87.3	7	12.7	0.162
	No	51	96.2	2	3.8	
Hypercalcemia	Yes	19	90.5	2	9.5	1.000
	No	76	91.6	7	8.4	

Bold value indicates statistically significant differences

Table 11 Bivariate analysis: urinary characteristics and mortality

Characteristics	Category	Mortality				p value
		Survived		Expired		
		Count	Row %	Count	Row %	
Acidic pH	Yes	44	93.6	3	6.4	0.504
	No	50	89.3	6	10.7	
Low specific gravity	Yes	31	96.9	1	3.1	0.268
	No	63	88.7	8	11.3	
Proteinuria	None	32	97.0	1	3.0	0.355
	Trace	12	80.0	3	20.0	
	1+	32	88.9	4	11.1	
	2+	15	93.8	1	6.3	
	3+	3	100.0	0	0.0	
Hematuria	Yes	50	94.3	3	5.7	0.310
	No	44	88.0	6	12.0	
Pyuria	Yes	64	91.4	6	8.6	1.000
	No	30	90.9	3	9.1	
Both hematuria and pyuria	Yes	48	96.0	2	4.0	0.162
	No	46	86.8	7	13.2	
Casts	Yes	15	88.2	2	11.8	0.640
	No	79	91.9	7	8.1	
Crystals	Yes	4	100.0	0	0.0	1.000
	No	90	90.9	9	9.1	

Serologic and urinary characteristics

Majority of patients presented with anemia (83.04%), while several exhibited leukocytosis (41.96%) and thrombocytosis (26.79%) (Table 4). Of the biochemistry data, hypoalbuminemia (58.10%) was the most common, followed by hyponatremia (50.93%), impairment of renal function (36.94%), hypercalcemia (20.19%), and hypokalemia (21.82%). Of those with urine samples, proteinuria (67.96%) and pyuria (67.96%) were the most common abnormal findings, followed by hematuria (51.46%), acidic urine (45.63%), and low specific gravity (31.07%) (Table 5).

Radiological findings

Two patients underwent intravenous pyelography (IVP), with one showing extensive calcifications throughout the urinary tract, while the other revealing non-functioning kidney. Table 6 shows the rest of the imaging findings observed in our investigation.

Treatment

Seventy-one patients (63.39%) were initiated on anti-Koch's treatment during their admission, while 29 individuals (25.89%) underwent surgery. Double J stent insertion (9.82%) and percutaneous tube nephrostomy (8.93%) were the most performed urologic operations (Table 7).

Short-term outcomes

In-hospital death occurred in 8.04% of the patients. The median hospital length of stay was 11 days, with a minimum hospital stay of 0.67 day to a maximum of 90 days. Fifteen patients (13.39%) required pressors and 1 patient (0.89%) needed renal replacement therapy in the form of hemodialysis throughout their hospital course (Table 8).

Characteristics associated with short-term outcomes

Mortality

Age, leukocytosis, and the need for pressors were all significantly associated with mortality (p values of <0.001, 0.010, and <0.001, respectively) (Tables 9, 10, 13). Other characteristics were not significantly associated with mortality (Tables 9, 10, 11, 12, 13).

Table 12 Bivariate analysis: treatments and mortality

Characteristics	Category	Mortality				*p* value
		Survived		Expired		
		Count	Row %	Count	Row %	
Anti-Kochs treatment	Yes	64	90.1	7	9.9	0.482
	No	39	95.1	2	4.9	
Underwent operation	Yes	29	100.0	0	0.0	0.167
	No	74	89.0	9	11.0	
Percutaneous tube nephrostomy	Yes	10	100.0	0	0.0	1.000
	No	93	91.2	9	8.8	
DJS insertion	Yes	11	100.0	0	0.0	0.595
	No	92	91.1	9	8.9	
Transurethralresection of bladder tumor	Yes	1	100.0	0	0.0	1.000
	No	102	91.9	9	8.1	
Bladder mass excision	Yes	3	100.0	0	0.0	1.000
	No	100	91.7	9	8.3	
Aspiration of abscess	Yes	1	100.0	0	0.0	1.000
	No	102	91.9	9	8.1	
Ureteroneocystostomy	Yes	1	100.0	0	0.0	1.000
	No	102	91.9	9	8.1	
Ureterotomy	Yes	1	100.0	0	0.0	1.000
	No	102	91.9	9	8.1	
Pelvolithotomy	Yes	1	100.0	0	0.0	1.000
	No	102	91.9	9	8.1	
Radial nephrolithotomy	Yes	1	100.0	0	0.0	1.000
	No	102	91.9	9	8.1	
Subcapsular nephrectomy	Yes	5	100.0	0	0.0	1.000
	No	98	91.6	9	8.4	
Cytoreductive nephrectomy	Yes	1	100.0	0	0.0	1.000
	No	102	91.9	9	8.1	
Nephrectomy	Yes	2	100.0	0	0.0	1.000
	No	101	91.8	9	8.2	

Table 13 Bivariate analysis: other outcomes and mortality

Characteristics	Category	Mortality				*p* value
		Survived		Expired		
		Count	Row %	Count	Row %	
Need for renal replacement therapy	Yes	1	100.0	0	0.0	1.000
	No	102	91.9	9	8.1	
Need for pressors	Yes	8	53.3	7	46.7	**<0.001**
	No	95	97.9	2	2.1	

Bold value indicates statistically significant differences

Table 14 Bivariate analysis: clinical characteristics and need for pressors

Characteristic	Category	Mortality				*p* value
		Survived		Expired		
		Count	Row %	Count	Row %	
Gender	Male	8	15.1	45	84.9	1.000
	Female	10	15.4	55	84.6	
Age	0 months to 1 year	1	100.0	0	0.0	**0.019**
	1–5 years	2	66.7	1	33.3	
	6–10 years	0	0.0	4	100.0	
	11–18 years	4	21.1	15	78.9	
	19–29 years	5	21.7	18	78.3	
	30–49 years	3	8.1	34	91.9	
	50–69 years	2	7.4	25	92.6	
	≥ 70 years	1	25.0	3	75.0	
Marital status	Single/widowed	13	17.6	61	82.4	0.436
	Married	5	11.4	39	88.6	
Occupation	Employed	3	15.0	17	85.0	0.762
	Unemployed	8	13.1	53	86.9	
	Not applicable	6	21.4	22	78.6	
	Unspecified	1	11.1	8	88.9	
Location	City	10	16.1	52	83.9	0.898
	Province	7	13.7	44	86.3	
	Unspecified	1	20.0	4	80.0	
Co-morbidity	Yes	8	14.5	47	85.5	1.000
	No	10	15.9	53	84.1	
Diabetes mellitus	Yes	0	0.0	5	100.0	1.000
	No	18	15.9	95	84.1	
Hypertension	Yes	0	0.0	13	100.0	0.214
	No	18	17.1	87	82.9	
Chronic kidney disease	Yes	2	33.3	4	66.7	0.227
	No	16	14.3	96	85.7	
History of urolithiasis	Yes	2	25.0	6	75.0	0.352
	No	16	14.5	94	85.5	
Malignancy	Yes	0	0.0	1	100.0	1.000
	No	18	15.4	99	84.6	
HIV/AIDS	Yes	2	15.4	11	84.6	1.000
	No	16	15.2	89	84.8	
Steroid use	Yes	3	33.3	6	66.7	0.139
	No	15	13.8	94	86.2	
Systemic lupus erythematosus	Yes	2	25.0	6	75.0	0.352
	No	16	14.5	94	85.5	
Nephrotic syndrome	Yes	1	100.0	0	0.0	0.153
	No	17	14.5	100	85.5	
Cerebrovascular disease	Yes	0	0.0	1	100.0	1.000
	No	18	15.4	99	84.6	
Coronary artery disease	No	18	15.3	100	84.7	No test*
Heart failure	Yes	0	0.0	2	100.0	1.000
	No	18	15.5	98	84.5	
COPD	Yes	0	0.0	1	100.0	1.000
	No	18	15.4	99	84.6	
Bronchial asthma	Yes	0	0.0	2	100.0	1.000
	No	18	15.5	98	84.5	

Table 14 (continued)

Characteristic	Category	Mortality				p value
		Survived		Expired		
		Count	Row %	Count	Row %	
Spina bifida	No	18	15.3	100	84.7	No test*
RTA Type 1	Yes	0	0.0	1	100.0	1.000
	No	18	15.4	99	84.6	
Previous TB	Yes	0	0.0	14	100.0	0.124
	No	18	17.3	86	82.7	
Other organ involvement of TB	Yes	15	21.4	55	78.6	**0.035**
	No	3	6.3	45	93.8	
Pulmonary TB	Yes	13	21.0	49	79.0	0.079
	No	5	8.9	51	91.1	
Gastrointestinal TB	Yes	10	32.3	21	67.7	**0.006**
	No	8	9.2	79	90.8	
Abdominopelvic TB	Yes	3	23.1	10	76.9	0.417
	No	15	14.3	90	85.7	
CNS TB	Yes	3	37.5	5	62.5	0.102
	No	15	13.6	95	86.4	
Bone TB	Yes	1	25.0	3	75.0	0.489
	No	17	14.9	97	85.1	
Cutaneous/Wound TB	Yes	3	100.0	0	0.0	**0.003**
	No	15	13.0	100	87.0	
TB Adenitis	Yes	1	10.0	9	90.0	1.000
	No	17	15.7	91	84.3	
Ear TB	Yes	1	50.0	1	50.0	0.283
	No	17	14.7	99	85.3	
Psoas TB	Yes	1	50.0	1	50.0	0.283
	No	17	14.7	99	85.3	
Dysuria	Yes	2	28.6	5	71.4	0.603
	No	16	16.7	80	83.3	
Hematuria	Yes	1	11.1	8	88.9	1.000
	No	17	18.1	77	81.9	
Urinary retention	Yes	0	0.0	1	100.0	1.000
	No	18	17.6	84	82.4	
Flank pain	Yes	1	8.3	11	91.7	0.687
	No	17	18.7	74	81.3	
Inguinal pain	Yes	0	0.0	1	100.0	1.000
	No	18	17.6	84	82.4	
Umbilical discharge	Yes	0	0.0	3	100.0	1.000
	No	18	18.0	82	82.0	
Fistula (uretero-cutaneous fistula)	Yes	0	0.0	1	100.0	1.000
	No	18	17.6	84	82.4	
Scrotal discharge	Yes	0	0.0	1	100.0	1.000
	No	18	17.6	84	82.4	
Double J stent reinsertion	Yes	0	0.0	1	100.0	1.000
	No	18	17.6	84	82.4	
Pedal edema	Yes	1	25.0	3	75.0	0.542
	No	17	17.2	82	82.8	
Fever	Yes	0	0.0	7	100.0	0.349
	No	18	18.8	78	81.3	

Table 14 (continued)

Characteristic	Category	Mortality				p value
		Survived		Expired		
		Count	Row %	Count	Row %	
Weakness	Yes	2	13.3	13	86.7	1.000
	No	16	18.2	72	81.8	
Abdominal pain	Yes	3	27.3	8	72.7	0.402
	No	15	16.3	77	83.7	
Abdominal/pelvic mass on diagnostic	Yes	0	0.0	4	100.0	1.000
	No	18	18.2	81	81.8	
Vaginal bleeding	Yes	0	0.0	2	100.0	1.000
	No	18	17.8	83	82.2	
Difficulty of breathing	Yes	4	30.8	9	69.2	0.235
	No	14	15.6	76	84.4	
Others	Yes	4	36.4	7	63.6	0.098
	No	14	15.2	78	84.8	

Bold values indicate statistically significant differences

*No test was done since all patients were classified under the *No* category

COPD chronic obstructive pulmonary disease, *HIV/AIDS* human immunodeficiency virus or acquired immunodeficiency syndrome, *RTA Type 1* renal tubular acidosis Type 1, *TB* tuberculosis, *y* year

Table 15 Bivariate analysis: serologic characteristics and need for pressors

Characteristics	Category	Mortality				p value
		Survived		Expired		
		Count	Row %	Count	Row %	
Anemia	Yes	16	16.2	83	83.8	0.734
	No	2	10.5	17	89.5	
Thrombocytopenia	Yes	1	16.7	5	83.3	1.000
	No	17	15.2	95	84.8	
Thrombocytosis	Yes	4	13.3	26	86.7	1.000
	No	14	15.9	74	84.1	
Leukocytosis	Yes	8	15.4	44	84.6	1.000
	No	10	15.2	56	84.8	
Leukopenia	Yes	1	16.7	5	83.3	1.000
	No	17	15.2	95	84.8	
Hypoalbuminemia	Yes	14	21.2	52	78.8	0.116
	No	4	8.9	41	91.1	
Renal function impairment	Yes	7	16.7	35	83.3	0.794
	No	11	14.7	64	85.3	
Hyperkalemia	Yes	2	22.2	7	77.8	0.628
	No	16	15.0	91	85.0	
Hypokalemia	Yes	4	16.7	20	83.3	1.000
	No	14	15.2	78	84.8	
Hyponatremia	Yes	12	20.3	47	79.7	0.204
	No	6	10.9	49	89.1	
Hypercalcemia	Yes	4	16.7	20	83.3	1.000
	No	13	15.1	73	84.9	

Table 16 Bivariate analysis: urinary characteristics and need for pressors

Characteristics	Category	Mortality				*p* value
		Survived		Expired		
		Count	Row %	Count	Row %	
Acidic pH	Yes	9	18.0	41	82.0	0.798
	No	9	15.3	50	84.7	
Low specific gravity	Yes	2	5.9	32	94.1	0.053
	No	16	21.3	59	78.7	
Proteinuria	None	4	11.4	31	88.6	0.727
	Trace	2	13.3	13	86.7	
	1+	7	17.9	32	82.1	
	2+	4	23.5	13	76.5	
	3+	1	33.3	2	66.7	
Hematuria	Yes	8	14.8	46	85.2	0.797
	No	10	18.2	45	81.8	
Pyuria	Yes	11	15.3	61	84.7	0.786
	No	7	18.9	30	81.1	
Both hematuria and pyuria	Yes	7	14.0	43	86.0	0.609
	No	11	18.6	48	81.4	
Casts	Yes	4	22.2	14	77.8	0.493
	No	14	15.4	77	84.6	
Crystals	Yes	0	0.0	4	100.0	1.000
	No	18	17.1	87	82.9	

Table 17 Bivariate analysis: treatments and need for pressors

Characteristics	Category	Mortality				*p* value
		Survived		Expired		
		Count	Row %	Count	Row %	
Anti-Kochs treatment	Yes	14	18.7	61	81.3	0.196
	No	4	9.3	39	90.7	
Underwent operation	Yes	1	3.3	29	96.7	0.095
	No	17	19.3	71	80.7	
Percutaneous tube nephrostomy	Yes	1	10.0	9	90.0	1.000
	No	17	15.7	91	84.3	
DJS insertion	Yes	0	0.0	12	100.0	0.209
	No	18	17.0	88	83.0	
Transurethral resection of bladder tumor	Yes	0	0.0	1	100.0	1.000
	No	18	15.4	99	84.6	
Bladder mass excision	Yes	0	0.0	3	100.0	1.000
	No	18	15.7	97	84.3	
Aspiration of abscess	Yes	0	0.0	1	100.0	1.000
	No	18	15.4	99	84.6	
Ureteroneocystostomy	Yes	0	0.0	1	100.0	1.000
	No	18	15.4	99	84.6	
Ureterotomy	Yes	0	0.0	1	100.0	1.000
	No	18	15.4	99	84.6	
Pelvolithotomy	Yes	0	0.0	1	100.0	1.000
	No	18	15.4	99	84.6	
Radial nephrolithotomy	Yes	0	0.0	1	100.0	1.000
	No	18	15.4	99	84.6	
Subcapsular nephrectomy	Yes	0	0.0	5	100.0	1.000
	No	18	15.9	95	84.1	
Cytoreductive nephrectomy	Yes	0	0.0	1	100.0	1.000
	No	18	15.4	99	84.6	
Nephrectomy	Yes	0	0.0	2	100.0	1.000
	No	18	15.5	98	84.5	

Table 18 Bivariate analysis: other outcomes and need for pressors

Characteristics	Category	Need for pressors				*p* value
		Yes		No		
		Count	Row %	Count	Row %	
Need for renal replacement therapy	Yes	0	0.0	1	100.0	1.000
	No	18	15.4	99	84.6	

Table 19 Comparison of mean hospital stay by clinical characteristics

Characteristic	Category	Hospital length of stay (in days)		*p* value
		Mean	**SD**	
Gender	Male	15.5	16.1	0.914
	Female	13.5	9.5	
Age	0 months to 1 years	23.0		0.444
	1–5 years	35.0	47.9	
	6–10 years	9.5	9.4	
	11–18 years	19.6	16.7	
	19–29 years	13.6	9.5	
	30–49 years	13.2	9.9	
	50–69 years	12.1	7.6	
	≥ 70 years	7.0	4.2	
Marital status	Single/widowed	17.2	14.8	**0.001**
	Married	9.6	6.2	
Occupation	Employed	12.2	11.7	0.506
	Unemployed	13.6	9.0	
	Not applicable	18.4	20.1	
	Unspecified	12.4	6.8	
Location	City	15.3	15.4	0.915
	Province	13.3	9.3	
	Unspecified	15.0	10.8	
Co-morbidity	Yes	15.3	12.4	0.338
	No	13.6	13.3	
Diabetes mellitus	Yes	7.8	4.8	0.143
	No	14.7	13.0	
Hypertension	Yes	13.3	9.4	0.897
	No	14.5	13.3	
Chronic kidney disease	Yes	16.5	9.7	0.333
	No	14.3	13.0	
History of urolithiasis	Yes	9.4	5.1	0.297
	No	14.8	13.2	
Malignancy	Yes	17.0		0.427
	No	14.4	12.9	
HIV/AIDS	Yes	14.5	10.9	0.740
	No	14.4	13.1	
Steroid use	Yes	28.7	18.5	**0.002**
	No	13.2	11.6	
Systemic lupus erythematosus	Yes	23.5	10.9	**0.008**
	No	13.7	12.8	
Nephrotic syndrome	Yes	70.0		0.091
	No	13.9	11.8	
Cerebrovascular disease	Yes	5.0		0.270
	No	14.5	12.9	
Coronary artery disease	Yes			No test*
	No	14.4	12.9	
Heart failure	Yes	19.0	18.4	0.669
	No	14.3	12.8	

Table 19 (continued)

Characteristic	Category	Hospital length of stay (in days)		*p* value
		Mean	SD	
COPD	Yes	11.0		0.953
	No	14.4	12.9	
Bronchial asthma	Yes	5.5	2.1	0.150
	No	14.5	12.9	
Spina bifida	Yes			No test*
	No	14.4	12.9	
RTA Type 1	Yes	11.0		0.953
	No	14.4	12.9	
Previous TB	Yes	9.9	5.6	0.204
	No	15.0	13.4	
Other organ involvement of TB	Yes	16.4	14.6	**0.030**
	No	11.5	9.2	
Pulmonary TB	Yes	17.1	15.3	**0.021**
	No	11.4	8.6	
Gastrointestinal TB	Yes	17.7	19.1	0.489
	No	13.2	9.6	
Abdominopelvic TB	Yes	16.0	10.4	0.273
	No	14.2	13.2	
CNS TB	Yes	22.5	27.7	0.309
	No	13.8	11.1	
Bone TB	Yes	34.5	37.8	0.157
	No	13.7	10.9	
Cutaneous/Wound TB	Yes	19.7	7.1	0.161
	No	14.3	13.0	
TB Adenitis	Yes	13.8	12.8	0.642
	No	14.4	12.9	
Ear TB	Yes	51.5	54.4	0.159
	No	13.8	10.9	
Psoas TB	Yes	61.0	41.0	**0.022**
	No	13.6	10.7	

Bold values indicate statistically significant differences

*No test was done since all patients were classified under the *No* category

COPD chronic obstructive pulmonary disease, *HIV/AIDS* human immunodeficiency virus or acquired immunodeficiency syndrome, *RTA Type 1* renal tubular acidosis Type 1, *TB* tuberculosis, *y* year

Need for pressors

Age, other organ involvement of MTB, gastrointestinal TB, and cutaneous or wound TB, were significantly associated with the need for pressors (p-values of 0.019, 0.035, 0.006, and 0.003, respectively) (Table 14). Other characteristics were not significantly associated with the need for pressors (Tables 14, 15, 16, 17, 18).

Mean hospital stay

Marital status, steroid use, systemic lupus erythematosus (SLE), other organ involvement of MTB, pulmonary TB, psoas TB, the presence of anemia, leukocytosis, hypoalbuminemia, hyponatremia, hypercalcemia, and anti-Koch's treatment had a statistically longer mean length of hospital stay compared to those without these characteristics (Tables 19, 20, 22). Other characteristics were not significantly associated with a longer mean length of hospital stay (Tables 19, 20, 21, 22, 23).

Table 20 Comparison of mean hospital stay by serologic characteristics

Characteristic	Category	Hospital length of stay (in days)		*p* value
		Mean	SD	
Anemia	Yes	15.7	13.5	**0.001**
	No	7.6	4.6	
Thrombocytopenia	Yes	14.2	14.3	0.708
	No	14.4	12.8	
Thrombocytosis	Yes	17.9	19.2	0.315
	No	13.2	9.7	
Leukocytosis	Yes	15.6	11.3	**0.027**
	No	13.4	14.0	
Leukopenia	Yes	16.7	14.1	0.690
	No	14.3	12.8	
Hypoalbuminemia	Yes	17.0	15.3	**0.029**
	No	11.3	8.0	
Renal function impairment	Yes	15.5	10.3	0.123
	No	13.9	14.1	
Hyperkalemia	Yes	10.2	5.2	0.411
	No	14.9	13.3	
Hypokalemia	Yes	11.4	6.8	0.373
	No	15.4	14.0	
Hyponatremia	Yes	16.0	13.5	**0.046**
	No	13.1	12.4	
Hypercalcemia	Yes	16.6	7.6	**0.015**
	No	14.3	14.3	

Bold values indicate statistically significant differences

Table 21 Comparison of mean hospital stay by urinary characteristics

Characteristic	Category	Hospital length of stay (in days)		*p* value
		Mean	Standard Deviation	
Acidic pH	Yes	14.3	11.8	0.745
	No	14.3	13.5	
Low specific gravity	Yes	13.3	9.9	0.724
	No	14.8	13.8	
Proteinuria	None	14.6	8.0	0.145
	Trace	8.5	5.5	
	1+	15.3	15.9	
	2+	14.4	8.7	
	3+	26.0	38.3	
Hematuria	Yes	12.9	8.2	0.709
	No	15.7	15.8	
Pyuria	Yes	14.0	12.7	0.679
	No	14.9	12.8	
Both hematuria and pyuria	Yes	12.7	8.2	0.609
	No	15.7	15.4	
Casts	Yes	15.6	16.7	0.722
	No	14.1	11.8	
Crystals	Yes	10.3	3.2	0.693
	No	14.5	12.9	

Table 22 Comparison of mean hospital stay by treatments

Characteristic	Category	Hospital length of stay (in days)		*p* value
		Mean	Standard Deviation	
Anti-Kochs treatment	Yes	17.1	13.9	**<0.001**
	No	9.7	9.1	
Underwent operation	Yes	13.0	9.8	0.666
	No	14.9	13.8	
Percutaneous tube nephrostomy	Yes	16.1	12.0	0.436
	No	14.2	13.0	
DJS insertion	Yes	14.4	9.8	0.762
	No	14.4	13.2	
Transurethral resection of bladder tumor	Yes	6.0		0.370
	No	14.5	12.9	
Bladder mass excision	Yes	5.3	3.1	0.074
	No	14.6	12.9	
Aspiration of abscess	Yes	18.0		0.347
	No	14.4	12.9	
Ureteroneocystostomy	Yes	9.0		0.724
	No	14.4	12.9	
Ureterotomy	Yes	5.0		0.270
	No	14.5	12.9	
Pelvolithotomy	Yes	11.0		0.953
	No	14.4	12.9	
Radial nephrolithotomy	Yes	11.0		0.953
	No	14.4	12.9	
Subcapsular nephrectomy	Yes	11.6	3.6	0.936
	No	14.5	13.1	
Cytoreductive nephrectomy	Yes	7.0		0.481
	No	14.5	12.9	
Nephrectomy	Yes	17.0	12.7	0.602
	No	14.3	12.9	

Bold value indicates statistically significant differences

Table 23 Comparison of mean hospital stay by other outcomes

Characteristics	Category	Hospital length of stay (in days)		*p* value
		Mean	Standard Deviation	
Need for renal replacement therapy	Yes	23.0		0.246
	No	14.3	12.9	
Need for pressors	Yes	20.2	24.0	0.790
	No	13.3	9.4	

Discussion

Genitourinary TB is the second and third most common form of EPTB in countries with high and low TB burden, respectively [9, 19, 25]. According to other registers, however, GUTB is only seen in 1.7–6.5% of the total TB cases reported [26]. In the Philippines, a 5-year retrospective study reported GUTB to have caused 3% of pediatric EPTB cases admitted in a tertiary government hospital [13]. It is important to emphasize that this infection is underdiagnosed in most health care centers, as GUTB remains a diagnostic challenge [9, 19, 25–27].

Diagnosis of GUTB is often delayed due to the insidious nature of the disease, non-specificity of symptoms, poor health-seeking behavior of patients, and lack of clinician awareness [28, 29]. In autopsy studies, only half of patients with renal involvement had symptoms, while only 18% were diagnosed clinically [30]. The four pillars to GUTB diagnosis are bacteriology, pathomorphology, radiology, and provocative test with therapy *ex juvantibus* [6, 19, 31], with culture as the gold standard [25, 29, 32]. In world literature, most cases of GUTB (64.2%) were diagnosed through identification of MTB

Table 24 Studies in the Asia–Pacific region involving patients with GUTB

Study (publication year)	Size	Setting (country)	Population	Outcomes	Method
Mishra [33] (2020)	53	Department of Urology, Indira Gandhi Institute of Medical Sciences (India)	Patients with confirmed GUTB	Demographic, clinical presentation Urinary profile, routine blood exams Urine AFB smear test, urine MTB culture Radiological examinations, cystoscopic examination, histopathological examinations	4-year prospective observational case series
Huang [10] (2019)	57	Chang Gung Memorial Hospital-Chiayi (Taiwan)	Patients with diagnosis of GUTB with at least one of the following: positive MTB culture or histologic evidence	Demographics, comorbidities, symptoms and signs Results of mycobacterial smears and cultures, histopathology CBCs, serum biochemistry profile Chest radiography GU tract operations, anti-TB therapy, complications, clinical outcomes	15-year retrospective study
Kim [35] (2018)	56	Severance Hospital, Seoul (South Korea)	Participants older than 18 years diagnosed with GUTB based on presence of any clinical finding plus a positive result for one of the ff: (1) urine AFB, (2) urine MTB culture, (3) urine MTB PCR, or (4) histopathology	Clinical and laboratory data Diagnostic methods, treatment modalities and outcomes	11-year retrospective study
Cao [36] (2017)	419	Peking University First Hospital (China)	All patients with clinical renal TB with microbiologic or histologic confirmation	Demographics, clinical data, complications, treatment Laboratory findings Imaging findings Pathologic features	15-year retrospective study
Krishnamoorthy [8] (2017)	110	Chennai, Tamil Nadu (India)	Patients with either (1) proven GUTB based on urine AFB smear, AFB culture, histopathological evidence of TB, and/or by serological methods; or (2) presumed GUTB who had ≥ 2 consistent features on urological imaging or endoscopic evaluation	Clinical history and examination Serum biochemistry Urine culture Imaging findings	3-year retrospective study
Ye [37] (2016)	193	West China Hospital, Sichuan University (China)	Cases with definite UTB based on results of comprehensive diagnosis, including clinical features, laboratory results (i.e., smear microscopy, MTB culture, real-time PCR, and histological patterns), radiological findings, and response to anti-TB therapy	Demographic data, clinical history, prognosis Radiological findings Selected laboratory results	5-year cross-sectional study
Singh [38] (2013)	117	Urology Department of Institute of Post Graduate Medical Education and Research and SSKM Hospital (India)	All cases clinically diagnosed as GUTB	Clinical presentation Urine AFB smear, urine MTB culture, urine PCR for MTB Radiological and histopathological examinations	13-year retrospective study

Table 24 (continued)

Study (publication year)	Size	Setting (country)	Population	Outcomes	Method
Chandra [39] (2012)	25	Himalayan Institute of Medical Sciences, Uttarkhand State (India)	Male patients with histopathologically confirmed GUTB	Occupation, socioeconomicstatus Clinical history Relevant radiological, laboratory and histopathology findings Treatment	13-year retrospective study
Hsu [40] (2011)	64	National Taiwan University Hospital and Taipei Medical University – Wan Fang Hospital (Taiwan)	All patients with urine culture-confirmed GUTB	Clinical features Laboratory characteristics Treatment outcomes Genotypic characteristics of MTB isolates	12-year retrospective study
Lee [17] (2011)	101	Department of Urology, Hanyang University College of Medicine (Korea)	Patients diagnosed with GUTB based on the presence of one or more positivities in terms of histopathological findings, urine AFB smear, urine MTB culture, and urine PCR for MTB	Yearly proportion, gender, patient distribution according to age, history of TB, and presence of other organ TB Urinalysis findings	10-year retrospective study
Karnjanawanichkul [41] (2010)	35	Prince of Songkla University, Hat Yai, Songkhla (Thailand)	Patients diagnosed with urinary tract TB by demonstration of AFB in urine smear, growth from urine MTB culture, or consistent histopathologic findings	Demographic data, clinical features Laboratory data Chest x-ray, intravenous urography, ultrasonography, or endoscopic findings	10-year retrospective study
Takahashi [42] (2007)	12	Urology clinics of six medical centers, Hokkaido (Japan)	Patients diagnosed with urinary TB based on NAAT or histopathology	Demographic data, clinical features Detection method for MTB Diagnostic findings Treatment, outcomes, and medication-related adverse events	5-year retrospective study
Hsieh [18] (2006)	31	Kaohsiunng Medical University Hospital, Kaohsiung (Taiwan)	Patients diagnosed with GUTB based on microbiological or histological findings plus compatible clinical and roentgenographic findings	Baseline characteristics, underlying diseases, treatment responses, and outcomes	11-year retrospective study
Buccholz [43] (2000)	55	Aga Khan University Hospital (Pakistan)	In-patients with GUTB proven either by urine culture positivity for MTB, or histopathology	Age, sex, concomitant diseases, medical history, symptoms, diagnosis, treatment and follow-up	13-year retrospective study
Ramanathan [34] (1998)	38	Sanjay Gandhi Post Graduate Institute of Medical Sciences, Lucknow (India)	All patients with either: (1) urinary TB based on positive urine or pus cultures for MTB or histopathology, or (2) presumed urinary TB with ≥ 3 consistent features on urological imaging or endoscopy	History and physical examination Serum chemistry Urine culture Chest x-ray and ultrasonography	8-year retrospective study
Dy [16] (1995)	61	Santo Tomas University Hospital (Philippines)	In-patients clinically diagnosed with GUTB	Demographic features Presenting manifestations, history of previous TB Diagnostic modalities (radiographic, bacteriologic, histopathologic) Therapeutic modalities	Case series

Table 24 (continued)

Study (publication year)	Size	Setting (country)	Population	Outcomes	Method
Tanchuco [15] (1987)	42	Philippine General Hospital and National Kidney Institute (Philippines)	Patients with discharge diagnosis of urinary tract TB based on the presence of one of the following: positive urine AFB smear, positive urine AFB culture, or consistent histopathologic findings	Clinical and laboratory parameters	6-year retrospective study

GU genitourinary, *MTB* Mycobacterium tuberculosis, *NAAT* nucleic acid amplification test, *PTB* pulmonary tuberculosis, *UTB* urinary tuberculosis

Table 25 Studies in the Asia–Pacific region describing the demographic features of patients with GUTB

Study (publication year)	Age	Male-to-female ratio	Demographic	Genitourinary organs involved (n)	Associated comorbidities (%)
Mishra [33] (2020)	Mean, 39.15 ± 12.62 y	1:1.21 (24:29)	Socioeconomic class: lower (88.7%), middle (9.4%), upper (1.9%)	Kidney (33; 18 unilateral, 15 bilateral involvement), ureter (16; 14 lower ureteral stricture, 1 middle ureteral stricture, 1 multiple strictures), bladder (13)	History of PTB (20.8%)
Huang [10] (2019)	Median, 71 years (range, 33–89 years)	1.85:1 (37:20)		Kidneys (8), kidney and ureter (4), epididymis (3), epididymis and testis (3), kidney and prostate (2), prostate (2), ureter (1), ureter and bladder (1), testis (1), epididymis and testis and prostate (1), scrotum and penis (1), uterus and cervix (1)	DM type II (35.1%), chronic renal disease (33.3%), underlying malignancies (hepatocellular, prostate, bladder, cervix, rectum, thyroid gland, lymphoma, and skin) (24.6%), adrenal insufficiency (24.6%), corticosteroid use (21.1%), chronic airway disease (19.3%), liver cirrhosis (17.5%), past history of TB (15.8%), alcoholism (8.8%), and autoimmune disease (3.5%)
Kim [35] (2018)	Mean, 52.8 y	1:1.15 (26:30)		Kidney or ureter (39, 69.6%), bladder (16, 28.6%), epididymis or testis (13, 23.2%), uterus or fallopian tubes (5, 8.9%), prostate (4, 7.1%)	History of TB (42.9%, PTB 37.5%), CVD (28.6%), immunocompromised state (21.4%), pulmonary disease (10.7%), liver disease (7.1%), DM (5.4%), history of gastrectomy (3.6%)
Cao [36] (2017)	Mean, 42.7 ± 13.4 years (range, 12–78 years)	1:1.29 (183:236)	Unemployed (24.6%), farmer (21%), civil servant (15.5%), worker (10.7%), retiree 9.1%), student (4.3%), other occupations (14.6%)	Left kidney (210, 50.1%), right kidney (171, 40.8%), both (38, 9.1%)	History of PTB (20.3%)
Krishnamoorthy [8] (2017)	Mean, 35.4 years (range, 11–67 years)	1.4:1 (65:45)		Kidney (70), ureters (30), bladder (18), testis and epididymis (6), prostate (4), penis (1)	History of PTB (22.7%), gastrointestinal TB (2.7%)
Ye [37] (2016)	Mean, 42.8 ± 14.95 y	1.64:1 (120:73)			Extra-urinary TB (36.3%)
Singh [38] (2013)	Third decade of life (63.2%)	1:1.51 (47:70)		Kidney (76; 56 unilateral, 20 bilateral involvement), ureter (32), bladder (20), prostate (4), scrotal swelling (6)	Past history of PTB (18.9%)

Table 25 (continued)

Study (publication year)	Age	Male-to-female ratio	Demographic	Genitourinary organs involved (n)	Associated comorbidities (%)
Chandra [39] (2012)	Mean, 37.7 y	NA; only males were included	Location: hilly region of state (68%), non-hilly region of state (32%) Occupation: farmer (56%), laborer (20%), shopkeeper (8%), student (8%), unknown (8%) Socioeconomic status: low (80%)	Urinary bladder (7, 28%), prostate (6, 24%), epididymis (3, 12%), testes (3, 12%), kidney (2, 8%), ureter (2, 8%), scrotum (1, 4%)	Previous history of TB (36%), alcoholism (28%), diabetes (12%)
Hsu [40] (2011)	Mean, 60.3 ± 16.1 y	1.46:1 (38:26)		Bladder (5), ureter (4), kidney (2), kidney/ureter (1), kidney/ureter/bladder (1), epididymis (3), testis/epididymis (2), testis/epididymis/prostate gland (2), epididymis/prostate gland (1), testis (1), prostate gland (1)	57.8% Disseminated TB (48.4%), PTB (43.8%), DM (23.4%), malignancy (14.1%), COPD (14.1%), previous TB (12.5%), CVD (12.5%), receiving steroids (12.5%), ESRD (6.3%), liver cirrhosis (4.7%), alcoholism (4.7%)
Lee [17] (2011)	Mean, 45.57 ± 12.55 years (range, 19–81 years)	1:1.53 (40:61)		Kidney and/or ureter (80.20%), epididymis and/or testis (14.85%), bladder (3.96%), prostate(0.99%)	Past history of PTB (21.8%), intestinal TB (0.99%), spine TB (0.99%)
Karnjanawanichkul [41] (2010)	Mode, 31–40 years (range,10–76)	1.3:1 (20:15)	Occupation: farmer (34.3%), housewife (20.0%), businessperson (14.3%), government service (14.3%), blue-collar worker (14.3%), and student (2.9%)	Kidney (7; 3 bilateral, 3 left, 1 right), ureter (7; 3 bilateral, 1 left, 3 right), bladder (4), testis (3; 1 left, 2 right), kidneys to urethra (2), kidney + bladder (2), ureter + bladder (1), bladder + urethra (1), urethra (1)	Active or past history of PTB (34.3%)
Takahashi [42] (2007)	Median, 68.5 years (range, 40–90 years)	1:1 (6:6)		Kidney (7), bladder (6), ureter (2)	Active PTB (16.7%)
Hsieh [18] (2006)	Mean, M: 54.4 years (range, 32–75 years), F: 61.8 years (range, 31–81 years)	1:1.21 (14:17)			History of PTB (25.8%)
Buccholz [43] (2000)	Mean, 39.9 ± 17.1 years (7–81 years)	3:1 (41:14)		Kidney (28), bladder (15), ureter (13), testes (5), urethra (1)	Active PTB or EPTB on Category I treatment (93%), on Category II (5.4%), on Category III (1.8%), history of EPTB (11%), DM (33%)
Ramanathan [34] (1998)	Mean, 38.8 years	1:3.22 (9:29)			History of PTB (43.2%)

Table 25 (continued)

Study (publication year)	Age	Male-to-female ratio	Demographic	Genitourinary organs involved (n)	Associated comorbidities (%)
Dy [16] (1995)	Mean, M: 48.4 ± 17.01 years (range, 21–72), F: 43.3 ± 17.58 years (21–78)	1:2.2 (19:42)		Kidneys (50.8%), kidneys + ureter (4.9%), kidneys + ureter + bladder (1.6%), kidneys + prostate (1.6%), pelvis (8.2%), bladder (1.6%), bladder + ureter (1.6%), epididymis (3.3%), epididymis + testis + vas deferens (1.6%), fallopian tube + peritoneum (1.6%)	Active PTB (47.5%), past history of TB (32.8%), hyperuricemia (13.1%), DM (1.6%), HTN (1,6%), DM + HTN (1.6%), hypertensive renal failure (1.6%), liver cirrhosis (1.6%), congestive heart failure (1.6%), myelofibrosis (1.6%), osteoarthritis and prostatic cancer (1.6%), rheumatoid arthritis (1.6%)
Tanchuco [15] (1987)	Mean, 39 years (range, 2 to 64)	1.3:1 24:18			Past history of TB or exposure (28.6%), malnutrition (4.8%), DM (2.4%)

COPD chronic obstructive pulmonary disease, *CVD* cardiovascular disease, *DM* diabetes mellitus, *ESRD* end-stage renal disease, *F* female, *HTN* hypertension, *M* male, *NA* not applicable, *PTB* pulmonary tuberculosis

Table 26 Studies in the Asia–Pacific region illustrating the clinical presentation of patients with GUTB

Study (publication year)	Time from symptom onset to diagnosis	Systemic symptoms	Genitourinary manifestations
Mishra [33] (2020)		Constitutional symptoms (28.3%)	Irritative voiding symptoms (69.8%), hematuria (56.6%), flank pain (56.6%), associated renal failure (13.2%), infertility and hematospermia (5.6%), scrotal mass (1.9%)
Huang [10] (2019)	Median, 4 m (range, 0.5–50 m)	75.4% Fever (56.1%), malaise/fatigue (36.8), weight loss (31.6%), night sweats (8.8%)	71.9% Gross hematuria (40.4%), frequency/urgency (33.3%), dysuria (29.8%), flank pain (26.3%)
Kim [35] (2018)		Nonspecific symptoms (fever, anorexia, weight loss, sweating, weakness, peripheral lymphadenopathy) (12.5%)	Urinary frequency or dysuria, urethral pain, or irritable voiding symptoms (55.4%); loin or abdominal pain (42.9%); gross hematuria (33.9%); scrotal pain/mass (19.6%); abscess or fistula (5.4%); vaginal bleeding (3.6%)
Cao [36] (2017)		Constitutional symptoms including weight loss, fever, night sweats, and/or fatigue (38.9%)	Lower urinary tract symptoms including frequency, urgency, and odynuria (65.2%); flank pain (37.9%); gross hematuria (26.3%)
Krishnamoorthy [8] (2017)			Loin pain (27.0%), storage symptoms (25.5%), hematuria (12.0%), stone disease (9.1%), palpable mass (8.2%), scrotal sinus (5.5%), infertility (2.7%), gastrointestinal symptoms (2.7%), urosepsis (1.8%), renal failure (1.8%), calcified kidney (0.9%), urinoma (0.9%)
Ye [37] (2016)		Fever (26.4%), night sweat (13.0%), weight loss (10.9%)	Urinary irritation (61.1%), lumbago (49.2%)
Singh [38] (2013)		32.6%	Irritative voiding symptoms (66.47%), hematuria (47.6%), flank pain (33.8%), recurrent urinary tract symptoms (18.9%), scrotal mass (5.1%), colocutaneous fistula (0.8%), nephrocutaneous fistula (1.8%), associated renal failure (14.7%), infertility or hematospermia (3.4%)
Chandra [39] (2012)		Fever and malaise (32.0%)	Urgency and increased frequency of micturition (56%), lumbar pain (56%), dysuria (52%), hematuria (44%), pyuria (40%), infertility (12%), renal failure (8%), recurrent abscess (8%), scrotal lump (8%), scrotal sinus (4%)
Hsu [40] (2011)	182.0 ± 311.1 d (range, 5 to 1245 d)	51.6% Fever (43.8%), fatigue (37.5%), body weight loss (12.5%)	62.5% Dysuria (31.3%), frequency (31.3%), flank pain (28.1%), hematuria (17.2%), scrotal pain or mass (10.9%)
Lee [17] (2011)		Fever (3.0%)	Frequency (40.6%), hematuria (33.7%), dysuria (16.8%), flank pain (16.8%), scrotal swelling (3%)
Karnjanawanichkul [41] (2010)	<6 m (65.7%), 6–12 m (17.1%), >1 years (8.6%), uncertain data (8.6%)		Frequency (48.6%), dysuria (42.9%), hematuria (31.4%), abdominal pain or mass (25.7%), urethral pain (20.0%), retention (14.3%), cutaneous fistula (14.3%), renal failure (5.7%)
Takahashi [42] (2007)	Median duration; between initial symptoms and clinic visit: 120 d (range, 3–360 d); between clinic visit and diagnosis: 14 d (7–150 d)		Chief complaint: frequency (58.3%), hematuria (25.0%), positive nuclear matrix protein 22 on screening test for bladder cancer (8.3%), incidental right renal tumor (8.3%)

Table 26 (continued)

Study (publication year)	Time from symptom onset to diagnosis	Systemic symptoms	Genitourinary manifestations
Hsieh [18] (2006)	Mean, 2 m (range, 5 d to 18 m)	Fever (29.0%), malaise/fatigue (12.9%), night sweats (3.2%), body weight loss (3.2%)	Frequency/urgency (61.3%), dysuria (58.1%), flank pain (35.5%), gross hematuria (32.2%), scrotal mass/pain (16.1%)
Buccholz [43] (2000)		Fever (36.0%), lassitude (13.0%), weight loss (13.0%)	Dysuria (49%), frequency (40%), flank pain (36%), gross hematuria (31%), urgency (15%), testicular swelling (13%), suprapubic pain (9%), renal colic (1%)
Ramanathan [34] (1998)			Pain (63.6%), hematuria (61.3%), lump (18.2%)
Dy [16] (1995)	Mean, M: 30.4 ± 42.09 m (range, 0.25–180), F: 27.8 ± 35.2 m (0.5–168)	Fever (29.5%), weight loss (18.0%), chills (9.8%), nausea/vomiting (6.6%), anorexia (6.6%)	Dysuria (32.8%), flank pain (27.9%), hematuria (19.6%), hypogastric pain (19.6%), nocturia (19.6%), frequency (18%), edema (14.8%), vaginal spotting (13.1%), costovertebral angle tenderness (11.4%), urgency (9.8%), hesitancy (6.6%)
Tanchuco [15] (1987)		Fever (52.4%), weight loss (26.2%), chills (21.4%), malaise (11.9%), night sweats (2.4%)	Dysuria (71.5%), hematuria (62.0%), flank pain (44.5%), turbid urine (47.6%), frequency (40.5%), hypogastric pain 23.8%), edema (4.8%)

Table 27 Studies in the Asia–Pacific region showing serologic and urinary profiles of patients with GUTB

Study (publication year)	Hematologic data	Biochemistry	Urinalysis
Mishra [33] (2020)			Acidic urine (98.1%), sterile pyuria (81.1%), pyuria (69.8%), hematuria (58.4%), alkaline urine (1.9%)
Huang [10] (2019)	Anemia (< 10 g/dL) (28.1%), thrombocytopenia (< 150 × 10^{12}/L) (26.3%)	Hypoalbuminemia (< 2.5 g/dL) (40.4%)	Pyuria + hematuria (29.8%), isolated hematuria (> 30/HPF) (17.5%), isolated pyuria (> 20/HPF) (12.3%)
Kim [35] (2018)			Pyuria (> 5 WBCs/HPF) (66.1%), hematuria (> 2 RBCs/HPF) (50.0%), proteinuria (19.6%)
Cao [36] (2017)			Pyuria (> 5 WBCs/HPF) (56.3%), hematuria (> 3 RBCs/HPF) (48.8%)
Ye [37] (2016)	Anemia (15.6%), leukocytosis (13.0%)	Increased BUN (23.3%), increased creatinine (20.2%)	Hematuria (63.2%), proteinuria (45.6%), pyuria (19.2%)
Singh [38] (2013)			Sterile pyuria (62.4%), hematuria (61.5%), proteinuria (57.4%)
Hsu [40] (2011)	Anemia (Hb < 12 g/dL) (46.9%), leukocytosis (WBC > 10,000/µL) (17.2%)	Hypoalbuminemia (albumin < 3.5 g/dL) (37.5%), renal function impairment (Cr > 1.5 mg/dL) (18.8%), liver function impairment (ALT > 40 IU/L) (17.2%)	Pyuria or hematuria (WBC > 10/HPF, × 400; RBC > 5/HPF, × 400) (64.1%), aseptic pyuria (53.1%)
Lee [17] (2011)			Proteinuria (57.4%), hematuria (51.5%), pyuria (42.4%)
Karnjanawanichkul [41] (2010)			Acidic urine with pyuria (80.0%)
Hsieh [18] (2006)	Anemia (Hb < 12 g/dL) (25.8%), leukocytosis (WBC > 10,000/µL) (25.8%), leukopenia (WBC < 4000/µL) (0%)	Poor renal function (Cr > 1.5 mg/dL) (58.1%), poor liver function (ALT > 40 IU/L) (16.1%), hyperkalemia (K^+ > 5.5 meq/L) (3.2%)	Pyuria + hematuria (51.6%), pyuria (WBC > 10/HPF; 400x) (25.8%), hematuria (RBC > 5/HPF; 400x) (12.9%)
Buccholz [43] (2000)			Pyuria (56%), hematuria (36%), sterile pyuria (6%)
Dy [16] (1995)			Hematuria (37.7%), proteinuria (32.8%), pyuria + bacteriuria (32.8%), sterile pyuria (26.2%), pyuria (8.2%), sterile pyuria + bacteriuria (3.3%), cylindruria (13.1%)
Tanchuco [15] (1987)	Anemia Hb < 12 g/dL (60.0%), leukocytosis (WBC > 10,000/µL) (37.0%)	Creatinine clearance < 30 ml/min (75.0%), elevated BUN (> 0.53 mmol/L) (38.9%), elevated serum Cr (> 176.8 mmol/L) (35.1%)	Alkaline urine (pH ≥ 6) (88.9%), pyuria (WBC ≥ 6/HPF) (82.4%), hematuria (RBC ≥ 6/HPF) (61.8%), albuminuria of 2 + or more (55.8%)

***ALT* alanine aminotransferase, *Cr* serum creatinine, *Hb* hemoglobin, *HPF* high-power field, *RBC* red blood cell, *WBC* white blood cell**

in the urine, mostly establishing the diagnosis via positive urine culture [9]. Similarly, most retrospective studies in the Asia–Pacific region diagnosed infection based on bacteriologic and histologic findings with consistent clinical history, while a few depended mainly on clinico-radiologic evaluation (Table 24). In our study, the lack of clinical registries of GUTB in our hospital prompted us to instead use laboratory registries for case finding, noting majority of cases being diagnosed based on positivity for urine AFB smear (50.00%). In contrast, one local study observed mycobacterial culture being sent in only 22.2% of urologic cases and in 11.1% of gynecology cases, relying more heavily on clinical, radiographic, and histopathologic assessment [16]. Despite being a recognized tool for diagnosis of GUTB, imaging is particularly useful only during the later stages of the disease when calcifications or cavernous forms have already developed [19, 33]. Nonetheless, this diversity in practice standards is expected in developing countries because of the disproportionate availability of medical facilities and services [34].

Many reviews of the world literature [28, 29] noted kidneys to be the most frequently organ, which is consistent with most studies done in the Asia–Pacific region (Table 25). In contrast, some reports observed the bladder to be the most frequently affected genitourinary organ [38, 40], similar to our investigation. Renal involvement of TB infection can either be a localized urogenital disease or a part of a disseminated infection [6]. In literature, up to 10% of affected individuals have concomitant active pulmonary TB, suggesting hematogenous or lymphatic spread to this highly vascularized organ [28]. The latent period between pulmonary infection and development of clinical GUTB is described to range from 1 to 46 years, averaging around 22 years [29]. Infection may also be acquired hematogenously from the gut [28]. Other genitourinary organs may become affected through ascent or descent of MTB from a source elsewhere in the genitourinary tract, or from contact with the bacilli shed into the urine [26]. They may also get involved from descending spread from the lymphatics [29] or from sexual intercourse [28].

Unilateral organ involvement is commonly shown in retrospective, clinical, and autopsy studies [28, 33, 36, 38, 41]. In our investigation, left laterality was observed in 60% of those with kidney and ureter involvement, consistent with other reports [36, 41]. Renal lesions are initially described to be bilateral attributing to hematogenous spread. They generally undergo a period of cicatrization then enter a latent phase of infection, only reactivating the moment an individual becomes immunocompromised. From a single focus, infection eventually progresses, affecting one kidney while sparing the other. This phenomenon accounts for the greater frequency of unilateral renal TB [9].

Patient characteristics

Our investigation noted several patients having chronic diseases (e.g., diabetes mellitus, hypertension, chronic kidney disease), immunocompromised conditions (e.g., HIV/AIDS, steroid use), history of tuberculosis, or presence of TB in other organs. Traditionally, risk factors for developing TB include malnutrition, immunosuppression, HIV infection, diabetes, chronic kidney or liver disease, smoking, and low socioeconomic status [25, 28]. Factors considered high-risk for GUTB include past or present TB infection, recurrent or resistant urinary tract infection, and fistulas involving the scrotum, perineum, or lumbar area [5]. Emergence of drug-resistant strains of TB as well as anatomical abnormalities of the urogenital tract from congenital conditions, renal cysts, and urolithiasis also predispose to its development [19]. In our study, a substantial number of patients were single or widowed (61.61%), lived in urban areas (53.57%), and were unemployed (51.79%). In comparison, several studies reported most patients to be living in the hilly region of the state (68%), working as farmers (21–56%) or unemployed (20.0–24.6%), and having low socioeconomic status (80.0–88.7%) [33, 36, 39, 41].

Worldwide, cases encountered between developed and developing countries exhibit different patterns. In developed countries, GUTB mainly affects the elderly, ethnic minorities, and immigrants [6, 9]. On the other hand, patients from developing countries are younger due to higher incidence and severity of TB disease. They present with more specific symptoms and complications which are further exacerbated by delays in diagnosis [9]. Our data demonstrated a mean age of 35.79 ± 18.29 years, with 22.32% belonging to the pediatric population. These findings are consistent with most studies in the region (Table 25). GUTB generally has the propensity to infect both men and women of child-bearing age (20–40 years old), with a mean age of 40.7 years (range, 5–88 years) [25, 29]. We also report a male-to-female ratio of 1:1.15 (52:60). A proper estimate is controversial since there is a lack of controlled epidemiological and clinical studies [28]. While some report more men to be affected than women (2:1) [29], others report women to be affected twice as many as men [28]. Even among past local data, sex distribution was inconsistent [15, 16]. Variation between geographical regions might reflect local TB endemicity or study bias, thereby making accurate epidemiological and clinical data on GUTB difficult to obtain [28].

Clinical manifestations

GUTB does not present with any specific clinical feature and may in fact be asymptomatic [6]. Up to 50% of cases are incidentally diagnosed when patients undergo work-up for other genitourinary disorders [28]. In those with symptoms, storage symptoms (e.g., urinary frequency, urgency, incontinence, nocturia) were the most common presentation on admission, followed by dysuria, hematuria, and lumbar pain [9, 26, 29]. In our study, we recorded 50.89% of patients to have genitourinary manifestations as their chief complaint, with 21.43% having flank or abdominal pain. Several studies also mentioned abdominal or hypogastric pain to be common (19.6%-42.9%) [15, 16, 35, 41].

We noted 21.43% of patients to have systemic symptoms such as weakness and fever as their initial complaints, while 12.50% manifested with difficulty of breathing. Such findings might be explained by the high rates of TB infection in other organ systems (57.14%), with lungs being the most common extra-genitourinary site (50.89%). In some literature, constitutional symptoms such as fever, weight loss, and night sweats are uncommon and, if present, are indicative of concomitant TB outside the genitourinary system. Some patients may initially present with a myriad of symptoms reflective of other concomitant infections like PTB and hence GUTB symptoms and signs are not always defined by the anatomical site of disease [28]. Moreover, secondary bacterial infections can concurrently occur in up to 50% of patients with GUTB [25, 28]. Our data is consistent with most studies in the Asia–Pacific region, with the exception of those done in South Korea where systemic symptoms are relatively uncommon (3–12.5%) [17, 35]. Systemic manifestations are otherwise present in many reports (28.3–75.4%), with fever being the most cited symptom (29–56.1%) (Table 26). Delays in diagnosis may result in disease progression and severe complications seen at presentation [28].

Hematologic abnormalities

Hematological and biochemical tests are considered non-specific and are instead utilized as adjuncts to GUTB management [28]. In our study, majority of patients presented with anemia (83.04%), while several exhibited leukocytosis (41.96%) and thrombocytosis (26.79%). This is similar to past local data, where anemia and leukocytosis were found in 60.0% and 37.0% of patients, respectively [15]. These estimates are higher than what is recorded in literature, where 15.6–46.9% of patients exhibited anemia and 13.0–25.8% had leukocytosis (Table 27). Thrombocytopenia (26.3%) occurred more frequently in some populations [10]. It is important to note that these studies applied different definitions of hematologic abnormalities, making comparison difficult.

TB infection is traditionally known to affect various cell lines. It can cause anemia attributed to four mechanisms: chronic disease, nutritional deficiencies, autoimmune hemolytic anemia, and marrow complications. It is described to commonly affect all subtypes of granulocytes during its course, predominantly affecting neutrophils either quantitatively or qualitatively. It may result in transient neutrophilia or, in extreme cases, leukemoid reaction. TB may also cause leukopenia, especially in females, elderly, or those with recurrent infections. Neutropenia may occur from direct suppression of granulopoiesis by activated T cells [44]. Lymphopenia and lymphocytosis are also commonly reported in active TB [45]. Lastly, TB may result in various platelet abnormalities. Thrombocytosis is frequently reactive in nature and is related to the degree of inflammation. It is mediated by increased levels of endogenous thrombopoietin produced as an acute-phase reactant. Thrombocytopenia, on the other hand, is usually from bone marrow infiltration, disseminated intravascular coagulation, immune thrombocytopenic purpura, thrombotic thrombocytopenic purpura, or drug-induced [44].

Biochemical abnormalities

Among those with laboratory results, hypoalbuminemia (58.10%) and impairment of renal function (36.94%) were commonly found, similar to those reported in literature, with estimates at 37.5–40.4% and 18.8–75.0%, respectively (Table 27). As plasma creatinine concentration is frequently described to be normal in the setting of unilateral renal involvement, increased levels may indicate bilateral renal involvement or presence of concomitant disorders such as interstitial nephritis or glomerulonephritis [46, 47]. In a review of 8961 cases, 5.7% of patients with GUTB were reported to develop end-stage renal disease (ESRD) [29]. Likewise, one retrospective study in South Korea reported occurrence of ESRD in 7.1% of GUTB patients, identifying acute renal failure and old age as independent risk factors for chronic kidney disease [35].

We also observed several electrolyte abnormalities, specifically hyponatremia (50.93%), hypercalcemia (20.19%), hypokalemia (21.82%), and hyperkalemia (8.18%). Mild hyponatremia has been reported in the setting of active pulmonary or miliary TB, with incidences ranging from 11 to 51% [27, 48]. Most cases are due to syndrome of inappropriate antidiuretic hormone secretion (SIADH), with a third having reset osmostat wherein the plasma sodium stabilizes at lower concentration levels. Mechanisms for such persistent ADH release are yet to be explored, but abnormalities in water handling are demonstrated to resolve following successful treatment of infection [27]. Hyponatremia in TB may also be attributed to adrenal insufficiency. Hyponatremia from this condition is accompanied by hyperkalemia and increased urinary potassium excretion. Cerebral salt wasting is another mechanism for hyponatremia, usually seen in patients with tuberculous meningitis [48]. Lastly, patients with kidney TB may also develop salt-losing nephropathy [49].

Tubulointerstitial nephritis (TIN) is one possible complication of TB which might contribute to the multiple electrolyte abnormalities seen in patients with infection. Several case reports described the development of chronic granulomatous TIN in patients with TB as evidenced by renal biopsy [50–53]. Unlike the other studies, one case series in west London found only 18.7% of those with granulomatous inflammation on renal biopsy to exhibit caseation necrosis [53], whereas another study in France raised the possibility of severe TIN in TB despite the absence of renal granuloma [54]. Although reports on this tubulointerstitial disorder are increasing, mechanisms for its development are poorly understood [55].

Hypercalcemia is another electrolyte abnormality commonly cited in patients with TB. Surveys from different countries show prevalence rates up to 11%-48%, noting that the actual estimates of prevalence are difficult to establish since concurrent serum albumin levels are not consistently reported [48]. Renal or extrarenal TB granulomas accounted for the non-physiologic synthesis of 1,25-dihydroxyvitamin D3 and the ensuing hypercalcemia [56]. Calcification is unusual in the early stages of infection, however, in the advanced stages, nearly all kidneys contains calcification [26].

Urinary abnormalities

Urinalysis is abnormal in up to 90% of patients with GUTB, with findings ranging from mild changes to extreme pyuria [6, 29, 57]. Pyuria with or without microscopic hematuria is seen in majority of patients, whereas heavy proteinuria and cellular casts are not generally observed [6, 26]. Persistent sterile pyuria, pyuria in an acidic urine without growth on routine culture, or symptomatic UTI unresponsive to standard antibiotics should prompt suspicion of GUTB [6, 25, 28, 58]. Our study showed proteinuria (67.96%) and pyuria (67.96%) to be the most common urinary findings, consistent with those cited in literature (Table 27). Low specific gravity was also found to be common (31.07%), possibly reflecting poor urinary concentrating ability especially in the setting of chronic kidney disease or tubulopathy.

Radiological findings

Various imaging modalities are used to support the diagnosis of GUTB, with findings dependent upon the extent of disease progression. Despite traditionally being used to suggest, and not to confirm or exclude, the presence of the disease, they are still paramount in management and can still be utilized to confidently diagnose GUTB by those with sufficient experience [59].

Intravenous urogram (IVU) is considered the gold standard for imaging in early renal TB [33, 59]. There might be no abnormalities present during early disease, but there usually appear moderate to severe urinary tract changes once patients become symptomatic [59]. Early findings include infundibular narrowing, calyceal erosion or blunting, and papillary necrosis with associated parenchymal scarring and calcification [27]. GUTB is considered if there is simultaneous involvement of both the upper and the lower urinary tracts, especially the kidney and the bladder [27, 29]. Later stages of the disease may demonstrate extensive cavitation, mass lesions, calyceal distortion, cortical scarring, calcification, autonephrectomy, perinephric abscess, fistula formation, ureteral strictures, and bladder fibrosis [25, 59]. In our study, both patients who underwent intravenous pyelography showed advanced findings of extensive stone formation and non-functioning kidney.

Triphasic computed tomography (CT) scan remains the mainstay imaging technique for cross-sectional imaging in GUTB [6]. It is the most sensitive modality to detect calcification, and is superior to IVU in detecting multiple small urothelial lesions [25, 60]. Findings suggestive of GUTB include the presence of lesions in other organs beyond the urinary tract, such as liver, lymph nodes, and vertebrae [29], as seen in our study.

Although IVU and CT scan are reported to be the more frequently used imaging modalities in GUTB [29], some investigations still heavily rely on ultrasonography [18, 36]. Ultrasonography may only give indirect evidence of GUTB, but it avoids exposure to ionizing radiation and can be conveniently used to guide fine needle aspiration biopsies [5, 25, 59]. In literature, two patterns of GUTB have been described: (1) the infiltrative pattern showing increased echogenicity from calcifications, infected debris, or abscesses; and (2) hydronephrosis or pyonephrosis, involving calyceal dilatation and a small renal pelvis. Another distinguishing feature for GUTB is the visualization of multiple abnormalities in different disease stages with various organ involvement [59]. All these changes were observed in our investigation.

Treatment

Medical treatment of GUTB should be initiated promptly when clinical, laboratory, and radiological findings suggest a presumptive diagnosis, even prior to the release of microbiologic and histopathologic results [26, 47]. Pharmacologic therapy for drug-sensitive TB consists of an intensive phase of quadruple therapy with first-line anti-TB agents (e.g., isoniazid, rifampicin, pyrazinamide and ethambutol) for 2 months, followed by a continuation phase with two drugs (e.g., isoniazid, rifampicin) for 4 months [28]. In our study, over sixty percent (63.39%) of patients were started on anti-TB therapy during admission, reflecting diverse in-hospital practices wherein several cases were discharged upon resolution of their reasons for encounter, with eventual treatment initiated on an out-patient basis after microbiologic and histopathologic confirmation.

Around half (54.9%) of patients with GUTB require surgery [28, 47]. Indications for surgery include diversion of urologic obstruction, drainage of abscesses, nephrectomy of non-functioning kidneys, reconstruction of affected ureters, and dilation of contracted urinary bladder [26, 28]. A quarter (25.89%) of patients in our study underwent an operation, lower than that observed in a previous local investigation (52%) [15]. This difference might be attributed to the higher proportion of younger individuals involved in our study, whose illness duration may not be long enough to develop complications that would warrant surgical therapy. This finding might signify a changing pattern of disease in the country.

Short-term outcomes

Deaths from tuberculosis are higher in developing (2–3 million deaths per year) than developed countries (40 thousand deaths per year) [9]. In GUTB, mortality rates vary (1.2–28.1%) [10], with most patients succumbing from disseminated infection [15]. In our center, all-cause in-hospital mortality occurred in 8.04% of the included patients. Age, leukocytosis, and the need for pressors were all significantly associated with mortality (p values of <0.001, 0.010, and <0.001, respectively). Several researches in Taiwan investigated risk factors for mortality in patients with GUTB. Fever was shown to be positively correlated with mortality (OR = 42.716; 95% CI 1.032–1767.569; $p = 0.048$), possibly attributed to its high prevalence in elderly patients, those with multiple co-morbidities, and those who had delays in diagnosis [10]. Other poor prognostic factors included genitourinary tract surgery (OR = 0.000; 95% CI 0.000–0.255; $p = 0.020$) [10], age older than 65 years old (HR = 4.03; 95% CI 1.27–12.76; $p = 0.02$), cardiovascular disease (HR = 5.96; 95% CI 1.98–17.92; $p = 0.001$), steroid use (HR = 10.16; 95% CI 2.27–45.47; $p = 0.02$), and no treatment (HR = 4.81; 95% CI 1.12–20.67; $p = 0.04$) [40].

It was observed that patients with longer mean lengths of hospital stay did not necessarily develop unfavorable hospital outcomes. Instead, prolonged admission duration seemed to have been influenced by management of co-morbidities (e.g., SLE, pulmonary TB, psoas TB) and correction of various clinically significant laboratory abnormalities (e.g., anemia, leukocytosis, hyponatremia, and hypercalcemia). Awaiting results of TB workups during admission for diagnosis of equivocal cases and for subsequent initiation of definitive therapy might have also contributed since anti-Koch's treatment had a statistically longer mean length of hospital stay ($p < 0.001$). These findings were reflective of the varying practices in our center, with many cases undergoing surgery for prompt treatment of symptoms and having medical therapy be initiated on an out-patient basis depending on the results of cultures and histopathology.

Limitations

Our study had several limitations. Its retrospective design which was affected by institutional limitations in recordkeeping made data collection restricted, as evidenced by a low chart retrieval rate (57.89%, 132/228). Given the absence of a unified clinical registry and data recording, our case finding was laboratory-based and was subject to selection bias, thereby rendering our results nongeneralizable to a broader patient population. It also proved to be a major barrier preventing inclusion of predictive modeling of study outcomes. Despite these limitations, our research is the largest study in the country to date, involving more accurate diagnosis of GUTB compared to past local studies since all reviewed cases had bacteriologic or histopathologic evidence of infection. It also involved more specific definitions of serologic findings adjusted per age and sex.

Conclusion

Our investigation observed a high prevalence rate of serologic and urinary abnormalities among admitted GUTB patients in the study. Apart from the commonly cited abnormalities in literature, multiple electrolyte abnormalities and urinary concentration defects were observed in many cases, possibly indicating tubulointerstitial involvement. Accordingly, we recommend future research be done on such complication to determine its correlation with disease activity and to possibly help with the diagnosis of infection particularly in low-resource settings. Mortality rate was also noted to be high among admitted patients with GUTB. Age, leukocytosis, and need for pressors were significantly associated with mortality. However, further research is recommended to explore predictive modeling.

Acknowledgements
We would like to thank the Philippine General Hospital and the Division of Nephrology for supporting us in this work. We would also like to thank Prof. Francisco N. de los Reyes for his assistance with our data analysis.

Authors' contributions
Conception and design of study: PNHS and ARTV. Acquisition of data: PNHS. Data analysis and interpretation, drafting of manuscript and critical revision, and approval of final version of manuscript: PNHS and ARTV. All authors read and approved the final manuscript.

References

1. World Health Organization: Global tuberculosis report 2019. 2019.
2. Mehta JB, Dutt A, Harvill L, Mathews KM. Epidemiology of extrapulmonary tuberculosis: a comparative analysis with pre-AIDS era. Chest. 1991;99(5):1134–8.
3. Das P, Ahuja A, Gupta SD. Incidence, etiopathogenesis and pathological aspects of genitourinary tuberculosis in India: a journey revisited. Indian J Urol. 2008;24(3):356–61.
4. Noertjojo K, Tam CM, Chan SL, Chan-Yeung MMW. Extra-pulmonary and pulmonary tuberculosis in Hong Kong. Int J Tuberc Lung Dis. 2002;6(10):879–86.
5. Kulchavenya E. Urogenital tuberculosis: definition and classification. Ther Adv Infect Dis. 2014;2(5–6):117–22.
6. Kulchavenya E, Yasuda M, Grabe M. Epidemiology, classification, clinical features, and diagnostics of urogenital tuberculosis. In: Bjerklund Johansen TE, Wagenlehner FME, Matsumoto T, Cho YH, Krieger JN, Shoskes D, Naber KG, editors. Urogenital infections and inflammations. Berlin: German Medical Science GMS Publishing House; 2019. https://doi.org/10.5680/lhuii000052.
7. Wildbolz H. Ueber urogenical tuberkulose. Schweiz Med Wochenschr. 1937;67:1125.
8. Krishnamoorthy S, Palaniyandi V, Kumaresan N, Govindaraju S, Rajasekaran J, Murugappan I, et al. Aspects of evolving genito urinary tuberculosis: a profile of genito urinary tuberculosis (GUTB) in 110 patients. J Clin Diagn Res. 2017;11(9):PC01–5.
9. Figueiredo AA, Lucon AM, Junior RF, Srougi M. Epidemiology of urogenital tuberculosis worldwide. Int J Urol. 2008;15:827–32.
10. Huang TY, Hung CH, Hsu WH, Peng KT, Hung MS, Lai LJ, et al. Genitourinary tuberculosis in Taiwan: a 15-year experience at a teaching hospital. J Microbiol Immunol Infect. 2019;52:312–9.
11. Porter MF III. Uro-genital tuberculosis in the male. Ann Surg. 1894;20(4):396–405.
12. Lansang MAD, Alejandria MM, Law I, Juban NR, Amarillo MLE, Sison OT, et al. High TB burden and low notification rates in the Philippines: the 2016 national TB prevalence survey. PLoS ONE. 2021;16(6):e0252240.
13. Santos R. Clinical profile of extrapulmonary tuberculosis cases admitted and diagnosed in a tertiary government hospital from January 2006 to June 2010. Pediatr Infect Dis Soc Philippines J. 2013;14(2):77–84.
14. Lim RG, Caro HP, Dominguez-Mejia AE, Yuhico MJ. The clinical profile of patients with sterile pyuria and recurrent urinary tract infection. Phillippine J Intern Med. 1996;34(3):89–92.
15. Tanchuco JQ, Lazo PO, King B. Urinary tract tuberculosis: local experience. Philippine J Nephrol. 1987;11:183–90.
16. Dy EER, Rosales LN, Lim EU. Genitourinary tuberculosis at the Santo Tomas University Hospital. Phillippine J Intern Med. 1995;33(2):47–52.
17. Lee JY, Park HY, Park SY, Lee SW, Moon HS, Kim YT, et al. Clinical characteristics of genitourinary tuberculosis during a recent 10-year period in one center. Korean J Urol. 2011;52:200–5.
18. Hsieh HC, Lu PL, Chen YH, Chen TC, Tsai JJ, Chang K, et al. Genitourinary tuberculosis in a medical center in southern Taiwan: an eleven-year experience. J Microbiol Immunol Infect. 2006;39:408–13.
19. Kulchavenya E. Best practice in the diagnosis and management of urogenital tuberculosis. Ther Adv Urol. 2013;5(3):143–51.
20. World Health Organization. Haemoglobin concentrations for the diagnosis of anaemia and assessment of severity. Geneva: World Health Organization; 2011.
21. Lo SF. Reference intervals for laboratory tests and procedures. In: Kliegman R, St Geme JW, Blum NJ, Tasker RC, Shah SS, Wilson KM, editors. Nelson textbook of pediatrics. 21st ed. Philadelphia: Elsevier; 2020. p. e6–7.
22. Longo DL, Fauci AS, Kasper DL, Hauser SL, Jameson J, Loscalzo J. Harrison's principles of internal medicine. 20th ed. New York: McGraw-Hill; 2018.
23. Berliner N. Approach to the adult with unexplained neutropenia. Uptodate, 2018. Accessed 3 Feb 2020.
24. Skorecki K, Chertow GM, Marsden PA, Brenner BM, Rector FC, et al. Brenner & Rector's the kidney. 10th ed. Philadelphia: Elsevier; 2016.
25. Abbara A, Davidson RN. Etiology and management of genitourinary tuberculosis. Nat Rev Urol. 2011;8:678–88.
26. Amaya-Tapia G, Aguirre-Avalos G. Urinary tract tuberculosis. IntechOpen. 2018. https://doi.org/10.5772/intechopen.76063.
27. Venyo AK, Venyo LK, Maloney DJL, Khan AN. Tuberculosis of the kidney and the genitourinary tract: a review of the literature. Hamdan Med J. 2015;8:345–60.
28. Muneer A, Macrae B, Krishnamoorthy S, Zumla A. Urogenital tuberculosis: epidemiology, pathogenesis and clinical features. Nat Rev Urol. 2019;16(10):573–98.
29. Figueiredo AA, Lucon AML. Urogenital tuberculosis: update and review of 8961 cases from the world literature. Rev Urol. 2008;10(3):207–17.
30. Medlar EM, Spain DM, Holliday RW. Post-mortem compared with clinical diagnosis of genitourinary tuberculosis in adult males. J Urol. 1949;61:1078–88.
31. Lewinsohn DM, Leonard MK, LoBue PA, Cohn DL, Daley CL, Desmond E, et al. Official American Thoracic Society/Infectious Diseases Society of America/Centers for Disease Control and Prevention clinical practice guidelines: diagnosis of tuberculosis in adults and children. Clin Infect Dis. 2017;64:1–33.
32. Mehta PK, Kamra E. Recent trends in diagnosis of urogenital tuberculosis. Future Microbiol. 2020;15(3):159–62.
33. Mishra KG, Ahmad A, Singh G, Tiwari R. Current status of genitourinary tuberculosis: presentation, diagnostic approach and management—single centre experience at IGIMS (Ptana, Bihar, India). Indian J Surg. 2020;82(817–823):2020.
34. Ramanathan R, Kumar A, Kapoor R, Bhandari M. Relief of urinary tract obstruction in tuberculosis to improve renal function. Analysis of predictive factors. Br J Urol. 1998;81:199–205.
35. Kim EJ, Lee W, Jeong WY, Choi H, Jung IY, Ahn JY, et al. Chronic kidney disease with genitourinary tuberculosis: old disease but ongoing complication. BMC Nephrol. 2018;19:193.
36. Cao Y, Fan Y, Chen Y, Zhao Z, Song Y, Shen C, et al. Gross hematuria is more common in male and older patients with renal tuberculosis in China: a single-center 15-year clinical experience. Urol Int. 2017;99:290–6.
37. Ye Y, Hu X, Shi Y, Zhou J, Zhou Y, Song X, et al. Clinical features and drug-resistance profile of urinary tuberculosis in south-western China. Medicine. 2016;95(19):1–8.
38. Singh JP, Priyadarshi V, Kundu AK, Vijay MK, Bera MK, Pal DK. Genito-urinary tuberculosis revisited: 13 years' experience of a single centre. Indian J Tuberc. 2013;60:15–22.
39. Chandra S, Chandra H, Chauhan N, Gaur DS, Gupta H, Pathank VP, et al. Male genitourinary tuberculosis: 13 years experience at a tertiary care center in India. Southeast Asian J Trop Med Public Health. 2012;43(2):364–9.
40. Hsu H-L, Lai C-C, Yu M-C, Yu F-L, Lee J-C, Chou C-H, et al. Clinical and microbiological characteristics of urine culture-confirmed genitourinary tuberculosis at medical centers in Taiwan from 1995 to 2007. Eur J Clin Microbiol Infect Dis. 2011;30:319–26.
41. Karnjanawanichkul W, Pripatnanont C. Tuberculosis of the urinary tract in southern Thailand. J Med Assoc Thai. 2010;93(8):916–9.
42. Takahasi S, Takeyama K, Kunishima Y, Hashimoto K, Miyamoto S, Ichihara K, et al. Current survey of urinary tuberculosis in Hokkaido, Japan. J Infect Chemother. 2007;13:105–8.
43. Buccholz NP, Haque R, Salahuddin S. Genitourinary tuberculosis: a profile of 55 in-patients. J Pak Med Assoc. 2000;50(8):265–9.
44. Balepur SS, Schlossberg D. Hematologic complications of tuberculosis. Microbiol Spectr. 2016. https://doi.org/10.1128/microbiolspec.TNMI7-0004-2016.
45. Oyer RA, Schlossberg D. Hematologic changes in tuberculosis. In: Schlossberg D, editor. Tuberculosis. New York: Springer; 1994.

46. Visweswaran RK, Pais VM, Dionne-Odom J. Urogenital tuberculosis. UpToDate, 2019. Accessed 9 Nov 2020.
47. Figueiredo AA, Lucon AM, Srougi M. Urogenital tuberculosis. Microbiol Spectr. 2017;5(1):1–16.
48. Vinnard C, Blumberg EA. Endocrine and metabolic aspects of tuberculosis. Microbiol Spectr. 2017;5(1):1–19.
49. Murphy FD, Settimi AL, Kozokoff NJ. Renal disease with the salt losing syndrome: a report of four cases of so-called "salt losing nephritis." Ann Intern Med. 1953;38(6):1160–76.
50. Mallison WJ, Fuller RW, Levison DA, Baker LR, Cattell WR. Diffuse interstitial renal tuberculosis: an unusual cause of renal failure. Q J Med. 1981;50:137–48.
51. El-Reshaid KA, Madda JP, Al-Saleh MA. A case of progressive tubulo-interstitial nephritis due to culture-negative renal tuberculosis. Saudi J Kidney Dis Transpl. 2001;12:534–7.
52. Sampathkumar K, Sooraj YS, Mahaldar AR, Ramakrishnan M, Rjappannair A, Nalumakkal SV, et al. Granulomatous interstitial nephritis due to tuberculosis: a rare presentation. Saudi J Kidney Dis Transpl. 2009;20:842–5.
53. Chapagain A, Dobbie H, Sheaff M, Yaqoob M. Presentation, diagnosis, and treatment outcome of tuberculous-mediated tubulointerstitial nephritis. Kidney Int. 2011;79(6):671–7.
54. Delafosse M, Teuma C, Miailhes P, Nouvier M, Rabeyrin M, Fouque D. Severe tubulointerstitial nephritis: tracking tuberculosis even in the absence of renal granuloma. Clin Kidney J. 2018;11(5):667–9.
55. Eastwood JB, Corbishley CM, Grange JM. Tuberculosis and tubulointerstitial nephritis: an intriguing puzzle. Kidney Int. 2011;79:579–81.
56. Pouchot J, Dreyfuss D, Gardin JP, Mier L, Remy P, Esdaile JM, et al. Ectopic production of 1,25-dihydroxyvitamin D3 in tuberculosis. Nephrol Dial Transpl. 1993;8:560–2.
57. Daher EDF, da Silva GB, Barros EJG. Review: renal tuberculosis in the modern era. Am J Trop Med Hyg. 2013;88(1):54–64.
58. American Thoracic Society. Diagnostic standards and classification of tuberculosis in adults and children. Am J Respir Crit Care Med. 2000;161(4 Pt 1):1376–95.
59. Merchant S, Bharati A, Merchant N. Tuberculosis of the genitourinary system: urinary tract tuberculosis: renal tuberculosis—part I. Indian J Radiol Imaging. 2013;23(1):46–63.
60. Merchant S, Bharati A, Merchant N. Tuberculosis of the genitourinary system: urinary tract tuberculosis: renal tuberculosis—part II. Indian J Radiol Imaging. 2013;23(1):64–77.

Permissions

All chapters in this book were first published by BioMed Central; hereby published with permission under the Creative Commons Attribution License or equivalent. Every chapter published in this book has been scrutinized by our experts. Their significance has been extensively debated. The topics covered herein carry significant findings which will fuel the growth of the discipline. They may even be implemented as practical applications or may be referred to as a beginning point for another development.

The contributors of this book come from diverse backgrounds, making this book a truly international effort. This book will bring forth new frontiers with its revolutionizing research information and detailed analysis of the nascent developments around the world.

We would like to thank all the contributing authors for lending their expertise to make the book truly unique. They have played a crucial role in the development of this book. Without their invaluable contributions this book wouldn't have been possible. They have made vital efforts to compile up to date information on the varied aspects of this subject to make this book a valuable addition to the collection of many professionals and students.

This book was conceptualized with the vision of imparting up-to-date information and advanced data in this field. To ensure the same, a matchless editorial board was set up. Every individual on the board went through rigorous rounds of assessment to prove their worth. After which they invested a large part of their time researching and compiling the most relevant data for our readers.

The editorial board has been involved in producing this book since its inception. They have spent rigorous hours researching and exploring the diverse topics which have resulted in the successful publishing of this book. They have passed on their knowledge of decades through this book. To expedite this challenging task, the publisher supported the team at every step. A small team of assistant editors was also appointed to further simplify the editing procedure and attain best results for the readers.

Apart from the editorial board, the designing team has also invested a significant amount of their time in understanding the subject and creating the most relevant covers. They scrutinized every image to scout for the most suitable representation of the subject and create an appropriate cover for the book.

The publishing team has been an ardent support to the editorial, designing and production team. Their endless efforts to recruit the best for this project, has resulted in the accomplishment of this book. They are a veteran in the field of academics and their pool of knowledge is as vast as their experience in printing. Their expertise and guidance has proved useful at every step. Their uncompromising quality standards have made this book an exceptional effort. Their encouragement from time to time has been an inspiration for everyone.

The publisher and the editorial board hope that this book will prove to be a valuable piece of knowledge for researchers, students, practitioners and scholars across the globe.

List of Contributors

Min Ji Kim, Dong Hwan Lee, Dong Ha Park and Il Jae Lee
Department of Plastic and Reconstructive Surgery, Ajou University School of Medicine, 164, World cup-ro, Yeongtong-gu, Suwon 16499, Republic of Korea

Cong Wang and ShouTong Wang
Department of Urology, Shanghai General Hospital, Nanjing Medical University, No.100, Haining Road, Hongkou District, Shanghai 200080, China

Jun Lu
Department of Urology, Shanghai General Hospital, Nanjing Medical University, No.100, Haining Road, Hongkou District, Shanghai 200080, China
Department of Urology, First Affiliated Hospital of Sun Yat-Sen University, Guangzhou 510080, People's Republic of China

Xuemei Wang
Department of Urology, Shanghai General Hospital, Shanghai Jiao Tong University School of Medicine, No.100, Haining Road, Hongkou District, Shanghai 200080, China

R. Pané-Alemany and A. Carralero-Martínez
Rehabilitación Abdomino-Pelviana (RAPbarcelona SL), Barcelona, Spain

E. Sánchez
Blanquerna School of Health Science-Universitat Ramon Llull, Barcelona, Spain

I. Ramírez-García
Rehabilitación Abdomino-Pelviana (RAPbarcelona SL), Barcelona, Spain
Servicio de Fisioterapia, Instituto Médico Tecnológico SL, Barcelona, Spain
Blanquerna School of Health Science-Universitat Ramon Llull, Barcelona, Spain
Universidad Internacional de Catalunya (UIC), Barcelona, Spain

L. Blanco-Ratto
Rehabilitación Abdomino-Pelviana (RAPbarcelona SL), Barcelona, Spain
Fundació Universitària del Bages (FUB), Barcelona, Spain

S. Kauffmann
Rehabilitación Abdomino-Pelviana (RAPbarcelona SL), Barcelona, Spain
Fundació Universitària del Bages (FUB), Barcelona, Spain
Servicio de Fisioterapia, Womens Salud Y Bienestar de La Mujer SL, Barcelona, Spain

Clemens Wiesinger, Emir Mirtezani and Walter Pauer
Department of Urology, Wels-Grieskirchen Medical-Center, Grieskirchner Straße 42, 4600 Wels, Austria

Dominik Stefan Schoeb
Department of Urology, Faculty of Medicine, Medical Center – University of Freiburg, Hugstetterstr. 55, 79106 Freiburg, Germany

Mathias Stockhammer
Department of Urology, BHB Salzburg, Kajetanerplatz 1, 5010 Salzburg, Salzburg, Austria

Lukas Mitterschiffthaler and Johann Knotzer
Department of Anesthesiology and Intensive Care II, Wels-Grieskirchen Medical Center, Grieskirchner Straße 42, 4600 Wels, Austria

Helga Wagner
Medical Statistics and Biometry, Institute for Applied Statistics, Johannes Kepler University Linz, Altenbergerstrasse 69, 4040 Linz, Austria

Ben Xu, Si-da Cheng, Yi-ji Peng and Qian Zhang
Department of Urology, National Urological Cancer Center, Peking University First Hospital and Institute of Urology, Peking University, 8 Xishiku Street, Xicheng District, Beijing 100034, China

Jung-Woo Shim, Yun Jeong Cho, Jaesik Park, Hyung Mook Lee, Yong-Suk Kim, Young Eun Moon, Sang Hyun Hong and Min Suk Chae
Department of Anesthesiology and Pain Medicine, Seoul St. Mary's Hospital, College of Medicine, The Catholic University of Korea, 222, Banpo-daero, Seocho-gu, Seoul 06591, Republic of Korea

Hyong Woo Moon
Department of Urology, Seoul St. Mary's Hospital, College of Medicine, The Catholic University of Korea, Seoul, Republic of Korea

Emily Heer
Department of Cancer Epidemiology and Prevention Research, Cancer Research and Analytics, Cancer Care Alberta, Alberta Health Services, 5th Floor, Holy Cross Centre, Box ACB, 2210 - 2 St. SW, Calgary, AB T2S 3C3, Canada

Lin Yang
Department of Cancer Epidemiology and Prevention Research, Cancer Research and Analytics, Cancer Care Alberta, Alberta Health Services, 5th Floor, Holy Cross Centre, Box ACB, 2210 - 2 St. SW, Calgary, AB T2S 3C3, Canada
Departments of Oncology and Community Health Sciences, University of Calgary, Calgary, Canada
Division of Public Health Sciences, Department of Surgery, Washington University School of Medicine, 600 S. Taylor Ave., 2nd floor, Rm. 208S, Campus Box 8100, St. Louis, MO 63110, USA

Jung Ae Lee
Agricultural Statistics Laboratory, University of Arkansas, Fayetteville, USA

Claire Pernar
Department of Epidemiology, Harvard T.H. Chan School of Public Health, Boston, MA, USA

Graham A. Colditz, Ratna Pakpahan and Siobhan Sutcliffe
Division of Public Health Sciences, Department of Surgery, Washington University School of Medicine, 600 S. Taylor Ave., 2nd floor, Rm. 208S, Campus Box 8100, St. Louis, MO 63110, USA

Robert L. Grubb III
Division of Urological Surgery, Department of Surgery, Washington University School of Medicine, St Louis, USA
Department of Urology, Medical University of South Carolina, Charleston, USA

Kathleen Y. Wolin
Coeus Health, Chicago, IL, USA

Adam S. Kibel
Division of Urology, Department of Surgery, Brigham and Women's Hospital, Boston, USA

Kellie R. Imm
Division of Public Health Sciences, Department of Surgery, Washington University School of Medicine, 600 S. Taylor Ave., 2nd floor, Rm. 208S, St. Louis, MO 63110, USA
Division of Health Behavior Research, Department of Preventive Medicine, Keck School of Medicine of the University of Southern California, 2001 N Soto St., Los Angeles, CA 90032, USA

Łukasz Nyk, Omar Tayara, Piotr Kryst and Wojciech Malewski
Second Department of Urology, Centre of Postgraduate Medical Education, Warsaw, Poland

Tomasz Ząbkowski
Department of Urology, Military Institute of Medicine, Warsaw, Poland

Aneta Andrychowicz
Urological Clinic, Warsaw, Poland

Jiwon Han, Yu Kyung Bae and Chang-Hoon Koo
Department of Anesthesiology and Pain Medicine, Seoul National University Bundang Hospital, Seongnam 13620, Korea

Young-Tae Jeon, Jung-Hee Ryu and Ah-Young Oh
Department of Anesthesiology and Pain Medicine, Seoul National University Bundang Hospital, Seongnam 13620, Korea
Department of Anesthesiology and Pain Medicine, Seoul National University College of Medicine, Seoul 03080, Korea

Hwanik Kim
Department of Urology, Seoul National University Bundang Hospital, Seongnam 13620, Korea

Xiao-Feng Chen, Jian-Ming Sun, Yi-Hua Zou and Wang-Long Deng
Department of Urology, The First People's Hospital of Chenzhou, 102 Luojiajing, Chenzhou 423000, Hunan, People's Republic of China
Department of Urology, The First Clinical College of Xiangnan University, 102 Luojiajing, Chenzhou 423000, Hunan, People's Republic of China

Jian-Jun Zhou and Guo-Can Cao
Department of Urology, The Fourth People's Hospital of Chenzhou, Chenzhou, Hunan, People's Republic of China

Gao Keyu, Li Shuofeng, Zhu Haitao and Wang Junqi
Department of Urology, The Affiliated Hospital of Xuzhou Medical University, Xuzhou 221000, China

Li Shuaishuai and Ashok Raj
Xuzhou Medical University, Xuzhou 221000, China

Liu Shuai
Xuzhou Central Hospital, Xuzhou 221000, China

Zhang Yuan
Xuzhou Children's Hospital, Xuzhou 221000, China

Masato Yanagi, Jun Akatsuka, Yuki Endo, Hayato Takeda and Yukihiro Kondo
Department of Urology, Nippon Medical School Hospital, 1-1-5, Sendagi, Bunkyo-ku, Tokyo 113-8603, Japan

Tsutomu Hamasaki
Department of Urology, Nippon Medical School Musashikosugi Hospital, 1-396, Kosugityo, Nakahara-ku, Kawasaki city, Kanagawa 211-8533, Japan

Zhouting Tuo, Ying Zhang, Jinyou Wang, Huan Zhou, Youlu Lu, Xin Wang, Chao Yang, Dexin Yu and Liangkuan Bi
Department of Urology, The Second Affiliated Hospital of Anhui Medical University, NO. 678 Furong Road, Hefei 230032, China

Anirban P. Mitra
Institute of Urology, University of Southern California, Los Angeles, CA, USA

Evalynn Vasquez, Paul Kokorowski and Andy Y. Chang
Division of Urology, Children's Hospital Los Angeles, Los Angeles, CA, USA

Hao Yang and Hang Zhang
Zhejiang University School of Medicine, Hangzhou, China
Children's Hospital, Zhejiang University School of Medicine, Hangzhou, China
National Clinical Research Center for Child Health, Hangzhou, China

Xiao-xiao Xuan, Qiang Shu and Jun-fen Fu
Children's Hospital, Zhejiang University School of Medicine, Hangzhou, China
National Clinical Research Center for Child Health, Hangzhou, China

Dong-lai Hu and Xiao-dong Guo
Department of Pediatric Surgery, Zhejiang University Jinhua Hospital, Jinhua, China

Jian-Hui Wu, Qing-Tong Ma and Shi-Qiang Yang
Department of Urology, Tianjin First Central Hospital, No. 24 Fukang Road, Nankai District, Tianjin 300192, China

Chun-Bai Mo
Department of Renal Transplant, Tianjin First Central Hospital, Tianjin 300192, China

Li Dong-Zhai
Department of Anatomy and Histology, School of Basic Medical Sciences, Tianjin Medical University, Tianjin 300070, China

Fei Luo
Department of Urology, Tianjin Union Medical Center, Tianjin 300121, China

Christina Oetzmann von Sochaczewski
Klinik und Poliklinik für Kinderchirurgie, Universitätsmedizin Mainz der Johannes Gutenberg-Universität, Mainz, Germany
Sektion Kinderchirurgie, Klinik und Poliklinik für Allgemein-, Viszeral-, Thorax- und Gefäßchirurgie, Universitätsklinikum Bonn, Venusberg-Campus 1, D-53127 Bonn, Germany

Jan Gödeke
Klinik und Poliklinik für Kinderchirurgie, Universitätsmedizin Mainz der Johannes Gutenberg-Universität, Mainz, Germany

Oliver J. Muensterer
Klinik und Poliklinik für Kinderchirurgie, Universitätsmedizin Mainz der Johannes Gutenberg-Universität, Mainz, Germany
Kinderchirurgische Klinik und Poliklinik, Dr. von Haunersches Kinderspital der Ludwig- Maximilians-Universität München, Munich, Germany

Se Young Choi
Department of Urology, Chung-Ang University Hospital, Chung-Ang University College of Medicine, 102, Heukseok-ro, Dongjak-gu, Seoul 06973, Korea
Biomedical Research Institute, Chung-Ang University Hospital, 102, Heukseok-ro, Dongjak-gu, Seoul 06973, Korea

Byung Hoon Chi
Department of Urology, Chung-Ang University Hospital, Chung-Ang University College of Medicine, 102, Heukseok-ro, Dongjak-gu, Seoul 06973, Korea

Wonchul Lee, Dalsan You, Bumjin Lim and Choung-Soo Kim
Department of Urology, Asan Medical Center, University of Ulsan College of Medicine, 88 Olympic-ro 43-gil, Songpa-gu, Seoul 05505, Korea

Jung Hoon Kim
Department of Urology, Hanil General Hospital, Seoul, Korea

Dan Li
Department of General Practice, The First Affiliated Hospital of Wannan Medical College (Yijishan Hospital of Wannan Medical College), Wuhu 241000, China

Zhou Shen
Department of Urology, Anhui Provincial Hospital, Anhui Medical University, Hefei, Anhui, China

Yujie Xu
Department of Urology, The First Affiliated Hospital of Wannan Medical College (Yijishan Hospital of Wannan Medical College), 2 Zheshan West Road, Wuhu 241000, Anhui Province, China

Yue He
Department of Urology, Suining Central Hospital, No. 127 Desheng W. Rd., Chuanshan District, Suining City 629000, Sichuan Province, People's Republic of China
Department of Urology, Institute of Urology, West China Hospital, Sichuan University, No. 37 Guoxue Alley, Wuhou District, Chengdu City 610041, Sichuan Province, People's Republic of China

You-Gang Feng, Jun He, Bo Liang, Ming-Dong Jiang, Jun Liu, Yong-Ming Kang and Tao Yang
Department of Urology, Suining Central Hospital, No. 127 Desheng W. Rd., Chuanshan District, Suining City 629000, Sichuan Province, People's Republic of China

Li-Ping Ma, Qin Zhang, Qi-Jia Peng and Yao Liu
Operation Room, Suining Central Hospital, No. 127 Desheng W. Rd., Chuanshan District, Suining City 629000, Sichuan Province, People's Republic of China

Li Luo and Min Zhang
Department of Anesthesiology, Suining Central Hospital, No. 127 Desheng W. Rd., Chuanshan District, Suining City 629000, Sichuan Province, People's Republic of China

Yaniv Shilo, Jonathan Modai and Dan Leibovici
Department of Urology, Kaplan Medical Center, 7661041 Rehovot, Israel

Ishai Dror and Brian Berkowitz
Department of Earth and Planetary Sciences, Weizmann Institute of Science, 7610001 Rehovot, Israel

Hongjie Gao
Department of Pediatrics, Qilu Hospital of Shandong University, Jinan, China

Jiawei Chen, Guowei Li, Xinhai Cui and Fengyin Sun
Department of Pediatric Surgery, Qilu Hospital of Shandong University, Jinan, China

Junjie Cen, Wenwei Wang, Pengju Li, Jiacong Mo, Zhenhua Chen, Yiming Tang, Jinhuan Wei, Junhang Luo and Yong Fang
Department of Urology, First Affiliated Hospital of Sun Yat-Sen University, Guangzhou 510080, People's Republic of China

Hongwei Zhao
Department of Urology, Affiliated Yantai Yuhuangding Hospital, Qingdao University, Yantai 264000, Shandong, People's Republic of China

Shiying Huang
School of Traditional Chinese Medicine, Southern Medical University, Guangzhou 510515, People's Republic of China

Teng Ma, Zhaoqin Huang, Qianqian Hua, Xiaojiao Li, Ximing Wang and Yunchao Chen
Department of Radiology, Shandong Provincial Hospital Affiliated to Shandong First Medical University, No.324, Jingwu Road, Jinan 250021, Shandong, China

Lin Cong
Department of Medical Imaging Interventional Therapy, Shandong Provincial Hospital Affiliated to Shandong First Medical University, Jinan 250021, Shandong, China

Qianli Ma
Department of Radiology, Taian City Central Hospital, Taian 271000, Shandong, China

Changhao Hou, Yubo Gu, Wei Yuan, Zeyu Wang, Jiahao Lin, Qiang Fu and Lujie Song
Department of Urology, Shanghai Jiao Tong University Affiliated Sixth People's Hospital, Shanghai 200233, China
Shanghai Eastern Institute of Urologic Reconstruction, Shanghai 200233, China

Lucas Mira Gon, Caio César Citatini de Campos, Brunno Raphael Iamashita Voris, Luís Augusto Passeri, Adriano Fregonesi and Cássio Luís Zanettini Riccetto
Division of Urology of Department of Surgery, Faculty of Medical Sciences, Hospital de Clinicas, University of Campinas - UNICAMP, Rua Vital Brazil, 250, Campinas, SP 13083-590, Brazil

Paolo Nikolai H. So and Anthony Russell T. Villanueva
Division of Nephrology, Department of Medicine, University of the Philippines Manila - Philippine General Hospital, Taft Avenue, Ermita, 1000 Manila, Philippines

Index

www.ingramcontent.com/pod-product-compliance
Lightning Source LLC
LaVergne TN
LVHW060058220926
848484LV00008BA/2164
9798887405469